Table of Contents

1.0 Introduction

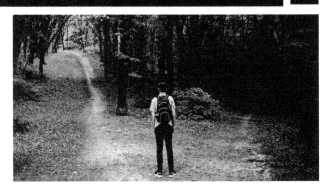

"Rock bottom became the solid foundation on which I rebuilt my life." (J.K. Rowling)

Congratulations on picking up this book and taking a leap toward creating an extraordinary life. By establishing coherent and self-reinforcing daily routines, you are about to put your life on an incredibly rewarding upward spiral of resilient intentional living.

1.1 Being at Choice: The Freedom of Intentional Living

The person who chooses alcohol or heroin to ease their emotional pain and the person who chooses running or powerlifting to ease their emotional pain are going to have two radically different outcomes and life trajectories. Both choices eventually create the inertia of habit. However, one places the person on a downward spiral towards self-destruction while the other goes in an upward, self-reinforcing direction toward healing and thriving. The decision for either path is merely the result of how we choose to think.

Mental toughness is actually a very teachable and learnable skill; and our society's failure to teach that skill condemns people to lives of misery. There are truly only two key differences

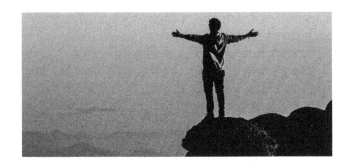

between creating an utterly miserable or an extraordinary life: what we choose to think about our circumstances and the habits we choose to implement in our lives as a result of how we think about our circumstances.

"The one thing you can't take away from me is the way I choose to respond to what you do to me. The last of one's freedoms is to choose one's attitude in any given circumstance." (Viktor E. Frankl).

We do not control our circumstances and horrible things sometimes happen by absolutely no fault of our own. However, our response to each event is still very much our most fundamental moral responsibility and the source of our true power.

When things happen we can separate fault and responsibility: an event can be entirely not our fault, but our response to that event is still **always** our most basic responsibility. Between every stimulus and our response exists a space where we make the choice of how we are going to respond to it. Within that choice, exists our responsibility, our sovereignty, our power, and our freedom.

Our response to any life event is entirely

dependent upon how we choose to think about that event. Before we choose the response, we either automatically or intentionally make a choice of how we think about the event.

Once aware, we always have the opportunity and thus responsibility to choose our thoughts.

While we do not control our circumstances, we can wholly control our thoughts and once we do that, we can also wholly control our responses to the circumstances. By taking control of our thoughts and then our actions, we can proactively affect, and thus often shape, our circumstances. Seeking control of our circumstances is dysfunctional and futile; but gaining total ownership over our thoughts and our actions is how we claim our sovereignty, our power and thus gain authorship of our lives. Own your mind, own your life and create an incredible future.

1.2 Hacking Your Way to a Healthy Mind

The way to own the mind is to optimize nutrition, sleep and daily core routines. When we talk about core routines, we mean the daily patterns we usually engage with little thought or intentionality. Each habit is a cycle of a queue – routine followed by reward – mostly done automatically.

Small changes in our routines cascade into truly profound impacts on all aspects of our lives. For example, simply fixing the all-too-common magnesium deficiency (up to 80% of Americans are deficient in this critical mineral) can result

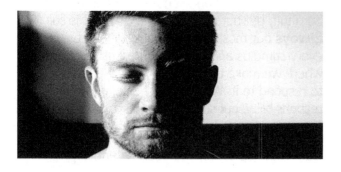

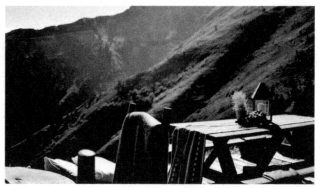

in suddenly getting exponentially more sleep, resulting in a happier emotional state and additional energy cascading through every other aspect of your life.

Many changes we suggest in this book are designed to reduce excessive inflammation, for example, resulting in greater overall wellbeing and a sharper mind.

Each positive change like this one that you make in your life is also inevitably a small step towards greater discipline, making every step that follows a little easier. The changes advised within these pages are thus self-reinforcing, putting your life on an upward spiral towards greater health and coherency.

Our culture tends to focus on our differences. The focus of this book and the principles that we teach, however, are based on universal commonalities which means that these are applicable to all human beings. Universal principles are certain things that every human being requires for optimum living, such as an abundant daily intake of water, a healthy balance of protein, fat and carbs, and regular access to wild nature.

This book intentionally covers a lot of ground on a diverse range of interconnected topics because a healthy life isn't something we create piecemeal. Every choice we make in each aspect of our Life affects everything else, creating a cascading series of changes. It's not the individual elements but the integration of our actions as well as the resulting reinforcing

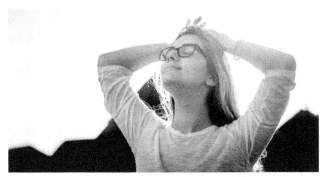

synergy that **causes** us to thrive. **Integration - rather than segregation - is the real magic.**

We're not interested in just going from negative to neutral as is the focus of most western medicine, but rather from negative to positive. The goal is not to barely survive, but to truly thrive. Combined with the principle of integration (rather than piecemeal segregation all too common in our culture), this is the fundamental uniqueness of the approach within this book.

1.3 Raising the Baseline of "Normal"

The goal of this book is to raise your day-to-day baseline of what feels "normal" by putting in place interconnected habitual routines, shifting upward the entire spectrum of feelings and emotions where you play and live each day.

Raising our baseline of normality causes life's lows to land proportionally higher, thus making them far more tolerable. It also means that our highs become proportionally higher. For some people, this spectrum shift can literally mean the difference between feeling suicidal and merely having a slightly bad day, all within the same exact life circumstances.

Far too many people in our society struggle with depression. Yet the focus is usually on numbing the lows, which only yields extremely limited results and has the negative effect of inevitably numbing the highs and everything else in-between. We can't just numb one part of ourselves without numbing all the other parts in the process.

Emotional stability and coherency come from correct nutrition and consistent optimum living habits, resulting in reduced inflammation and consistent blood sugar levels. It is entirely unreasonable to expect to feel good while eating shit food, going to bed at 3 am, not getting sufficient exercise and abusing your body with toxic poisons like alcohol. We can, however, create healthy routines and climb our way out of the hell that is the "average" life.

Whether it is improving digestion, the quality of our sleep, reducing our sugar intake, or any other changes suggested in these pages, every habit and hack we teach in this book fundamentally reduces inflammation, which is the critical key to mental health, emotional well-being, and mental clarity.

A disease is always either caused by or aggravated by excessive inflammation. Reducing inflammation is the key to health. Gut health, reduction in toxin intake, consistent and stable blood sugar levels, proper nutrition, regular intermittent fasting, and consistent sleep are the keys to reducing inflammation. When we reduce the excess inflammation, we allow our bodies to come back into balance.

Moreover, everything is interconnected. Health is the natural balance of life, and nature always seeks to restore balance. Likewise, our bodies always seek a state of homeostasis. By consistently simplifying our lives and our nutritional intake, we avoid paralysis by analysis and are able to prioritize actions that restore health.

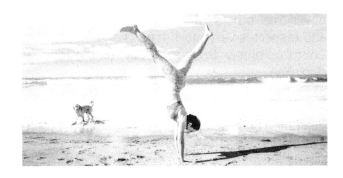

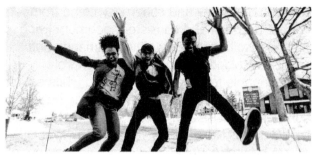

When we take care of the simple things, we allow nature to take care of the complicated and the complex. Life always seeks and inevitably finds balance of what we call "normal". The goal is to move that balance point upward, shifting the entire spectrum of our day-to-day reality.

1.4 Self-Respect + Purpose + Progress = Happiness

"Love fiercely. Because this all ends." (Unknown)

Self-respect is the mandatory foundation of a healthy and coherent life. It is also the inception point to falling madly in love with the world. The way we treat ourselves is always going to reflect how we treat everything and everyone in our lives. It is our individual moral imperative to thrive – that is what we are here to do. When people thrive, the land will thrive with us. We are the keystone species and this is the fundamental law of interconnection.

Self-respect begins with healthy core routines, because trust in yourself starts with doing small things with great consistency. The private victories must always happen first, before any public victories can become possible. We can never trust others until we trust ourselves; and respect is very much a function of trust. Discipline breeds trust, and daily routines enable discipline.

Millions of words have been written since the beginning of human history about finding meaning in life. There is, however, a profoundly simple universality across virtually all patterns of meaning in our culture. When we serve other beings, we find meaning. To be human inherently means that we find our greatest purpose, our greatest meaning and our greatest satisfaction in service. Don't overcomplicate life. Find a way to serve and you will find yourself.

That brings us to the last ingredient within the equation: progress. When we observe nature, we quickly come to recognize the fundamental reality that everything is either growing or dying, with the dead quickly becoming compost and thus soil for new life. Life is always moving, shifting, flowing, and evolving. We rejoin life in movement.

It doesn't really matter where you are in life right now. It's actually entirely irrelevant. What matters is figuring out where you want to go and making consistent steady movement towards that goal. As long as your goal is rooted in self-respect, involves other beings, and as long as you keep moving and thus making progress, you will find yourself feeling more satisfied with your life. We're either growing or we're dying. Start growing and keep moving.

1.5 Your Universal Bedrock Foundations for Coherent Living

Emotional stability and coherency come from correct nutrition and consistent optimum living habits resulting in reduced inflammation and consistent blood sugar levels. It is entirely unreasonable to expect to feel good while eating shit food, going to bed at 3 am, not getting sufficient exercise and abusing your body with toxic poisons like alcohol. You can, however,

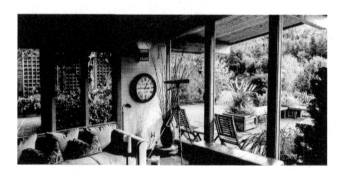

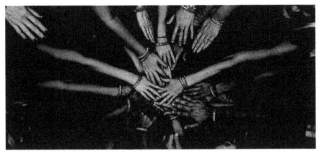

create healthy routines, and you can climb your way out of the hell that is an "average" life. Keep it SIMPLE and always focus on the root cause. Numbing symptoms without treating root causes, which is what our entire allopathic mainstream medical system is designed to do, creates much larger problems by allowing the root causes to continue to deteriorate.

Everything is interconnected, health is the natural balance of life, and nature always seeks to restore balance, and our bodies always seek a state of homeostasis. By consistently simplifying our lives and our nutritional intake, we avoid paralysis by analysis and are able to prioritize and execute actions that restore health.

Context is everything. Understanding the present requires a coherent understanding of our factual history going back to the beginning of life on this planet. All of us come from ancient tribes that since the beginning of time held true an understanding of the universe as a profoundly wise living system, with our own destiny being inherently interconnected with the web of life.

It is toward a relationship of respect and interconnection that we must turn today, and that relationship begins with self-respect. We cannot truly respect other humans and we cannot respect all life unless we first and foremost respect ourselves.

Changing our relationship with the world requires first and foremost changing our relationship with ourselves from human doings to human beings. Self-respect within the context of the past is the magic key that unlocks everything because it gives us the compass by which to orient our lives.

While we live in profoundly uncertain times, this uncertainty has been around from the beginning of time. It is only now that we have been given the chance to evolve into a radical consciousness that we can give a meaningful answer to that uncertainty.

When we're fully prepared to meet each challenge as it comes, calmly prioritizing and executing with a forward-sight focus, grounded in an understanding of our lives in the context of history, our ability to truly be present heals the anxiety of uncertainty. Managing uncertainty and complexity are the two core skills most necessary for these times, and yet often they are also the ones least taught and therefore so little understood.

Underneath all the dust and static noise of the stories we have accepted without questioning, exists literally everything we need to create powerful, meaningful, beautiful lives. The key to our power as a human being exists in unlearning the blatantly false stories about life that we have been handed by other people in our families, communities, and countries. Our individual perceptional reality is simply the net sum of those stories. This is true for each and every human being.

When we learn to hear our own truth, to trust our own voice, and to create our own story, we claim our inherent place on this planet and we begin to turn back toward life. Now is the time for each of us to take authorship of our individual life story and perceptional reality. When we thrive, the planet thrives with us, and we thus have a moral responsibility to learn to thrive.

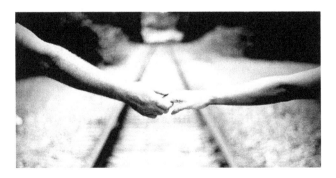

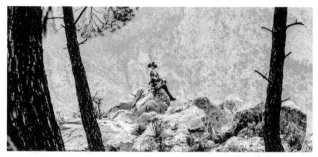

Unlearning is far more powerful than learning, and everything we need to thrive is already within each of us. Our bodies are the most ancient and advanced technology on this planet and we are each born with the answers we seek. Now is the time to learn to truly listen to your own inherent wisdom. Own your story, own your life.

There are five universal balance points that enable human beings to thrive. To be clear, life certainly doesn't boil down to just these five things, but rather these patterns are the foundations that enable growth in life. Get these things right, and growth becomes not only possible but inevitable:

1) **Daily nature connection, ecologically-coherent decision-making, and movement.** The prime directive must be interconnection with nature, trust in its wisdom, including the inherent wisdom of our bodies. **Nature always seeks balance, and we are nature.** Stability in an increasingly complex and uncertain world is defined by our capacity to remain in balance. We learn to trust the inherent balance and wisdom of our bodies - and thus life - through the many movement practices (running, yoga, dance, etc.) that shift our awareness out of our heads and into our bodies. Reconnection with the trust in the balance and wisdom of life then enables for coherent decision-making, which cascades throughout our lives.

2) **Discipline of gratitude, radical presence, and intentional life design.** When things get hard and yet we choose to feel gratitude for our lives, everything

changes because our story about our circumstances changes. Gratitude is both the cure to the poison of entitlement and the inception point to meaningful happiness. It moves us from the false concept of how life "should be" and places us into radical presence and mindfulness. The discipline of gratitude as our inner dialogue leads us to presence, and presence leads us to living meaningful and fulfilling intentional lives. We honor ourselves and our lives by cultivating mastery of our full emotional spectrum and intentionally growing the depths of our intellectual capacities.

3) **Clean plant-based nutrition:** low-carb (40%), adequate fat (30%) + protein (30%), with regular intermittent fasting, and avoidance of toxins such as pesticides and alcohol. While there are many ideas about optimum nutrition, our focus is on basic universal principles and self-respect. The optimized human diet is neither complicated nor expensive.

4) **Consistently optimizing sleep pattern with our natural circadian rhythm.** The quality of our sleep affects absolutely every aspect of our lives, including our emotional state and inflammation levels, so optimizing our sleeping environment, routine and ensuring proper nutritional basis for optimum sleep is one of the most important aspects of optimum wellbeing.

5) **Relationship fabric that supports positive life choices, woven within effective communication.** Our quality of life is largely the product of the stories

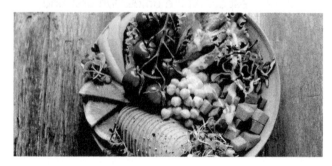

of our internal dialogue combined with learnable communication skills to produce the social fabric of our relationships. By choosing healthy inner stories and building effective communication skills, we begin to weave a thriving social fabric with people who resonate with our life choices.

1.6 Your Optimized Plant-Based Nutrition Done Right

We suggest universal nutritional principles rooted in cutting-edge science that create optimum living conditions for most people by eating a clean, balanced, plant-based diet.

1) **Clean up your diet** by replacing all animal products, gluten, soy, processed, artificial, fried foods and alcohol. There are exponentially better choices available for each of these. Always hack your dietary habit loop by replacing foods with better options, or the inevitable cravings will make your changes unsustainable.

2) **Eat a consistent diet by choosing the same simple** plant-based whole foods each week, and optimize your diet with food-based nutritional supplements. Following a consistent diet creates simplicity and stability, while nutritional supplementation helps ensure proper micronutrient intake, optimizing your digestion, blood sugar levels and general wellbeing.

3) **Drink abundant water, replacing all sugary drinks and juices.** It's quite

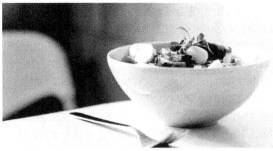

astounding how many entirely pointless calories are consumed each week in drinks. Replace your sodas, lattes and juices with water and unsweetened teas. For an extra jolt of energy, discover Yerba Mate and Matcha teas. For flavor, check out all the different herbal teas, most of which are also great cold. While you're at it, get yourself a metal water bottle, so you're not sipping up plastic toxins with your water.

4) **Choose a correct macro-nutrient balance at each meal.** Prioritize healthy fats and proteins, minimize carbohydrates and optimize digestion with daily probiotics, enzymes, ginger, and turmeric. The balance between macro-nutrients (40% carbs / 30% fat / 30% protein) is just as critically important as the quality of the food itself. Eating more healthy fats (avocado and coconut are always good choices) and proteins will help you feel more full, thus preventing carb/sugar cravings.

5) **Follow a daily or weekly intermittent fasting schedule** appropriate to your life's flow. Whether you choose a limited daily eating window or abstain from food one specific day each week, you're going to experience a huge boost to your health.

1.7 Own Your Story, Own Your Life: Purpose, Small Victories and the Cookie Jar

"He who has a why to live for can bear almost any how." (Friedrich Nietzsche)

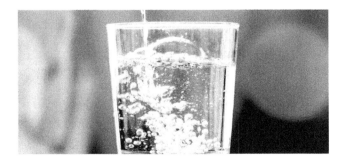

We live in a culture of positivity hype, and that hype is slowly killing us. Motivational hype without grounding in life purpose is destructive bullshit. While our attitude in any given moment determines our reality, without alignment with our highest purpose, positivity hype is the shortest route to depression. It's unreasonable to expect to be happy while living a life void of meaning. Create your meaning by aligning your life with service.

There are three keys to sustainable excellence in every aspect of our lives:

1) having a foundational purpose (your why) by being clear on how you serve others
2) generating ongoing motivation from a daily flow of small victories
3) having an accomplishment inventory – the mental cookie jar

Life meaning often gets either overcomplicated or entirely ignored in our culture, whereas it is both radically simple and superbly necessary if you want to be happy. Purpose always boils down to the simple question of "how am I serving the world to my absolute highest ability?". Life purpose is simply the question of how we choose to make the world a little better for other people, plants and animals.

This simple question is the ultimate reality check. If you do not have an instant answer, you need to redesign your life. If you aren't living your life in a way that coherently improves the lives of other people or animals, you will always find yourself unsatisfied and trying to fill an unfillable void and you're never going to find sustainable happiness or satisfaction. There isn't any way

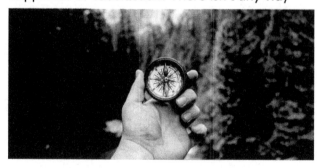

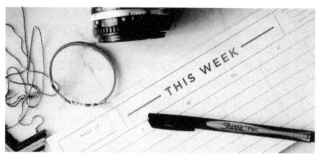

around this. Alignment with core purpose - our service in the world - and then making consistent progress towards fulfilling that purpose is the magic secret to happiness in life.

If you don't know how you can best serve, get curious and find ways to experiment. Curiosity is one of the most important tools available to us, as human beings. If you're not getting the answers you're seeking, get curious about how you can ask better questions because we only truly ever get better answers by asking better questions. Learn to reframe responses to events by making curiosity the default primary response to every challenge. This choice, alone, will completely change your life.

If you're not willing to die for your goals, you need better goals. The worthwhile achievements in life are likely to be challenging. When we're handed anything on a silver platter, those things don't have anywhere near the same meaning to us as if we earn them. Quit seeking the easy life and start seeking the meaningful life of service, meaning and purpose. If you choose to walk a life path aligned with your highest calling and consistently expect and seek out challenge, not only are you going to orient yourself toward growth, but you're also going to become more resilient because challenges that come your way will become reframed as simple opportunities for growth.

When you align with service and choose to live a life of meaning and purpose, you choose a life filled with challenges that enable your growth. Everything in life is either growing or composting: this is a fundamental law of the natural universe. Truth be told though, no

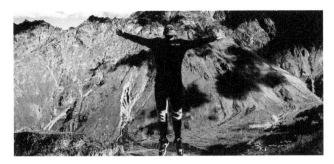

matter what path we choose (even if we choose the "easy" road), sometimes life inevitably kicks our proverbial ass, and this is the time where basic routines become most essential. Daily routines, when designed right, create a sequence of small victories that build confidence which enables the larger victories.

Focus on the small victories. Eating dinner early, so you get to bed on time, so you get up early in the morning, so you get to walk outside is a series of small cascading victories. Start designing and paying attention to these small sequences. Be reasonable by working with the basic laws of nature, rather than against them. Don't set yourself up for failure by setting a goal of waking up early without preparing the night before by eating dinner early, getting to bed early, and getting enough sleep to enable you to jump out of bed when the time comes.

The small victories also matter the most when things get hard and the big victories become temporarily harder to score due to circumstances outside of your control. Because the small victories are things you choose for yourself and that are within your full control, they allow you to own the foundation where the locus of control for your life is internalized. An internal locus of control has consistently been shown in study after study to be the single most important factor for success in life across a wide range of metrics.

Finally, create a mental "cookie jar" of your big life achievements and then grounding your confidence in those achievements. When things are difficult and you're running out of steam, take the time in your mind to inventory all the past things you've achieved or overcome. That

inventory is much akin to a cookie jar into which you can reach for inspiration, grounded in your own life experience, to keep going.

1.8 The Six-Month Roadmap to Optimizing Your Life

There are many moving pieces to the puzzle of optimum living. However, it doesn't have to be complicated. Here is your step-by-step guide:

Month 1: Daily Routines: Hack the Morning, Then Add Nature, Movement, Gratitude, and Mindfulness
Month 2: Drink Water, Dump the Sugar and Alcohol
Month 3: Easy Win: Subtract the Home Toxins, Add Air and Water Filter and Supplements
Month 4: Own Your Sleep Routine and Environment to Get Consistent Good Sleep
Month 5: Transition to a Clean and Consistent Plant-Based Whole Foods Diet
Month 6: Integrate a Consistent Intermittent Fasting Routine

Month 1 Goal) Daily Routines: Hack the Morning, Then Add Nature, Movement, Gratitude, and Mindfulness.

Start every day right with a routine of small victories. Your morning routine, which is what you do within the first hour when you wake up, dramatically impacts the quality of your day, and thus your life. Small victories build upon each other, creating momentum for bigger successes. Equally important, these small steps give you the embodied experience of being

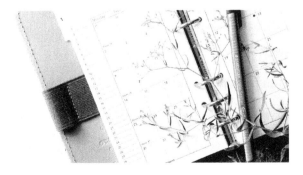

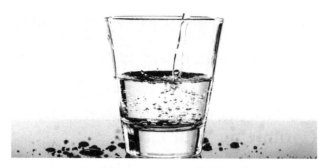

pro-active and being in control of your actions. An internal locus of control and a pro-active mindset are correlated to variety of positive metrics including happiness, higher income, etc., and this daily routine, which allows you to earn a set of relatively easy victories every morning, is your first step toward feeling in control of your actions.

Start your morning by drinking a glass of water with lemon juice and a pinch of salt, followed by a very simple physical routine such as fifty pushups, followed by twenty to thirty grams of protein.

If you can't do fifty push-ups yet, start by doing literally just one, and increase the number by one additional pushup every other day, eventually doing them in sets of five or ten with thirty seconds rest in between. Before you know it, within a few months you'll be doing fifty straight without a problem.

Then find a way to spend 30 minutes every single day outside, in the **wildest** place easily available to you, and gradually increase the time to one hour each day. Choose a place where you are fully surrounded with nature, off-pavement and away from human-built structures. This is ideally going to be part of your morning routine, but your schedule may dictate a different time of day; just be sure to do this daily.

Trail running is a great way to combine exercise and nature connection time, but if running isn't your cup of soup, make this time a daily hike routine, or do yoga.   Your goal is one hour every day outside and moving your body.

Complete your nature run, hike or yoga routine with at least five minutes of complete silent stillness, with your eyes closed and focusing on simply breathing. Count to four as you breathe in, count to four as you hold your breath, count to four as you breathe out, count to four again, then repeat the cycle at least five times. This is called box breathing, and it is taught to first responders and military snipers as a tool to break the stress cycle.

Close your routine by acknowledging one thing for which you are grateful today (and we can always find one thing, even on our worst days – and in fact, especially on our worst days). Gratitude is most important not when we're sitting at the banquet with the love of our life, but when seemingly nothing is going right and we can still find gratitude for our lives.

Month 2 Goal) Replace 100% of your sugary drinks with water, and cut processed sugars and alcohol. Start carrying around a metal water bottle and start ordering unsweetened tea instead of lattes. Juices are hugely potent punches of sugar with all the fruit fiber (which normally slows down sugar digestion) removed, guaranteed to cause your energy levels to spike and then crash. Consider a variety of teas, especially green teas and herbals, if you want yummy flavor.

Go through and check every food you eat, including condiments such as catchup, and if they include high fructose corn syrup, replace that food from your diet. Also remove anything that has artificial colorings and flavors. If it says

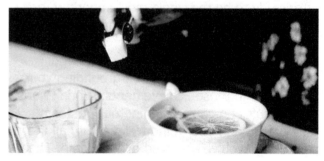

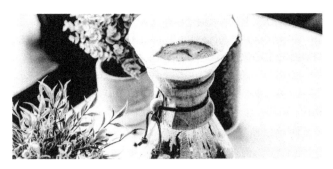

something like "artificial flavoring" or "food color #7" it doesn't belong in your belly.

Alcohol has no place in a healthy person's life. It is a carcinogen and a crappy substitute for real vulnerability as a social lubricant. Cut it out.

Month 3 Goal) Easy Win: Subtract the Home Toxins, Add Air and Water Filters, Add Supplements Lower your household toxin exposure by replacing your shampoo, toothpaste, personal products and household cleaners with biodegradable options, which generally are the healthiest choices available on the market.

Improve your air quality by installing a HEPA air filter appropriately sized for your living space (or at least the bedroom where you sleep), and keep that filter running around the clock. In addition, you can also purchase some houseplants that improve indoor air quality (but the filter should definitely be your first step).

Please install a kitchen faucet water filter that removes fluoride. We specifically highlight fluoride because if a filter is rated to remove fluoride it will also remove the other most critical toxins.

Add in probiotics, nopal cactus, turmeric, omega 3s and ginger in the morning and magnesium at night. Due to poor farming practices and soil depletion, the foods we eat today contain only a fraction of the minerals and vitamins our bodies need. Take full advantage of the extraordinary option of superfood supplements from across the planet now available to us, such as ginseng, maca, etc.

Eighty percent of the American population are deficient in magnesium, for example – and supplementing this one key mineral can dramatically improve the quality of your sleep. Taking probiotics, nopal cactus and ginger is likely to rapidly improve your gut health, resulting in a clearer mind and a higher emotional baseline, as well as a slew of other benefits. Nopal cactus will also help stabilize your blood sugar, reducing inflammation and creating its own cascade of benefits. Adding turmeric and omega 3s will further help reduce inflammation.

Be sure to take the supplements every single day for at least three months minimum before evaluating the impact on how you feel. The changes may or may not be instant.

Month 4 Goal) Own Your Sleep Routine and Environment to Get Consistent Good Sleep Your sleeping space must be 100% dark. Get yourself blackout curtains, place tape over any blinking LED lights, and eliminate other light sources. Replace fluorescent or LED "bright white" light bulbs, which disrupt your circadian rhythms and your ability to fall asleep, with "soft/warm white (yellow)" LED bulbs. Get all the electronic gadgets out of your bedroom, including TVs, cellphones, tablets, etc.

Ensure that your sleep area is not ever used for anything other than sleep and sex. Create a very clear mental separation between your sleep area and the rest of your home.

Create a consistent evening sleep ritual that

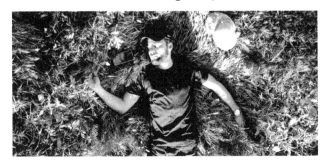

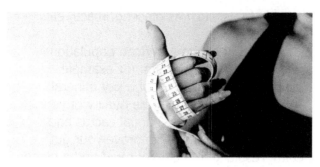

starts with an early dinner at least four hours before your bed each night, as eating early will help you sleep better. Make sure your dinner is focused on fats and proteins, thus lowering carbs. Before the time you intend to fall asleep, begin a routine of at least an hour of no-screen time and avoid fluorescent white lights.

Get a sleep app for your phone to figure out the correct time for you to fall asleep, depending on the time you want to wake up. It's important to sync your sleep with the natural REM cycles, and the apps can help you figure out the optimal time you should fall asleep.

For falling asleep, you can try supplements that include low doses of melatonin. If you have trouble staying asleep, be sure you add a magnesium supplement. If you are waking up early, try sleeping on a far-infrared heating biomat.

Month 5 Goal) Transition to a Clean and Consistent Plant-Based Whole Foods Diet

Create a Consistent Weekly Menu. If you cook most of your own meals, create a weekly menu for yourself that prioritizes fats (avocado, coconut, olive oil), followed by protein and minimizes carbs. If you eat out for most of your meals, then pick certain cuisines (such as Indian and Ethiopian) and order the same items each time, for example, skipping the rice.

Clean out your kitchen cupboard and fridge. Donate or toss **all** the junk food, replacing it with plant-based whole foods.

Remember that you do not ever want to give up any food or you will inevitably crave it, so replace foods with yummier options that also happen to be healthier. Stock up on snacks that are plant-based, high in healthy fats, high-protein and low-carb to replace your junk choices.

Perfect your fat - protein - carb balance. Every time you eat, maximize healthy fats like avocado and coconut and clean plant-based proteins like seeds, nuts, lentils, and beans while omitting needless carbs like rice and breads. Simply prioritize fats and proteins at every meal, and you will have fewer carb cravings as your blood insulin level stabilizes.

Month 6) Integrate a Consistent Intermittent Fasting Routine. Just as important as what we eat is when we choose to eat. We did not evolve to have abundant food at all times, and our bodies are hardwired to make use of fasting periods when our cells clean out toxins and our insulin/sugar balance stabilizes. Intermittent fasting is also a superbly simple way to create a caloric deficiency and lower your weight, if that's a goal. Whether you choose to limit your eating window each day to eight hours, skip a day of food entirely, or utilize any number of other fasting patterns, you are certain to dramatically improve the way you feel. Drink unsweetened teas and add electrolytes to your water and fasting won't be very hard, especially after the first few weeks.

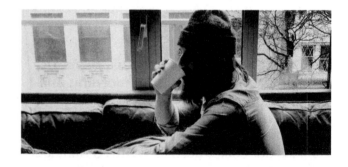

2.0 Habit Psychology: Thoughts + Actions + Habits Determine Your Life

"We are what we repeatedly do. Excellence, then, is not an act, but a habit." – Aristotle

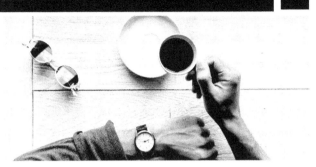

2.1 What is a Habit?

What is a habit? Is it something that just happens to you, forcing your hand, creating your outlook, and demanding that you conduct yourself in a certain way throughout your life?

Sort of.

The *American Journal of Psychology* defines a habit as "a more or less fixed way of thinking, willing, or feeling acquired through previous repetition of a mental experience."[1]

A habit isn't something we have no control over. It is largely the work of the subconscious mind. We become "primed" to act in certain ways based on our conception of things.

For instance, if we see a briefcase in a room, we're more likely to work harder, and if exposed to a picture of a cheetah, we'll tend to run faster than if we see a picture of a turtle.

It is too much work for the brain to keep everything in the focus of the conscious mind – to take in the trillions of pieces of information about our environment that tell us when to

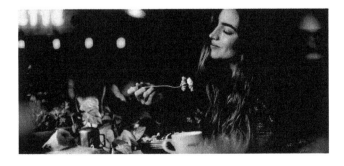

move, when to sit, when to think, who to talk to, etc.

As a coping mechanism for this informational onslaught, the brain relegates certain thoughts and actions to the subconscious mind. It puts certain chunks of information into a basket and dumps them in auto-pilot.

A study published in the journal *Proceedings of the National Academy of Sciences*, found that we can process sentences and solve equations before we're even aware of the words and numbers in front of us. That's due to "priming" or your brain putting certain information in the auto-pilot category.[2]

If we can read and do arithmetic non-consciously, how many other habitual thoughts and actions are happening on auto-pilot?

Think about how many daily, repetitive tasks you perform. You brush your teeth, ride the train to work, or have a cup of coffee. Maybe you have certain conversations even, almost as a matter of habit.

You do most of these tasks without much thought. You've already taught your brain that it is helpful and safe to put these tasks in the subconscious mind.[3]

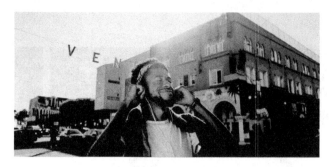

Now ask yourself, how many of these habitual tasks are positive and provide you with a sense of accomplishment?

A positive habit is formed exactly as a negative habit is formed. Going for a run, eating fresh food instead of fast foods – these are all positive habits we may want to incorporate into our lives, yet how many of us concentrate on positive habits?

If you haven't already made positive actions rote, the default, "bad" habit of eating cake at the office party will always take precedence over a better choice.

The process by which patterns of behavior are repeated until they become imprinted in your brain is known as habit formation. New actions become less conscious and more automatic.

When an action is frequently repeated, you learn to respond to a similar situation in a specific, automated way.

We can choose a new way to respond to a habit that isn't serving us by realizing it will need to be traded out for a new, subconscious set of behaviors. This starts in the *conscious* mind.

You can start to unravel an unproductive habit by noticing how you respond or what happens directly after you indulge in it.

On average, it takes approximately two months for a new action or behavior to become automatic and for the action to become a habit. Reconditioning ourselves for a more efficient life will take time, but it is worth the journey.

2.2 How Habits Are Triggered

"If you want something you have never had, you must be willing to do something you have never done." – Thomas Jefferson

The habit formation process involves three parts: the *cue*, the *behavior* or routine, and the *reward*.

The cue is the mechanism that acts as a trigger for the habitual behavior – like feeling hungry. The behavior or routine (eating a cookie) is the habit, and the reward is the positive or good feeling – the satisfying feeling of a warm cookie in your mouth and the subsequent dump of glucose in your blood which leads to a temporary high.

With time, the reward may not be present, but the habit continues as this becomes an automatic action.

Let's look at another example.

One day your child comes home from school exhausted and upset. You offered the child a piece of chocolate, and your child suddenly feels better. The next time your child feels tired or upset, your child asks for the same piece of chocolate to feel better again. This will eventually become a habit.

This habit is obviously a negative habit, as you have conditioned your child to see the chocolate as the source for dealing with exhaustion or sadness, instead of other habits that might help them cope with worldly challenges, like talking to a friend, getting some exercise, or even choosing a non-sugary snack.

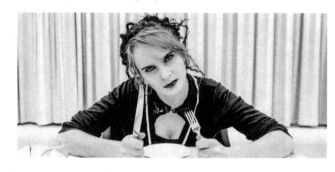

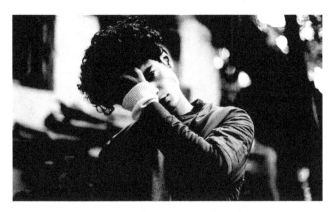

2.3 Reformatting Old Habits to Create Better Ones

"We become what we repeatedly do." – Sean Covey, motivational speaker and author of *The 7 Highly Effective Habits of Teens and The 7 Habits of Happy Kids*

The pattern of behavior must be changed to change a bad habit. The best way to eliminate an undesirable habit is by replacing it with a good one.

A moment of temporary bliss typically follows a routine habit, and that is why it is difficult to change it. You need to identify that cause and effect, and replace the routine you feel is unhealthy with a better, healthier one with similar benefits. Otherwise, your brain has no reason to tuck the new habit away as an automated response to life.

You cannot just order your body to stop doing something. It is equally challenging to order yourself to do something new, unless there is an associated reward that satisfies your brain.

To change your current routine and to stick to a new one is only possible if you believe that you can do it. Armed with this information, you can essentially hack your brain to develop a better subconscious reaction to life.

Believe in yourself and follow these suggestions below to change a bad habit:

- Plan ahead, and decide how you will respond if a trigger situation arises
- Surround yourself with supportive people to help you achieve the desired change
- Try to avoid trigger situations as much as possible as these will only reinforce the habit you are trying to change
- Use the power of rewards to help you enjoy a new routine

It's easiest to do what is easiest, so make your new habit is as easy as possible.

Meet Joe, our friendly example.

Joe wants to stop eating highly processed foods. He currently has half a bag of cookies left in his cupboard from his nightly I-have-one-cookie-for-dessert-every-night routine.

To replace the cookie-habit with a whole food, plant-based-diet-habit, Joe gives away his remaining cookies to someone else who wants them, and isn't trying to eat better.

This removes the temptation from his environment and suddenly makes the desired behavior (ditching the cookies from Joe's diet) an easier task to perform.

This tip has two parts:

1. *Remove the temptation to engage in the bad habit. As Joe did, get rid of the cookies.*
2. *Make it easy to do something better instead.*

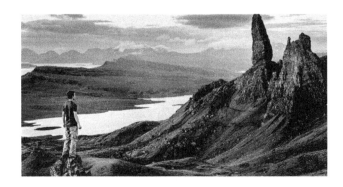

After getting rid of the cookies, Joe filled his freezer with frozen fruit so he could enjoy an after-dinner smoothie. This helped to ease him out of the cookie routine and take up a much healthier one. By keeping healthy snacks around instead of cookies, Joe isn't depriving himself of something, he's giving himself something different and better.

2.4 Five Stages of Habit Formation

Mahatma Gandhi taught that strength comes not from physical strength, but an indomitable will. Our will is simply the set of habits we create.

New habit formation includes five distinct stages. These stages follow a model called the Transtheoretical Model.[4] This model observes intentional behavioral changes and helps to establish your readiness for behavioral change.

2.4.1 Precontemplation

In the first stage, you do not intend to take action in the foreseeable future. Being uninformed or under-informed about the consequences of your behavior places you in the precontemplation stage. You tend to be stuck between making a change and not making one. There is no established time when the change will occur.[5]

In the precontemplation stage, it is imperative to observe your daily habits and identify them as positive or negative in your life. Being conscious of the negative habits you currently have is the first step.

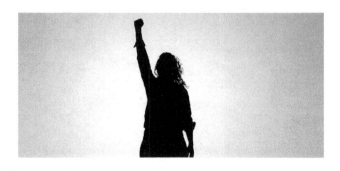

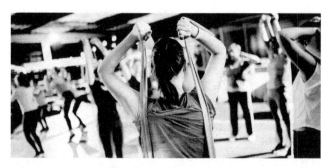

2.4.2 Contemplation

In this stage, you have identified the bad habit and you understand that changing this habit will improve your life. In contemplation, you understand that a change can be for the good and may even make plans to make a change in the near future.

The goal here is to make a change within the next six months – adhering to a timeline or goal will spark a change in your behavior.

2.4.3 Preparation

In the preparation stage, you make plans. Your mind is ready to take the required action. In some cases, you may already have attempted to make real changes and are in the process of refining your goals.

While in this stage, it is important to seek extrinsic assistance (social support) to break the habit. If your goal is to lose weight, then join a gym. Just keep in mind that a personal trainer will enable you to feel more motivated and provide a social structure to assist you in the long term, than if you were to attempt your goals alone.

2.4.4 Action

It is in the action stage that you implement change. Progress may come quickly, or it may take time. The important thing to remember during the action stage is that you are making a positive change just by your personal attempt.

This is a critical stage in making a behavioral change, so be patient here. Many people move into the action stage, fail to make the change

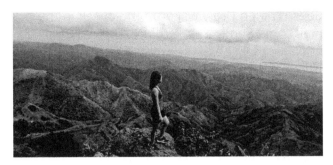

they want to see and then regress back into the preparation stage. While this may happen many times, the key is not to give up.

Continuous action is the greatest determinant in your overall success in altering habits.

2.4.5 Maintenance

The maintenance stage is where your behavior becomes routine. The only threat to your new, positive habit at this point is if you don't keep it interesting. You will be far less tempted to relapse to your old habit at this point, but identifying new goals and new potential actions will enable additional growth and habit change to occur.

2.5 Understanding the Cue-Routine-Reward Cycle

Habits are shortcuts that reduce the number of decisions we need to make throughout the day. We teach ourselves to take a certain path automatically as soon as we recognize we have the option. It's the cue that tells us we are at that point of choice.[6]

The routine is the path we have taught ourselves to take.

The reward is what makes our brains light up, in an area called the amygdala. That creates the sensation of pleasure.

Meet Pat, another friendly example.

When Pat gets home, she always puts her keys on the table, pours some apple juice and drinks

it while she thumbs through the mail. Then, she starts to feel relaxed and allows her mind to transition from thoughts of work to her home life.

* *The Cue:* arrive at home
* *The Routine:* lay the keys on the table, pour juice and sip while browsing the mail
* *The Reward:* a relaxing, calming sensation; the sweet taste of juice, and the anticipation of possibly finding her favorite magazine in the mail

To alter our habits, we can interrupt an automated response or rote way of thinking when there is a cue. Only then can we change our routine.

Pat decides to anticipate the cue and skip her routine. One day, she arrives at home as always, but this time, her new routine will be to drop everything on her bed and take a warm shower as soon as she walks in her front door. She is replacing one routine with another for a similar reward - a relaxing, calming sensation and a sense of closure to the workday.

Pat can tweak her routine. She decides to do everything as usual, except that now she decides to replace the large glass of apple juice that has no fiber, and high calories, with a fresh apple containing all the sweetness of her normal juice habit, but which also contains lots of fiber to fill her up with fewer calories as it slow the sugar's entry into her bloodstream.

This tiny change, from drinking apple juice to eating an apple as soon as she arrives home is one building block toward her larger goal of getting into a new bikini by summer.

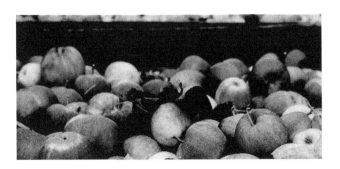

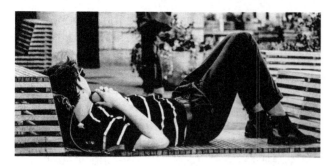

Making small changes like this may seem redundant, and in some cases futile, yet these new habits will enable you to live a healthier life and allow you to practice reforming small habits before you commit to larger ones.

2.6 Tips for Taking Your Old Habits Head On

2.6.1 External Accountability Rocks, For Some People

Lots of us perform better when we know others are watching. This is true in our work and athletic lives, and it goes for our habits too. Tell someone about the change you intend to make and set up an accountability plan with them.

Perhaps you check in with them daily or weekly to tell them how it's going. Better yet, find someone who wants to make similar changes and be accountability buddies for each other.

Try this external accountability trick:

Lee wants to make a big change to an old habit. She picks an organization she feels diametrically opposed to. The organization or person could be anyone or anything, so long as she would never give them a cent, not one.

Now, she writes a check to that organization for $5 or $500. That's how much she disagrees with the organization: she'll do anything not to send that $5. She asks her buddy Drew to hold it for her. Lee bets that she will exercise for 10 minutes on four different days this week. If she

doesn't, then Drew will drop the check in the mail come Sunday.

If Lee gets her 10 minutes of exercise 4 days this week, then Drew will give her the check and Lee can proudly and gleefully rip it to shreds.

This external accountability will allow anyone to seek assistance and collaborate with others to install new habits and success in life.

This is also a form of negative motivation, which we discuss below.

2.6.2 Leverage the Power of Positive Reinforcement

This is commonly known as a reward: you do a good thing, you get a good thing. We're using "good" and "bad" here for the sake of demonstrating these principles as simply as possible.

For many of us, food is our go-to reward. But you can also use non-edible things to celebrate and reward yourself, and you may eventually find that they nourish you at a deeper, more satisfying level than food does.

For example, a massage, a long walk, a book you can't wait to read, an in-person date with a good friend, a trip to an exciting destination, or an extra round of golf this week might all feel like even bigger rewards than a bowl of ice cream.

2.6.3 Leverage the Power of Negative Reinforcement

There's a common misconception that negative reinforcement is the same thing as punishment.

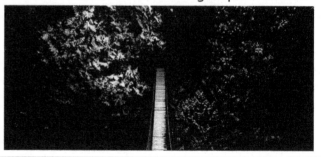

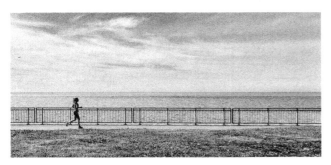

It isn't. Instead, negative reinforcement means that, if you don't do the desired thing, you don't get a reward. That is, if you don't do a good thing, you don't get a good thing (punishment = you do a bad thing, you get a bad thing). Make a bet you can't stand to lose. This can bring a little fun into the mix.

2.6.4 Experiment with Your Rewards

It is extremely difficult to say which reward will work for you. Experimenting with various rewards will enable you to determine what works best - after all the most effective reward may be hiding in plain sight.

Think of yourself as a scientist, and you are the experiment. When you want to install a new habit, such as going for a workout - experiment with various rewards. It could be anything from a post-workout smoothie, to 10 min of TV time. Finding the right reward for each goal will enable you to effectively determine your own success.

The purpose of experimenting with various rewards is to determine which specific craving is driving your routine. If you have a habit of getting a cookie every day at 10:30 a.m., is it the cookie you crave or the brief break from work?

Can you get that same break by simply taking a 5-minute walk outside? This is a healthier and more productive reward for your goal.

As you test various rewards, record your observations. Use a simple three-point observation. Using the example of going for a walk rather than eating a cookie, three observations could be; saw flowers, not hungry, felt relaxed.

Writing down the rewards forces you into momentary awareness. If your reward was, in fact, the cookie and your three observations were still, "I felt hungry, felt sedentary, and I ate too much sugar," it becomes obvious that this reward is not proactive. Writing the observations down will help you keep track of the actual effects of the various rewards.

2.6.5 Isolate the Cue

Years ago, researchers at Western University in Ontario, Canada wanted to discover why some crime scene witnesses could recall events exactly, while others completely forgot or misinterpreted information.

When eyewitness were questioned with a friendly tone and demeanor, they were more likely to provide false information. Why is this?

Researchers theorized that subconsciously, those friendship cues triggered a habit to please the questioner. Others hypothesized that this occurred due to overstimulation, or too much information.

Ask yourself, do you eat breakfast at a certain time each morning because you are hungry? Because the clock reads 8:30? Or perhaps because you're dressed and that's when the habit kicks in?

To decipher the code and understand/isolate your habitual cue, we can use a five-step model diagnosis. These are location, time, emotional state, other people, and immediate preceding action. Let's move back to the cookie at work example.

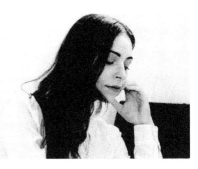

Location (sitting at your desk)
Time (2:35 p.m.)
Emotional state (bored, tired)
Other people (no one in sight)
Immediate preceding action (answered a phone call)

Use this 5-step model every time you have the cookie urge and try to pick up on cues. Chances are, you will notice that the time and social structure (other people) are consistent. Understanding the trigger can help you to create a new cue and change your habit loop.

2.6.6 Execute a Plan

Now that you have established the reward driving your behavior, the cue triggering it, and the routine itself - you can begin to make sustainable change.

The best way to execute a plan is to use a system called "Implementation Intentions".

Use the example of the afternoon cookie. Using the above framework, you learned that your cookie cue was at about 3:00 p.m. You identified your routine as going to grab a cookie and chatting with friends. Through experimentation, you now understand that it was not actually the cookie you craved, but rather the social interaction.

Solving this issue becomes as simple as writing out a plan and using a cue. The reward will follow.

Plan: At 3:00 p.m. every day, I will go to a friend's desk and talk for five minutes.
Cue: I have set an alarm on my watch.

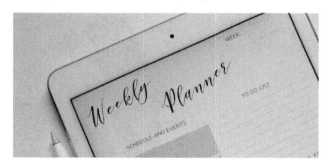

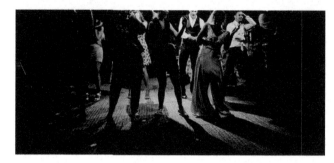

Reward: Social structure of chatting with a friend.

Over time, you will notice that you will not need the watch. In many cases, the cue has become a routine. At the same time every day, you go and chat with a coworker, avoiding the cookie and negative habits. You now have a better understanding of your own rewards system.

Creating change will take time and will require repeated experiments and failures. Once you understand how a habit operates – once you diagnose the cue, the routine and the reward – you obtain the power over it. Now you can change it for good.

2.7 How to Implement Healthier Routines

Now that we understand the basics of habits and routines, let's break down how we can install new, healthier habits into our routine structure.

2.7.1 Example #1: Jane

Jane enjoys a Friday night out with coworkers. After a long day at work, all the ladies from work go out for a drink and do some dancing.

This is by no means a bad habit or negative routine, yet it could be improved into a healthier one.

With Jane's night out there are two things at play:

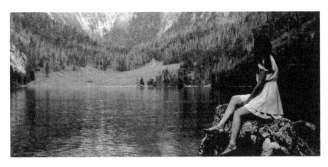

(1) The environment of socialization and being with friends after work
(2) The relaxing effects of alcohol on her central nervous system

If Jane makes a change that is too drastic, she may fall back into a different stage, or simply not enjoy the change. The trick here is to keep her cue and rewards, yet change her routine.

In this case, a simple solution would be to convince a coworker to start exercising with her - running, yoga, or rock climbing (a sport where a social structure can occur). She could even suggest keeping the dancing portion of the evening, but moving it to a local activity center where no booze is available.

If Jane simply replaces the unhealthy drinking routine with a healthy, positive exercise routine, accompanied by the social reward of relaxing with friends, there's no downside.

She's creating a healthier life and still getting all the rewards, without a morning hang-over that might come from drinking – not to mention a whole bunch of empty calories, unwanted advances by men who've had too much beer, and the damage alcohol does to her liver over time.

2.7.2 Example #2: Massimo

Every evening Massimo comes home after work and watches television, eats chips, and relaxes by himself to de-stress from a tough day at work surrounded by demanding customers and an irate boss.

In this situation, we can pinpoint two significant rewards:

(1) The enjoyment of peace and quiet
(2) The relaxing effect of eating junk food and vegging out in front of the television

In this case, the solution requires a simple rewiring of Massimo's habits. If he enjoys being isolated from people after a long day at work, all he needs to do is alter his reward.

In this case, Massimo has created the reward of food. Altering his consumption of something equally satisfying, yet that is unprocessed and natural can enable Massimo to enjoy some alone time while becoming healthier.

If Massimo wanted to make his new habit even more beneficial, he could quit the television habit, have a quick healthy snack, and if weather is permitting, take a long walk in solitude outdoors before the sun goes down.

With this new habit, he satiates his hunger, spends time in nature, and gets the endorphin rush of exercise, all while avoiding the chaos of constant interaction with others which leaves him feeling burnt out.

Simply by choosing a different reward – and one that can scientifically change his neuronal connections resulting in higher levels of dopamine, serotonin and other healthy endorphins – his reward is now euphoria!

When he anticipates all those positive effects, he'll further rewire his brain to seek out the reward, and the new behavior with solidify.

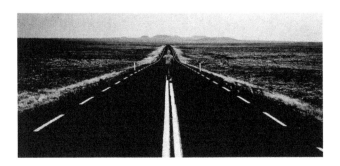

If you're like Massimo, and you need to fit more exercise into your busy life, then choose a cue (going to the gym) and a reward (a great tasting post-workout smoothie). You could also choose a non-food reward, like sitting in your favorite café and reading through a magazine you never have time to read.

When you allow yourself to enjoy both the cue and the reward - working out can be euphoric, and a post-workout shake will taste great. Set yourself up for success by thinking about the smoothie and allowing the euphoria to push you through the workout.

Sometimes this is easier said than done. That's the result of the brain wanting to stick to its well-worn, tried-and-true, subconscious ways of doing things.

By moving back to our original definition of a habit: "a more or less fixed way of thinking, willing or feeling acquired through previous repetition of a mental experience," we see that new habits can only become your "new norm" with practice.

Studies have also shown that a cue and reward are not enough on their own. In order for you to install a new, positive habit, your body must start to crave the sense of accomplishment that comes from those new behaviors. Sometimes the reward in and of itself is enough, but if it isn't on the first try, give your brain a chance to *shift the new behavior from a conscious decision to a subconscious habit.*

Your goal is to crave the reward as much as we crave the accomplishment of success that is inherent in the new behavior.

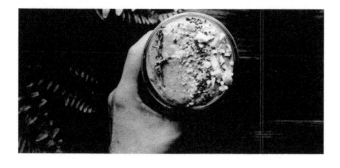

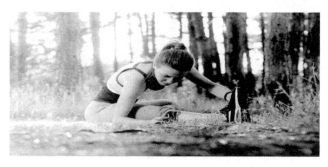

2.8 Crave-Worthy Rewards

Incentives have been used as a reward system for millennia. They help us to achieve a task, knowing we will be rewarded. The thought of receiving a reward, in most cases, is enough to motivate work.

It becomes ever more important to define your reward as something that is emotionally stimulating to you to receive the maximum benefit of using a reward.

The incentive of exercise is getting healthier and losing weight, yet the reward for that work can be a great tasting smoothie, along with the adrenaline rush that comes from learning a new dance move, or tackling a yoga pose with success that you've never done before.

During the course of your run/workout, you may constantly feel like quitting - as if the goal is too difficult. That's where your reward kicks in.

Having a predefined reward or incentive will help you push through the cue/task you are having difficulty in. It also gives your mind something else to focus on aside from its aversion to doing the new task. Would you rather spend an hour-long workout thinking, "I can't wait to have that smoothie" (or some other reward that is meaningful to you), or "This sucks, when is it over?"

2.9 Believe You Can Change

"Belief consists in accepting the affirmations of the soul; unbelief, in denying them." – Ralph Waldo Emerson

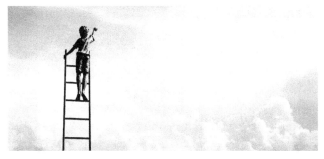

Research has shown that the most powerful determinant in habitual change comes from an intrinsic belief in change. In plain English, you need to believe at a core level that you are capable of making a change and that it will benefit you.

When people learn to believe in something, new positive habits will become easier to create. Intrinsic belief - belief in oneself - is the greatest determinant in reworking the habit loop so that you can create permanent change.

Belief is so important, in fact, that it can even change deterministic genes in your body. Scientists have long believed that if your parents and their parents had a certain type of cancer, for example, you were more likely to have that cancer too.

Cell biologist and researcher in epigenetics, Bruce Lipton, has determined that just changing your mind about something, or altering your environment, can change how your cells and DNA communicate.

This can turn the cancer switch "off" or "on," in ways scientists never understood until very recently. This is the foundation of a revolution in cellular health, but it can also be your revolution to change bad habits.

NOTHING is written in stone, unless your mind tells you it is.[7]

If belief can do all that, what's stopping you from achieving just about anything you put your mind to?

2.10 What To Do If Negative Habits Persist

Stop. If you are beating yourself up because you weren't instantly successful in changing a habit, you don't need to beat yourself with a wet noodle.

Making a change is not as simple as thinking, "Here goes, I'm just going to do it". If it were, everyone would live a happy, blissful, rich life. Breaking a habit requires constant attention, a conscious effort, and a little help from science.

Researcher and writer Mel Robbins discovered an amazing method to help rewire the brain and support change effectively. This method is called the 5-Second Rule.

2.11 The 5-Second Rule

Every morning you wake up and smack the alarm clock to snooze for another 10 minutes. You reward yourself by getting another 10 minutes of sleep, tricking your body into a habit that is not necessarily productive. Changing this habit is not as simple as just deciding that you won't hit snooze anymore.

The 5-Second Rule enables you to effectively rewire your habit, understand the negative effects of continuing the same behavior, and then change it. The habit works like this: next time you want to hit the snooze button, stop and count backwards from five - 5,4,3,2,1 - then get up.

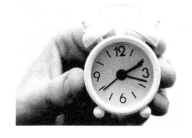

The act of counting backwards breaks your bad habit by using a little-known brain-hack. This seemingly useless act of counting engages the prefrontal cortex in the brain – one region that plans complex cognitive behavior, personality expression, decision making, and social behavior.

The 5-Second Rule enables you to make a change at the exact time when a previous negative habit would occur.

This method can be implemented in any aspect of your life. For example: the next time you are thinking of ordering some unhealthy comfort food, use the 5-Second Rule, count down, and then go to your kitchen for some fresh and healthy alternatives that you've already pre-stocked.

2.12 Psychological Mechanisms at Work: The Science Behind the 5-Second Rule

"Self-control is the chief element in self-respect, and self-respect is the chief element in courage." – Thucydides, ancient Greecian philosopher

2.12.1 Loss of Control

There are two types of people: those who control their lives and those who believe that life controls them. We have learned over the years that, on average, people who think that they control what is happening in their lives are happier, more successful, and live a more fulfilling life.

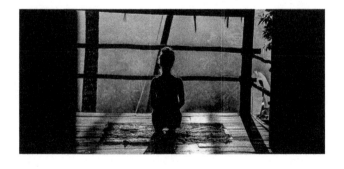

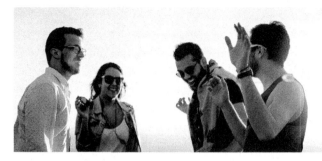

Having control of your life – more acutely, having a perception – that you have control, will lead to greater success in life, and will enable you to successfully change habits. How do you gain control –well, there are some strange ways, and some scientifically proven ones.

Henry Ford's favorite power-lunch consisted of "roadside greens."

Benjamin Franklin would sit in the nude for hours at a time to take "cold air baths". He swore they refreshed his mind and enlivened his spirit.

Yoshiro Nakamatsu believes that he can overcome a feeling of having no control by tempting death. He routinely dives into deep water, holds his breath, and waits until he is 5 seconds from passing out before rising to the surface.[8]

Why do people do these things?

2.12.2 Behavioral Flexibility

There used to be a general belief that the brain stopped growing and learning at around age 25. We now have concrete evidence demonstrating that the brain is always growing, always learning, and always installing new habits.

Understanding behavioral flexibility, and using the 5-Second Rule at any time throughout your life will enable you to adapt your habits.

2.12.3 Do Good, Be Good

Many clinical psychologists have come to a common observation – action is better than just talking about something or thinking about it.

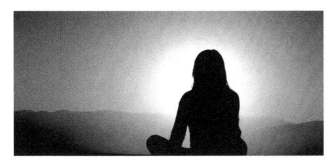

It's an age-old theory that you need to walk your talk. When it comes to creating new habits and taking control of your life, you need to actually take action – and lots of it.

Thinking about changing something in your life can only take you so far. In many cases, you'll experience a very high relapse rate into your old behaviors.

Taking action enables you to effectively break old habits and install new ones. Using the 5-Second Rule is the first action in changing your habits. 5,4,3,2,1 - GO. Or as the famous psychologist Carl Jung would say, "You are what you do, not what you say you'll do."

2.12.4 Habit Change

To change a habit, you must use a starting ritual, though it doesn't have to be as extreme as Nakamatsu's diving until near-death practice.

This will enable you to break old habits and adopt new ones with greater ease. The 5-Second Rule is a starting ritual that interrupts your subconscious reaction and starts a new, conscious act. Over time, this 5-Second Rule becomes its own habit which cues new behavior.

2.12.5 Activation Energy

Getting started is the hardest part. Have you ever noticed how hard it is to get started at the gym, to get out of bed first thing in the morning, or to start to walk out the door to enjoy a new pastime when it would be easier just to stay at home?

Activation energy is the mechanism at work that can create change and activate your new habits - awakening the prefrontal cortex to do some serious reprogramming of your current habits.

It may feel strange to think that in five seconds you could change your life for the better, but consider this. How long does it take for you to become worried about rent, or skip out on the gym, decide to eat comfort food, or decide to say hello to a stranger? Less than five seconds.

If you are anxious or scared to make decisions don't worry - this is completely normal. Powerful mechanisms reside in your brain that inhibit you from making changes, but you can take control of these mechanisms. Use the 5-Second Rule to activate your prefrontal cortex, diminish your old habits, and start new ones.

2.13 How to Break a Habit for Good and Succeed in Life

"Without action, the best intentions in the world are nothing more than that: intentions." – Jordan Belfort

There are many ways to break habits, move toward success, and bring bliss to your life, but they all require *action*.

Breaking bad habits will require constant dedication, and you might fail at first. The only thing that is worse than failing though, is not continuing. Not taking another action. That's what divides the world between people who are wildly successful, serial achievers, and those

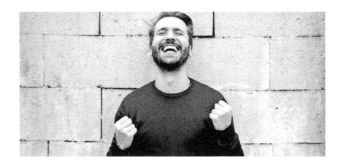

who just don't even both to start a new project or tackle a new goal.

Only after constant repetition, understanding the habit loop and applying the constant use of the 5-Second Rule can you diminish old habits and reprogram powerful new ones.

The reality of a habit is that each is unique. There is no quick fix habit hacker, only careful attention to detail and use of techniques that work with action. But there are physiological hacks that will help you achieve your goals a little easier.

2.14 Take Ownership of Your Mind: Breathing & Meditation

2.14.1 Box Breathing

Ever heard of the fight-or-flight mechanism? This is the physiological reaction of your body when it perceives any type of stress, danger, or attack on its survival. Maybe changing a habit doesn't seem like an attack on your very survival, but the brain will often treat it as if it is.

You can use the breath to change this physiological response.

Every day, we take over 20,000 breaths - yet how many of those are conscious? Breathing can be a very strong action to decrease stress and to improve the overall quality of life.

Most of us breathe with what is called a stress breath pretty much every second of every day.

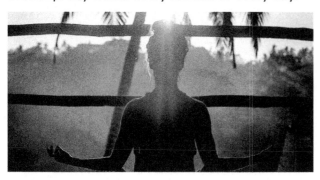

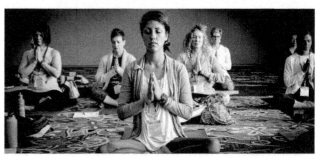

Or worse, we don't breathe at all. We hold our breaths, even if it is for only a few seconds, any time we feel uneasy. This might be when we're sitting in traffic, having an argument with a loved one, or yes – trying to change a bad habit.

The rest of the time that we're not holding our breath, we breathe very shallowly. We deprive our bodies of oxygen, and the positive physiological effects of deep, slow, repetitive breathing.

Being conscious of our breath by using the *Box Breathing method* is a life hack taught to first responders, military snipers and across numerous other high-stress professions.

This method of Box Breathing is literally a way to create space between a stimulus and response, giving you the full power to choose the most appropriate response. Instead of reacting to a stressful situation, you are then empowered to snap your mind out of fight-or-flight mode.

The method is simple. You just train your body to do three complete breaths each minute.

Inhale (3-5 seconds)
Hold breath (3-5 seconds)
Exhale slowly (3-5 seconds)
Hold breath (3-5 seconds)
Repeat for 5-10 cycles.

Many meditative practices used around the world employ this very same breathing technique, because it allows you to concentrate on what is, not what you are afraid of happening in the future, nor what you will lose if you stay stuck in the past.

2.14.2 The Science Behind Breathing and Meditation

"The goal of meditation isn't to control your thoughts; it is to stop letting your thoughts control you." – Anonymous

For millennia, Eastern medicine has been aware of the positive effects of meditation and breathing techniques on stress, quality of life, and happiness. In meditation, you connect with yourself on a deeper level, find your center, and promote a sense of wellbeing.

But can science back up the benefits of meditation?

Some research has shown that meditation and breathing help to promote mental health by increasing overall personal well-being, lowering mental disability and emotional distress, while improving the regulation of certain behaviors.

Science does not fully understand the internal mechanisms at work yet, but we do know that engaging in meditation and breathing techniques lights up the prefrontal cortex of the brain - a system responsible for deep thought and intrinsic motivation.

Meditation also changes your brain wave state from a harried, wakeful, analytical thinking state (beta) to one of relaxed concentration (also called the alpha state).[9]

When your brain wave activity slows down to between 7 and 14 Hz (cycles per minute), you are in the alpha state.

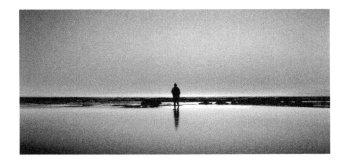

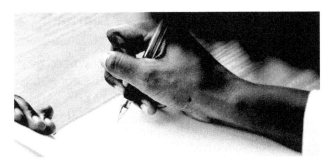

This state is also associated with daydreaming or the "a-ha" moment that so many artists, painters, inventors and out-of-the-box thinkers maintain. It makes change more relaxed and new thoughts easier to implement.[10]

Use the simple method to slow down, relax, and destress all while connecting with yourself on a more physical level. Meditation can be a powerful tool for your mental & physical health. Slowing down the mind and body brings its own rewards. This method can be used every morning, after a workout, or after a long day at work.

2.15 Summing it Up

In an ever-intensifying digital age, it can be easy to find short-term solutions to break a bad habit.

A simple internet search will show you thousands of ways to lose weight, stop drinking coffee, and stop eating food that is bad for you; yet few of these search results will prepare you for long term change.

You will need to do the work to change your behaviors. There is no way around doing that work, but you can use the "Cliff's Notes" of change by applying what you've just learned.

You can take control of your habits and engage in a new and proactive life by taking control of understanding the habit loop, applying persistent action and implementing the 5-Second Rule, whenever the need arises.

Record your observations, understand your habits, and focus on making new and positive changes.

2.15.1 Here's What You've Learned:

- Habits are actions that we perform repeatedly over time until they become second nature (move from the conscious mind to the subconscious mind).
- To break habits, you need to find new, more proactive habits.
- You can't just ditch a bad habit, it must be replaced with a new, rewarded behavior.
- The more you perform a new habit, the sooner the old habit will vanish.
- Remember the stages: precontemplation, contemplation, preparation, action and maintenance. Which stage are you in?
- Don't become discouraged if you move backwards in the steps of change. Just keep trying.
- Write down the habits you need to change and work on them one at a time. Remember to set a due date for yourself to make these potential changes concrete.
- Make sure you understand the cue-routine-reward cycle system.
- Share your new habit goals with your family, friends, and co-workers. Accountability will assist you in forming new habits.
- Isolate the cue. What does it mean to you?
- Be kind to yourself. Beating yourself up about not succeeding fast enough is just another bad habit.

- Your habit did not form in a day, so undoing that habit will take longer than a day.

Remember, a habit is the constant repetition of a particular task. You will not change your habits tomorrow, or next week necessarily. However, constant work creates consistent results.

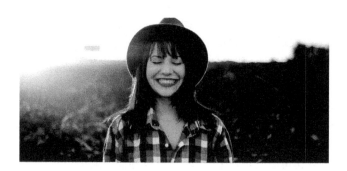

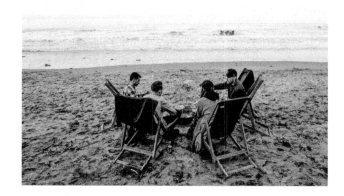

3.0 Successful People Always Think Differently

"I don't care that they stole my idea. . . I care that they don't have any of their own."
– Nikola Tesla

Successful people are rarely gifted. They just work hard, create amazing habits, and repeat the process.

They think differently.

Ever noticed that people who live extraordinary lives think in ways that make you scratch your head?

Super successful people can seem like a spotted unicorn, rare and mysterious in the making. These individuals aren't a mythical meme. They are real. History is littered with examples.

They don't necessarily come out of the womb with genius intelligence or super-human strength, but it can look that way from the outside.

Successful people aren't a magician's trick. They follow very specific steps to become someone others aspire to be.

J.K. Rowling, Steven Spielberg, Pele, Michael Phelps, Yo-yo Ma, and Steve Jobs aren't anomalous freaks that only come along once

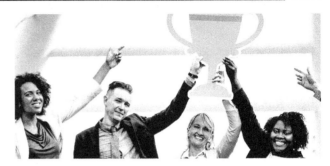

every few decades. If you want to breathe the rarified air of people this influential, you need to develop the habits of a successful person.

If you're going to be "one of them", you need concrete, actionable steps to succeed with the most grandiose dream or the most nerve-wracking or even racking works new project. Get ready to demystify the process.

3.1 Fifteen Core Habits of Successful People

Here are fifteen habits that the spotted unicorns use to live extraordinary lives:

3.2 Make a Big Goal and Then Forget It

With all the bad advice about making 'smart' goals, let's talk a little about making a goal and forgetting it.[11]

A smart goal is defined mnemonically as specific, measurable, achievable, results-focused and time-bound. An example would look like this: you want to get in shape.

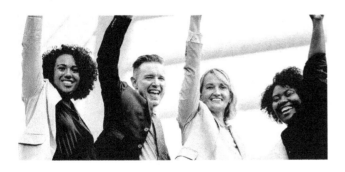

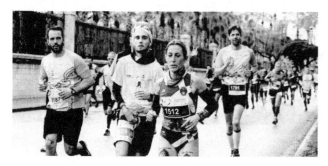

You would never say, "I am going to run the Boston Marathon next April," if you are currently forty pounds overweight and the last thing you lifted was a stack of pizzas.

It's too grandiose. It isn't broken into achievable, time-stamped parts. At least according to smart goal nonsense.

Here's the problem with smart goals, though. They aren't goals. They are tasks, or guideposts along the way. They don't inspire you or push you out of your comfort zone.

If you want to run the Boston Marathon, make that goal even if it seems impossible. Then figure out a specific plan about how to make it happen, and forget about your goal.

Get to work on the plan, and don't even think about running 26 miles and 385 yards. If you think about the 26-plus miles you'll feel discouraged. You'll feel defeated before you even start.

However, any amazing accomplishment starts out feeling impossible. Ask Edmund Hillary and Tenzing Norgay,[12] the first men to ever climb Mount Everest or Michal Jordan, the first athlete to make a billion dollars.

Focus on the first step of your plan, which might simply be: buy running shoes. Then focus on step two: walk 1 mile before Monday's morning meeting. Step three: Do five yoga stretches for runners on Tuesday, etc.

3.3 Self-Identify with the Process

To quote Nassim Taleb, we are all fooled by randomness.[13]

Outcome is a result; it might be due to skill, or intelligence, but it is often also the result of luck, or a multitude of other random factors.

Outcomes are also like a poker hand. You may be dealt four aces, or you could end up with a 3/2 offsuit. Even if you're great at poker, you can't control the game.

If you are obsessed with outcomes, you won't find true happiness or personal fulfilment. This is true whether you are a high-powered attorney, a stock trader, or an elite athlete competing at the highest levels.

Outcomes – something you can't control – eat into exhilaration.

The outcome-obsessed will need more positive outcomes over time to feel the same level of euphoria they once felt with a small, seemingly inconsequential achievement.

Outcomes are a crack habit as much as they are a poker hand.

Conversely, if you fall in love with a process, and constantly tweak it to make it better no matter the result, you will not only achieve higher levels of fulfilment, but as a by-product your outcomes are likely to improve, too.

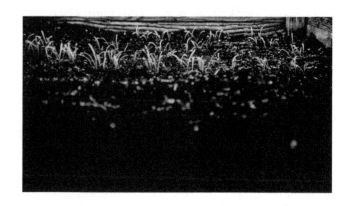

3.4 Innovate

Elon Musk, the CEO and owner of SpaceX, the Boring Company and Tesla doesn't believe in process. Yes, this totally contradicts what we just told you, but read on.
Unproductive meetings cost US companies an average of $37 billion per year. Many of these meetings discuss process.[14]

Musk runs his business based on a philosophy called First Principles instead. It's a genius problem-solving method developed by Aristotle with these major tenets:

- Forget what has been and start with a core question. I.e. Identify the problem you want to solve.
- Make a list of all the reasons the problem is unsolvable.
- Make a list of all the things that might solve the problem, but do it inadequately. Ask yourself what you would do if the problem didn't exist, and you could just create out of desire.

The crux is that you innovate by putting aside your personal beliefs and expanding your perspective.

If a process isn't working, ditch it. If you apply "fall in love with the process," as well as "ditch the process," you'll be certain to never stagnate creatively.

3.5 Overcome the Motivation Myth

We've all been suckered by the motivation myth. When the Gods at Mount Olympus strike us with

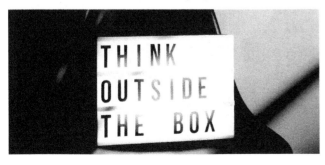

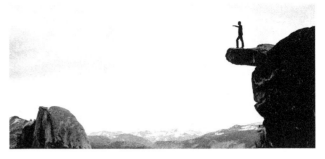

lightning, we'll get right to work on our most important goals – right?

Only, true motivation doesn't work that way.

Motivation is the result of steady, consistent action, and the thrill of achieving small goals, not the Sisyphean push of a 1000-pound boulder up a hill.

Financial planners often suggest paying off the smallest bill you have, even if it has the lowest interest rate because in so doing, you'll feel motivated to pay off bigger ones. This small action creates confidence.

That monstrous bill with the ridiculous interest rate will then seem easier to tackle.

True motivation isn't an urge. It is created by action. It is the result of this action, not a sugar rush that leaves you high for ten minutes, and then depleted and angry.

You don't wish, sulk, hope, or save up for Anthony Robbins' next seminar, and then wait for inspiration to strike. Motivation is a repeatable exploit that you can do every single day.

When you are first learning a new language, you revel in the ability to be able to ask for coffee in a restaurant or count to ten. You don't wait for "motivation" to learn those simple first words. Yet, you are more motivated to learn more with this small accomplishment.

Successful people are always surprised by their success because they don't wait for motivation to act. They get excited about the

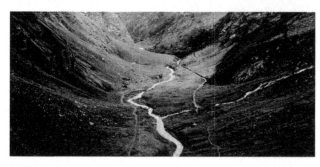

little successes, and soon they pile up to create bigger ones.

A tiny success today leads to the motivation to do something small again tomorrow, and the joy of achieving that success.

3.6 Find Flow

Mihaly Csikszentmihalyi has talked about "finding flow" in numerous books over the past several decades, using in-depth psychological studies to support his findings.

In a nutshell, Csikszentmihalyi found that what makes life worth living is a very specific level of engagement and challenge.

He suggests that to experience "ecstasy," which comes from the Greek word meaning "to stand beside something," you must step outside of a mundane consciousness that comes from doing every-day, ordinary things.

You don't need to achieve some incredible, far-flung goal. Quite the contrary. You engage completely with what you are doing moment-to-moment.

You must give so much interest and attention to what you are doing (because it is challenging, but not infuriating) that you don't have enough cognitive power left to monitor how your body feels, what is happening at home while you are at work, or any other distraction that would normally impede achievement.

If you find that you are not engaging with this level of attention, you need to do one of two things:

- Find something that challenges you more.
- Break a very challenging goal into smaller steps.

This is because the brain-wave state (alpha, primarily) that causes ecstasy is most often achieved with relaxed concentration.

As you begin to release neurotransmitters like serotonin, norepinephrine, and dopamine because you are thoroughly engaged, you will be internally rewarded to create this state again. It's a recipe for high productivity.

3.7 Own Your Attention

Most people waste a minimum of 25 minutes every day. Some of us waste much more. Many of these moments are wasted mental energy.

How much progress could you make toward your goal by eliminating just 25 minutes of wasted attention? 9,125 minutes per year.

How do you own your attention? You eliminate all distractions. If you think you aren't squandering your attention, think about the time and mental energy you spend on the following:

- Worrying about what other people are achieving or what others think of you

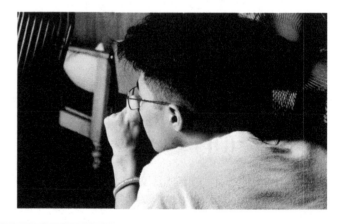

- Sitting in traffic
- Answering emails
- Sitting in agenda-less meetings
- Doing things that could be outsourced (and often inexpensively)
- Doing stuff you hate that could be delegated
- Focusing on things that don't bring you closer to achieving your goals

Owning your attention is more than just proper time-management.

You need to train your attention like a muscle. If you were starting from absolute zero and wanted to get in shape, you wouldn't throw yourself into an advanced training class. You'll just psyche yourself out. The mind and attention work in the same way.

You need to start slow.

Start with these distraction-busting tasks:

Create a distraction check-in list. How often do you check social media, or pick up your smart phone to text someone?

It takes an average of 25 minutes to get your mind refocused on a moderately challenging task once you break away to do something mindless like check your Facebook feed.

Be brutally honest with yourself, and then post this list where you will see it. Every time you find yourself engaged in one of these activities, stop.

Build Willpower. Willpower and attention are inextricably linked. Every time you refuse to stop

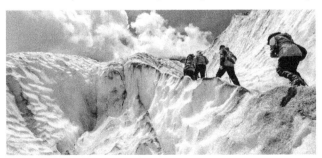

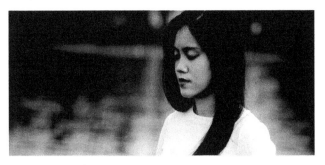

at Krispy Crème to get a donut or take the stairs instead of the elevator, you are increasing your willpower. This, in turn, increases your ability to focus.

Meditate. Wildly successful entrepreneurs meditate. So do famous athletes. Jeff Weiner, CEO of Linked In takes time out of his schedule every day to meditate.

Ray Dalio, one of the most successful hedge fund managers of all time has been meditating for more than 40 years.

LeBron James and Derek Jeter meditate. So does Oprah.

Meditation improves concentration in many ways, but a distinct way it does so is through improving attentional blink – the lag in our brain's cognitive function after you focus on something.

Exercise. This single act can increase your attention 10-fold. A study conducted by University of Illinois found that physical activity gives us greater cognitive control.

3.8 Prioritize Better

Prioritizing falls in line with owning your attention. We all know we need to do it better, but how?

Rank everything.

Stephen Covey of 7 Habits of Highly Effective People suggests ranking tasks across four metrics: important/not important and urgent/not urgent.

This will keep you from writing down endless lists of unimportant things just to get the thrill of crossing them off. Though this gives you a quick little dopamine dump, make sure your list is laser-focused.

Focus on what will deliver exponential success.

Some tasks might create small to moderate success, but what would propel you into the next stratosphere in your life or career if you did them right now?

Yes, you can write in a gratitude journal, but would making a substantial donation or raising funds for a worthy cause inspire massive gratitude and pride? Do those things that excite you and create massive success, first.

Do the hardest stuff first.

We tend to avoid the things we find most challenging. Don't let that one thing that you dread pull you down for the rest of your day.

Take a small bite out of it, and then you'll feel charged to do everything else that is a priority on your list.

Don't put out fires, give your people fire-extinguishers.

If your day consistently consists of putting out fires, then empower your people to prevent them from happening, or give them their own way to put them out.

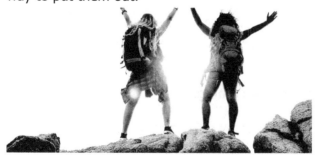

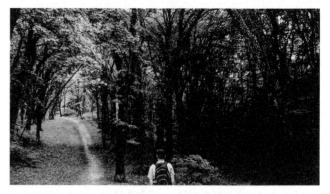

Also, be careful that you aren't creating false urgency because you like the adrenaline rush or you just want to feel wanted. These are productivity killers.

3.9 Create a Bias for Action

Not many successful people are procrastinators. They have a bias toward getting things done. An ability to make decisions quickly and move on them is essential to becoming faster, stronger, more influential, richer, and yes – happier.[15]

Many of us get caught in finding the "best' way to do something, but this can be a self-sabotaging way to not do anything at all.

Let's go back to the Boston Marathon example. If you are a beginner, you don't even know which fitness program will be best for you, but you might search Google for days wondering which of the dozens of training schedules or diets you should follow.

You wring your hands in confusion and don't make a decision at all. Day one of your action plan comes, and you haven't walked, let alone run a single mile. You need a bias for action.

Maybe you aren't internally motivated to be action-oriented. You don't have to be. Here's how you create the mindset to get things moving, instead of sitting on your butt:

1. **Do something that makes you un-comfortable**. Don't rob a bank or tag

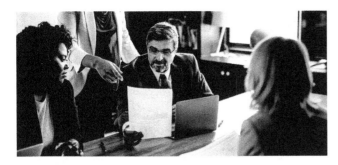

your kid's school with neon yellow graffiti, but do step outside of your comfort zone. If you have always dreamed of painting a portrait, sign yourself up for a painting class. Even if it makes you feel ridiculous, and the first picture you paint looks like pea-soup spilled across a canvas, you're moving toward your goal. And that feels amazing.

2. **Take a commission based job.** People who make a living based purely on results can't be complacent. Their daily grind consists of action, action, and more action. They know that there are no immediate gains from making cold calls, or researching a client's favorite golf course, but by making steps every day toward their target, they eventually win. It is an excellent model of how you should conduct business in every aspect of your life.

3. **Go big**. Once you've flexed your action-muscles, use them. Tackle a big project that you've been putting off, or start planning that trip around the world you've always wanted to take.

3.10 Execute Like a Boss

30% of Americans working full time say they're engaged and inspired by their work according to a recent poll. That leaves 70 million of us who are unplugged, cut-off or just bored silly between the hours of 9 and 5 every day.[16]

The executives that manage these 70 million people are contributing to their apathy.

Not everyone loves their career just because of the money it puts in their pockets. Cash can assure a certain level of health and financial freedom, but many people are looking for engagement.

They are looking for love, acceptance, respect, recognition, or reward and self-actualization. If you manage people and you aren't giving them these things, you will never reach your biggest goals.

Execute a means for people to have acceptance, recognition, and self-actualization and you'll be the boss of bosses.

3.11 Prep It Now to Nail It Later

Yo-Yo Ma, the world-famous cellist can teach us a few things about over-preparation. He's been playing cello since before he could talk, but when he has a concert on his schedule, he'll prepare as if he is playing a piece for the very first time.

Or as the acting coach Constantin Stanislavakin says, "Rehearsals are the work. Performance is the relaxation."[17] Once Yo-Yo steps into the green room just before a performance, he isn't sweating. He just chills out. He's spent countless hours working. Now it is time for him to play.

When we prepare so much that we can play a piece backwards, or give a presentation or speech in our sleep, we can relax into the performance. We've already worked out the awkward spots, the mistakes, the gaps in information.

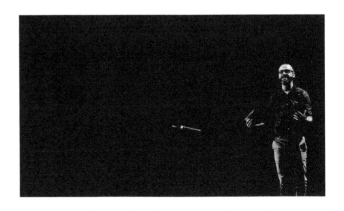

Want a new job opportunity? Practice like you have a killer performance to give in a few months. Then relax into the interview.

3.12 Realize You Can't Hack Your Way to Success

The four-day work week is a joke. Supposedly by cramming everything into four days you'll magically have more time to do the things you love.

But success takes hard work. Self-made millionaires say they work an average of 95 hours a week, or around 14 hours a day.[18]

You can't hack your way to a Fortune 500 company or the Olympic record for snow-boarding. The trick is to work hard in the right ways so that you become successful instead of spinning your wheels.

To work hard, you need to do what you love so that you are less likely to get sick of it. If you aren't working in a field that lights you up, you are likely never going to put in the hours it will take to become truly successful.

3.13 Don't Bother to Be Better Than Others

We can compare ourselves to others all day long, but what you should do is compare you – to you. Comparison will kill the joy of achievement. Knowing you just beat your all-time best financial quarter, running time,

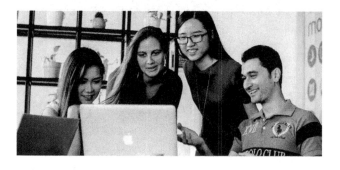

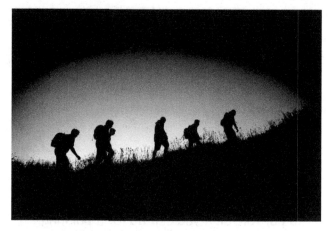

or that you learned 200 phrases in a foreign language this year is priceless.

3.14 Those Who Think They Are, Are

If you think that you can achieve something, your brain starts to find ways to make that thing achievable. Schwarzenegger swore by the power of visualization techniques, and his hunch is now scientifically proven.

The brain doesn't know the difference between actually nailing a presentation that scores a billion-dollar contract and imaging it. The brain uses the pretend presentation to prepare you for the real thing.

If you think (or imagine) something is possible, it is. You start laying down the neurological pathway to create the probable from the inconceivable.

3.15 Develop Influence

As a CEO, Amy is in crisis. For the seventh quarter in a row, her company's manufacturing numbers are down and people are starting to question her leadership.

She decides to call a meeting with 40 of her top managers. She discovers that there is a chasm of seething hatred between the top leaders.

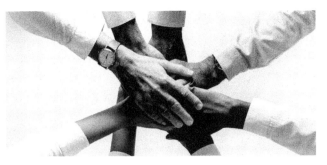

Some are trying to lead the company in one direction, with a desire to expand into new markets, and the other half want to focus on serving the clients they already have, feeling that the company's resources are thin.

The answer, Amy realizes, is that she needs to influence these people to cooperate. To take the vision for the company's future and marry it with core business practices that won't leave their current clients behind. The problem is, she's new to the company. No one trusts her. Her word means mud until it's proven. Without influence she'll be dead in the water.

Here's what Amy started to do:

Connect with people emotionally. When people get to share a part of their emotional selves with you they get a dopamine in their brains. This makes them feel more open and receptive to suggestions.

Use confident body language. People respond to our body language almost more than to what we say. Stand tall. Expand your chest. Hold your head high.

Tell stories of success. Instead of numbers and bottom lines, she started talking to her executives like she was telling an Aesop's tale. She found they related more, and their actions changed.

3.16 Be Humble

"The true artist is not proud: he unfortunately sees that art has no limits. He sees darkly, how far he is from the goal, and though he may be admired by others, he is sad not to have reached that point to which his better genius only appears as a distant, guiding sun." – Ludwig van Beethoven

Great composers like Beethoven or Mozart lost themselves in their work. It was never good enough, even when packed audiences gave them a standing ovation, and patrons poured money into their next masterwork.

No matter what you achieve, stay humble. Stay wide-eyed with curiosity. The answer to the question of what you can do next is infinite.

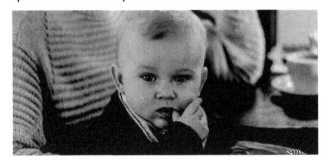

4.0 Food is Medicine: The SimpleOptimum Nutrition Blueprint

4.1 Why Your Diet Is Killing You: Preventable Disease and Early Death Are Inevitable Until You Change

"We are a nation of food addicts, not metaphorically but literally. Americans eat 146 pounds of sugar and 152 pounds of flour every year. That's almost a pound of sugar and flour for every man, woman, and child in America every single day! It has led to an epidemic of unprecedented obesity and disease." Mark Hyman, MD, functional medicine physician and best-selling author of several books, including *The Blood Sugar Solution.*

If you are anything like the average American, you often feel run-down, restricted by chronic symptoms, are overweight, and barely have the energy to get out of bed every morning, let alone tackle bigger goals that nag at your soul.

Maybe you just want to lose ten pounds, or your problem is more serious. Perhaps like so many Americans (and people increasingly around the world) you're suffering from a growing obesity epidemic. You may wonder how you got to be one of *those* people.

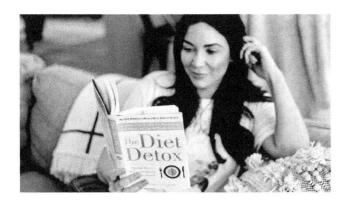

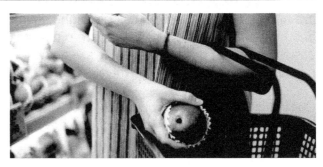

We've been trained to write off these unpleasant red flags as an unavoidable result of aging. Once we graduate from our teenage years to adulthood, we're supposed to put up and shut up.

Simple changes to our grocery store list or daily lunch order at the café surely can't make that much of a difference ... or can they?

More of us are finding ourselves feeling run-down in our early twenties now, so what the heck is going on? Obesity, lack of drive, and a lack of energy are for old farts, not people barely out of their adolescent urges.

We no longer need to run from saber tooth tigers as our ancestors did, modern life is increasingly demanding in other ways. Our attention is pulled like a deranged spider on a web with no end.

After we walk the dog, drop off the kids at school, work a full day, reply to emails and calls once we leave the office, pick up the kids – you are then expected to pay the bills, survive a killer commute on jam-packed freeway or public transit system.

Then, of course your significant other expects quality time with you, and you'd love to give it to them, but you're just plain pooped. Who has time or energy left to take exquisite care of themselves?

What's more, we are confronted with over 200 food and beverage-related decisions every day. This drains our finite energy and attention.[19]

Food is more accessible than ever, and our culture encourages us to eat anytime, anywhere, whether it's mealtime or not, and whether we are hungry or not. The high-calorie, high-sugar, and high-sodium packaged snacks are often the easiest to find in our office building's vending machine, the corner store, or the local café.

Our workplaces, the environment where we easily spend most of our waking hours, are rarely supportive of self-care practices and healthy eating habits. The workplace culture is changing with a growing popularity of workplace wellness programs, but still too many of us work in a job that requires us to remain seated, eyes glued to a computer screen, and working hours meant only for those with no prospects for a life at all, let alone a quality, healthful one.

Caffeine, soda and other sugary sweetened drinks, and high-sugar snacks and desserts usually dominate the vending machines. Cafeterias or snack shops in or near our workplace don't offer much better. Convenience understandably wins out.

It can be incredibly hard to set and stick to our health priorities with so much stacked against us.

But there is a way to revitalize your health and well-being – and it is easier than you think. Remember that glow and radiance we mentioned? How envious have you been of others that seem to have some genetic

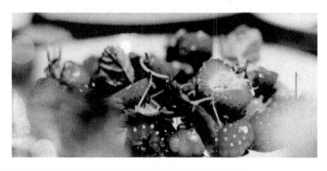

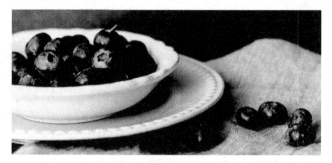

magic trick up their sleeves to look and feel so amazing? You're about to find out that there *is* no trick. There are actionable steps you can take to achieve the best health you've ever experienced.

All it takes is your willingness to explore and experiment to discover what works for you and your unique body. Once you understand that the quality of your food has real consequences for both your day-to-day vitality as well as long-term disease prevention and management, you won't turn back.

That glow and radiance come naturally when you eat as close to the source of life as possible – whole, plant-based foods, as fresh and minimally processed as possible, brimming with vitamins, minerals and other nutrients will do wonders for your health.

At every meal, you have a choice. You will soon find that making more choices from the world of whole, plant-based foods leaves you feeling more energetic, healthier, and lighter than ever.

You will train your body to crave these foods instead of the nutritionless junk it has been forced to live on.

4.2 The Standard American Diet (S.A.D)

But first, let's discuss our current food environment. What does the average American diet look like? Where is there room for improvement, and why is it so important that we

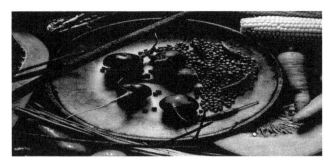

make those improvements? How can you benefit from a new way of eating, and ditching the S.A.D. way that most people eat?

Depleted by demanding and stressful lifestyles, many of us find ourselves faced with the task – not the chore – of filling our fuel tank. Yep, it's time to eat.

The Standard American Diet, sometimes called S.A.D., encompasses our contemporary food environment. The S.A.D. often features calorically dense foods that offer little nutrition (think vitamins, minerals, and other key nutrients) in return.

This way of eating supports your indulgence in bagels, muffins and cookies, burgers, side dishes like French fries or dinner rolls, multi-layer sandwiches with generous portions of highly processed and salted meats and cheeses, sweetened and caffeinated beverages from soda to mocha to energy drinks, and frozen pizzas and pastas.

Vegetables and fruit are more often seen as garnishes and side dishes, less often as the main attraction. When plants do make an appearance on our plates, they are often canned or underneath high-calorie, high-sugar dressings and sauces, and rarely in their fresh and unadulterated form.

If the way we feed our children is any reflection of our national food culture, recall the recent controversy in the funding of our national school lunch program that concluded that ketchup on French fries and tomato paste on pizza do in fact count as a serving of vegetables.[20]

Famous chef, Jamie Oliver, visited kids in suburban and rural schools to teach them about eating well, and more than half didn't know the difference between a tomato, and a potato. No joke.[21]

Visit the average American grocery store's snack aisle, and you'll find products that are high in refined flours and sugars – corn syrup and white flour are the main, if not only, ingredients in pastries and other baked goods. But they are also hiding in chips, crackers, and snack bars.

As you will see in the next sections, this reliance on refined flours, refined sugars, and an overall high intake of sugar, salt, and unhealthy fats lead to poor blood sugar management and sluggish metabolism.

In the short term, these "dead" foods affect many aspects of our daily life from sleep quality to energy and mood. The long-term effects of the S.A.D. are also discouraging, as evidenced by the ballooning rates of heart disease, high cholesterol, type 2 diabetes, neurodegenerative diseases, high rates of adolescent depression, so-called attention deficit disorders, autism, and other chronic conditions.

No longer hunting and gathering for our daily caloric needs, we now enjoy 24/7 access to food. Remember when all you could buy at a gas station was gas? Or, when the only thing available at a bookstore was, well, books?

Now, locations like these are round-the-clock opportunities to eat, and eat badly. Gas stations come complete with mini-marts, and no bookstore is complete without a cute café

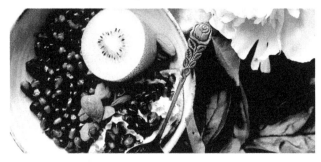

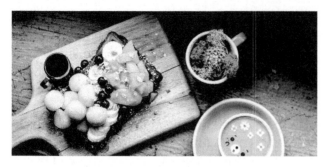

offering fancy coffee drinks and pastries, cookies, sweetbreads, and more.

Whether it is mealtime or not, whether we feel genuine hunger in a given moment, this is not the point. Implicit messages reach our conscious and subconscious awareness on a daily basis through printed billboards, food industry commercials on radio, TV, and magazine ads.

Restaurants and coffee shops are open at all hours. We are encouraged to grab a bite here, sip on a sweetened coffee drink or soda there, and treat ourselves to something tasty after a hard day. We nibble on refreshments during business meetings, slip into a drive-thru for a quick snack on the way home for work too exhausted to seek out high quality, plant based foods, and the rest is history.

Even our cars reflect our sad food environment. Remember when cars came without drink holders inside? The auto industry knows we eat in our cars, and they responded. In Michael Pollan's 2008 *In Defense of Food*, he indicated that we eat about 20% of meals in our cars.

At three meals a day, seven days a week, that comes to more than 4 meals a week completely on the go and on the road. Considering what is usually available on the interstate, that's astounding!

Increasingly, "food products" dominate today's food environment. Notice the word product.

In contrast to whole foods, relatively unchanged from their original state in nature, food *products* are highly processed with gobs of sugar, fat,

and salt (MSG), all designed and engineered to generate cravings. That's right folks, this is food "stuff" created by chemists in labs, not by Mother Nature.

Packaged and processed food products trigger both blood sugar spikes and blood sugar crashes, creating a vicious cycle of mood and energy swings often accompanied by insane cravings. Food products are cheap, easy to overeat, high on calories, low on vitamins and minerals, and quite convenient.

They're made that way so that you want more of them, and often. They were never designed to nourish your body.

4.3 The Effects of S.A.D. on Health

Unfortunately, this way of eating has consequences that are not so convenient. The Standard American Diet combined with a high-stress and hectic lifestyle that most of us are used to is a recipe for disaster.

Lifestyle and diet are the most influential determinants of health, and there's no getting around that fact. **There is a better way, and it comes down to two words: nutrient density.**

What most of us accept as food – really food *products* – are low nutrient-density foods. They are engineered, packaged stuff that has fewer nutrients (vitamins, minerals, and phytonutrients) per calorie than just about any whole food. Typically, they are not very satiating,

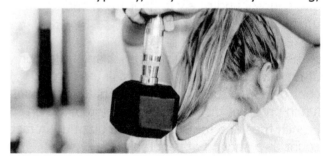

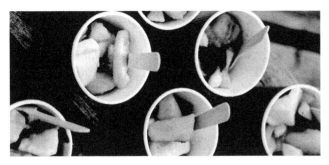

or, satisfying. So, we eat, eat, and eat, and then wonder why we don't feel full.

The side effects of this disastrous diet are not surprising, exposing you to a number of degenerative diseases. Today, even youngsters are diagnosed with diseases that were once considered "old age" diseases, with type 2 diabetes being the most eye-popping.

Because processed foods associated with S.A.D. are far lower in nutrients per calorie than whole foods, they don't stop us from feeling hungry.

We keep munching on these foods without ever feeling satiated because they offer our bodies no real nutrients – and so we're compelled to eat more.

This grave habit has caused severe metabolic and cardiovascular disorders, like never before.

Whether you realize it or not, you are putting your health at risk because of your diet.

Here are some of the shocking statistics related to the causes of death from diseases and their relation to food consumption:[22]

- One in three Americans die from cancer.
- Nearly one in ten Americans die from diabetes annually.
- Heart problems are extremely common. Someone has a heart attack every 25 seconds, and a person dies from a heart attack every 45 seconds. Heart disease is the most common cause of death in the U.S.
- The risk of a heart attack for an average American on a S.A.D. can be reduced

from a whopping 50% down to 4% if they are on a plant-based diet, eliminating dairy, eggs and meat from the diet.
- The risk of fatal prostate cancer in men and fatal ovarian cancer in women is higher for those who consume animal products than those on a plant-based diet.

Thanks to S.A.D., you are more vulnerable to the following health problems:

- Acne
- Acidosis
- Heart attack
- Lower back problems
- Reduced breast cancer survival rates
- Obesity
- Higher cardiovascular mortality risk
- Alzheimer's disease
- High cholesterol levels
- Enlarged prostate and prostate cancer
- Inflammation and unhealthy oxidation
- Inflammatory bowel disease
- Kidney malfunction
- Constriction of blood vessels
- Asthma
- Pancreatic cancer

Once you realize how horrid the S.A.D. way of eating is for your health, vitality, and mental fortitude, you'll be compelled to eat differently. Knowledge is power, right?

Let's now turn our attention to eating like a boss, not a tired, sick, prematurely old person.

Cancer, diabetes, and heart disease are some of the leading causes of death in the world, and multiple studies suggest they have a common underlying factor: inflammation.[23]

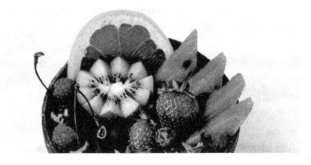

simple + optimum
core routines for extraordinary living

simpleoptimum.com

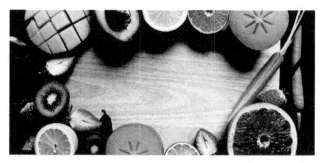

Chronic inflammation can make you feel uncomfortable in your own skin. It can zap your energy in a hurry and cause you to pack on the pounds so you can't fit into your favorite clothes.

Studies have found that the Standard American diet, full of starch, carbohydrates and excessive refined sugar, is the leading cause of this inflammation and the consequential rise of inflammatory diseases. In fact, an average adult eats more than 60 pounds of added sugar in foods every single year, and that doesn't even include sugar from fruit juices.[24,25,26,27,28,29]

Besides chronic inflammation, this extreme sugar and starch intake is leading to what doctors and dietitians call an "astronomical obesity epidemic". A whopping 31% of adults are obese, and this number continues to rise thanks to the widespread use of added sugar, high fructose corn syrup, and other sweet additives. According to researchers, manufacturers add extra sugar to 74% of the foods you'll find in the grocery store.

It's time to take control of your health by returning to whole foods, reducing sugar, and stabilizing blood sugar naturally. This is key if you want to get inflammation under control, maintain a healthy weight, reduce your risk of chronic disease, and restore your health and wellness. By shifting to a more holistic approach to food, you can help your body to naturally moderate its blood sugar levels.

Are you ready to reset your mind and body, free yourself from a sugar-laden diet, and experience renewed vitality and lowered inflammation?

To be successful, you need to identify the habits that can help you to succeed. For example, if

you want to lose weight, get disciplined with your eating habits. Healthier eating will not only help you drop pounds, but it will also help to boost your energy, making you more active, healthier, and thus happier about your improved life. We are now going to discuss the guiding principles of a balanced diet and healthy lifestyle.

The following are ten guiding principles that can be adopted as habits to banish inflammation, lose weight, and feel your best. By incorporating these ten basic principles of holistic nutrition, you'll immediately begin to see health benefits like reduced weight, fewer signs of indigestion (e.g., bloating, gas and cramping), fewer sugar cravings, increased energy and vitality, and an improved mood.

Over time, stabilizing your blood sugar by eating fewer carbohydrates and more healthy whole foods rich in protein and fat can stabilize your blood sugar and reduce your risks of common diseases like diabetes.

4.4 Five Guiding Principles

These five principles are easy to implement and accessible to anyone. Starting on them as soon as possible is a good way to kick off your healthy lifestyle.

We'll present these principles briefly here, and then talk about them in more detail throughout the rest of this chapter.

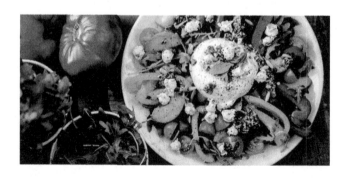

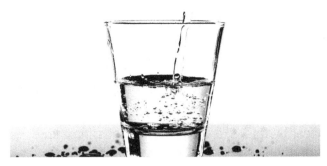

4.4.1 Clean up your diet by replacing all animal products, gluten, soy, processed, artificial, **fried foods and alcohol. There are** exponentially **better choices** available for each of these. Always hack your dietary habit loop by **replac**ing foods with better options, **or** the inevitable cravings will make your changes unsustainable.

4.4.2 Eat a consistent diet by **choosing the same simple** plant-based whole **foods each week**, and optimize your diet with food-based nutritional supplements. Following a consistent diet creates simplicity and stability, while nutritional supplementation helps ensure proper micronutrient intake, optimizing your digestion, blood sugar levels and general wellbeing.

4.4.3 Drink abundant water, replacing all sugary drinks **and** juices. It's quite astounding how many entirely pointless calories are consumed each week in drinks. Replace your sodas, lattes and juices with water and unsweetened teas. For an extra jolt of energy, discover Yerba Mate and Matcha teas. For flavor, check out all the different herbal teas, most of which are also great cold. While you're at it, get yourself a metal water bottle, so you're not sipping up plastic toxins with your water.

4.4.4 Choose **a correct macro-nutrient balance** at each meal. Prioritize healthy fats and proteins, minimize carbohydrates and optimize digestion with daily probiotics, enzymes, ginger, and turmeric. The balance between macro-nutrients (40% carbs / 30% fat / 30% protein) is just as critically important as the quality of the food itself. Eating more healthy fats (avocado and coconut are always good

choices) and proteins will help you feel more full, thus preventing carb/sugar cravings.

4.4.5 Follow a daily or weekly intermittent fasting schedule appropriate to your life's flow. Whether you choose a limited daily eating window or abstain from food one specific day each week, you're going to experience a huge boost to your health.

Now. Let's get down to the details of these guiding principles so you can understand exactly how they'll change your life for the better.

4.5 The Fat-Protein-Carb Ratio Makes or Breaks Your Life

4.5.1 It's Carbs, Not Fats that Are Making You Unhealthy

The controversial topic of carbs shouldn't dissuade you from learning more about why they can be so dangerous. There are many opinions about carbs, but one thing seems to be agreed upon by everyone in the medical field, and certainly by nutritionists. Carb consumption can cause wild blood sugar swings.[30] When they are restricted, somehow people "magically" experience healthy blood glucose levels and all the health benefits that come with those levels.

Whether you choose to use the entire menu we provide at the end of this book, or portions of it, you'll be cutting carbs. Before we discuss why the fat-protein-carb ratio is so important to your health, let's talk about carbs vs. fats more specifically.

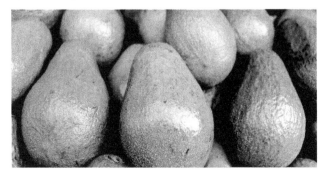

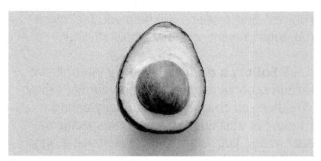

A Harvard epidemiologist describes the problem most aptly. Dr. Frank Hu told the LA Times, "The country's big low-fat message has backfired. The overemphasis on reducing fat causes the consumption of more carbohydrates and sugars. That shift may be the cause of some of the biggest health problems in America today."[31]

This projection and demonization of fats – including healthy ones – has made us very unhealthy overall.

Moreover, if you want to be a high-performance person (and this isn't just for athletes) once you increase carbohydrate consumption above the levels that you need for survival or periods of intense physical activity, you lose your ability to rely on fat burning mechanisms.

You also begin to experience the damaging effects of chronically elevated blood sugar levels, including neuropathy (nerve damage), nephropathy (kidney damage), retinopathy (eye damage), increased cardiovascular disease risk[32], potential for cancer progression (tumor cells feed on sugar) and bacterial or fungal infection.[33]

While we don't advocate eating animal products, you also shouldn't fall into the trap that so many vegetarians and vegans succumb to – of becoming a carb-o-holic.

Carbohydrates are an important element of your overall diet, but the amount and type is very important. Getting the ratio right, while making sure not to over-indulge in simple carbohydrates can mean the difference between a sustained energy level, stable glucose over a 24-hour period, and easy weight maintenance.

Weighing in too heavily on carbs – especially processed carbs – can lead to your worst nightmare: wild weight fluctuations, gut health issues, unstable blood sugar levels, mood swings, and more. Getting your fat-protein-carb ratio right is vital.

Healthy fats, like those in avocados, flax seed, hemp and camelina oils, etc. can replace carbs to help boost your health. Of course, we advocate a plant-based diet. Plants contain carbs too but they are the right kind. They provide massive amounts of vitamins, minerals and fiber, whereas simple carbs only cause unstable blood sugar levels.[34]

Ideally, plant-based foods offer a high level of nutrition, which will ultimately fuel your body, but we need the right kinds of nutrients from varied sources of foods to live in good health and with overflowing energy. What we eat every day will determine, to a large degree, the quality of our lives.

4.5.2 Getting Macronutrients Right

We consume three main types of nutrients on a daily basis.

They are called macronutrients and are sourced from fats, proteins and carbohydrates. Nearly every food you eat from rice (carbohydrate) to lentils (protein) can be sorted into a particular macronutrient profile.

More important than the respective macronutrients are the ratios in which we eat them. A high fat, low-carbohydrate style diet would see ratios of 50% fat, 30% protein, and 20% carbohydrates.

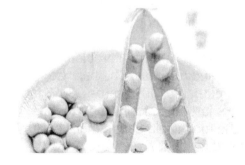

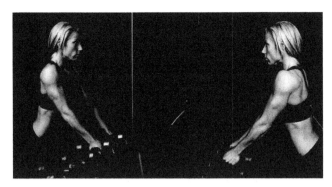

This type of diet has been shown to promote fat oxidation and improve the profile of distance runners who run more than 80km/day (ultra running).

In contrast, a high carbohydrate diet would see ratios of 60% carbohydrates, 20% protein, and 20% fat. This is a typical profile for athletes who rely on short bursts of power, such as strength training or weightlifting.

Macronutrients play a large role in your physiology and overall body composition. Body composition is a term we use to describe multiple aspects of your overall health, including weight, body fat percentage, waist-hip ratio, and more.

When it comes to health and fitness, body composition is far more important than overall weight as it provides a much more detailed perspective on your overall health.

For example, if Jessica, who's under a weight training, resistance-based program only looks at the scale as a health measurement, she may feel discouraged as the weeks go on since her weight might increase due to increase of muscle mass.

We know that muscle density plays a large role in our overall weight, which means even if Jessica is lowering body fat through diet and training, she may be gaining muscle - and not moving the scale.

Observing your health from the perspective of body composition enables you to monitor true progressions in body fat loss, waist-hip ratio, muscle density, and more.

Depending on your specific goal and current body composition, you can eat a variable amount of each macronutrient to attain a specific goal. Keep in mind that all three, carbohydrates, fats, and proteins are important to your health and vitality.

For example, a diet that is high in protein has been shown to promote weight loss and reduce the amount of time spent recovering from workouts. If your goal is similar to that of strength athletes and bodybuilders, a diet that is high in low fat protein is essential to your success.

It is also important to note that a diet with a constant surplus of any nutrient, including protein, may be detrimental to your health.

A diet that has an excess amount of protein on a consistent basis has been shown to increase the risk for coronary heart disease and even cancer.

For more information on the amount of protein you should consume, see the protein section below.

In contrast, if you fall into obesity spectrums, or have chronic high blood pressure which can lead to diabetes, or obesity caused illnesses, a diet that is high in vegetables has been shown to be very effective in lowering blood glucose levels and effectively reversing diabetes and obesity caused illnesses.

This is why your macronutrient split becomes a very important factor in your overall health. Understanding how each macronutrient works,

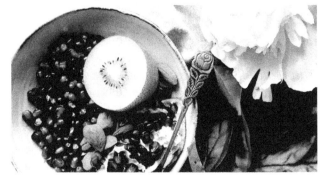

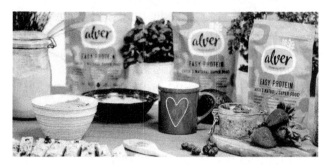

its benefits and downsides can help you determine the best macronutrient profile for your goal(s).

Let's break down each macronutrient to better understand nutrition.

4.5.3 Protein

It's the most talked about nutrient in the health and fitness industry, but what is it all about?

Protein is a macronutrient that is broken down into amino acids. These amino acids are then metabolized by the body and used for various roles. For example, L-glutamine is an amino acid regularly found in the proteins of meat based products. When consumed, L-glutamine has been shown to assist in immune function and promote recovery of type 1 muscle fibers - perfect for endurance based athletes.[35]

Each macronutrient, including protein, can be categorized by the amount of energy it provides the body. Energy in the human body is measured in calories - this is our main source of burned fuel.

Protein contains, on average, 4 calories/gram (relatively low). This low caloric value means we can eat a lot of protein based foods and not become overly concerned with overeating.

Therefore; finding clean sources of protein becomes essential to your success.

How Much Protein Should I Eat?

Protein is a staple in your diet, and depending on your goal you should eat around 30-40% of your daily calories from protein based sources. For most people, this means eating about 600-800 calories from protein sources.

If you exercise on a regular basis and have goals of weight loss and gains in muscular strength, you can use the chart below to determine how much protein you should eat on a daily basis.

WEIGHT	ACTIVITY LEVELS	MULTI-PLIER	TOTAL
100 kg (220 lbs)	**High** (4-5x/ week)	1.5-1.8	160g Protein/ day
80 kg (180 lbs)	**Moderate** (3-4x/week)	1.2-1.4	105g Protein/ day
60 kg (130 lbs)	**Low** (1-2x/ week)	0.8-1.1	55g Protein/ day

4.5.4 Fat

For years, fat has been the enemy. You have been told that fat makes you fat when, truth be told, the real enemy is sugar.

Fats, also known as triglycerides, are esters of three fatty acid chains and the alcohol glycerol. This sounds a bit complicated but basically a fat is any calorie that contains lipids and are insoluble in water (they don't mix).

Over the years, fat has received a bad reputation for promoting weight gain and assisting in obesity caused illnesses. The fault

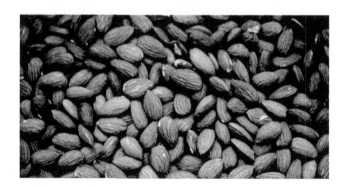

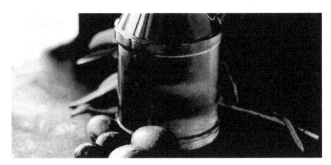

does not lie with fat, rather the type of fat we are consuming.

Good fats and bad fats?

Good fats and bad fats co-exist, and we must remember that fat is essential to our diet and physiology. Fats, better known as triglycerides, store energy, insulate us, and protect our vital organs.

They act as messengers, helping proteins do their jobs. Without a regular amount of fat in our diet, we would struggle to maintain energy levels, fight infection, and perform athletically.

As stated before, we have two types of fat, good, and bad. Good sources of fat are those that contain unsaturated and polyunsaturated fat - these come mainly from plant-based sources, vegetable oil, avocado oil, etc. Eat lots of these.

Eating a diet rich in unsaturated and polyunsaturated fats has been shown to reduce the risk of heart disease.[36]

Bad fat comes from fat sources that are heavily processed, such as the trans fats you find in baked goods. Over the years, saturated fats have been given a bad reputation for causing heart disease and other illness.

However, recent research has shown saturated fats to be an inclusive part of a wholesome diet. It should be noted that all types of nutrients should be consumed, but moderation is most important.[37]

Saturated fats can be consumed, but you should limit the amount - just as you would limit the amount of processed sugar in your diet.

Fats are also very high in calories. At more than double protein, fats contain on average 9 calories/gram. Fats are an integral part of your diet and health, but you should eat less fat than protein and carbohydrates.

So, is sugar the reason we put on weight?

In many cases, eating a diet high in processed sugar (fast food, highly- processed goods, baked goods, etc) that are high in calories and contain high amount of trans fat is the reason that many people put on weight.

Conflicting evidence on what promotes weight gain makes it difficult to identify the specific culprit. For decades, large corporations who produce sugar filled products such as soft drinks and baked goods have paid research teams to influence data towards fat as the primary cause of obesity and heart disease.

This misinforms the public leading them to eat a copious amount of sugar filled food causing an imbalance in their diet.

Complete nutrient profile means getting food from all sources. Moderation is key. Keep in mind that a diet high in processed sugar has been shown to promote obesity which can lead to several illnesses.

For optimal health try to maintain a diet that contains 10-15% of its calories from unsaturated and polyunsaturated fats.

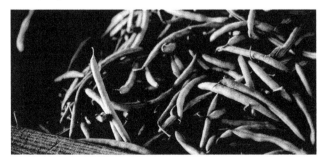

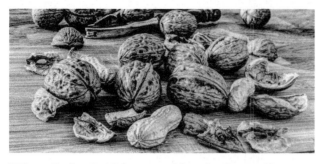

What Role do Omegas Play in Overall Health?

We are concerned with two main types of Omegas, Omega 3 and 6. Both play a crucial role in the overall success of your macronutrient split, yet one should be eaten more than the other.

Omega 3

An integral part of cell membranes, Omega 3s work as a precursor to regulate blood, heart, and genetic function. Omega 3 can be found in many food, including walnuts, flax, cauliflower, Brussels sprouts, and fish.

How much Omega should I eat?

Omega 6 is great for brain function and muscle growth but can also promote inflammation. Currently, dietary recommendations for Omega 6 are skewed due to the large amount of oils and fats in everyday foods. Companies add these fats into our food because they are cheaper to produce. This throws our ratio off and can lead to chronic inflammation and illness.

It's essential to balance your diet. The easiest way to balance out your Omega 3/6 is to avoid eating processed foods, especially if they contain hydrogenated oils (trans fats) and move towards healthier alternatives like walnuts, flax, and seeds.

4.5.5 Carbohydrates

Although vilified as a culprit for weight gain over the past couple of years, carbohydrates are misunderstood. They are the body's primary fuel source throughout the day and are the main source of fuel for the brain and muscle.

The type of carbohydrates you consistently indulge in can make or break you, though.

To be considered a carbohydrate, food must be broken down into a starch, sugar, or cellulose. Some examples of carbohydrates are rice, grains, potatoes, vegetables, fruit.

Each carbohydrate is broken down into starch or glucose. From a performance perspective, glucose is metabolized into glycogen and used to fuel muscular contractions.

Glucose is also a primary fuel source for the brain; nearly 60% of brain function runs on blood glucose concentrations.

Carbohydrates fall into a similar spectrum as fats - they are essential to your diet, yet some sources of carbohydrates may push you further from your goal, promoting unwanted weight gain and even heart disease.

From a general perspective, we want to avoid eating foods that contain high amounts of sugar, especially processed sugar. This is how you run into obesity caused illnesses such as diabetes.

The best carbohydrate sources are natural and have not gone through any type of processing to alter their organic structure. This brings us to the conversation of simple and complex carbohydrates.

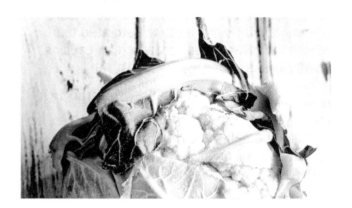

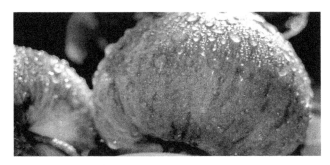

Simple Carbohydrates

These carbohydrates are sugar-based. Some examples are candies, baked goods, cereals. They are the type of carbohydrates that you want to avoid because absorption rate is low and insulin sensitivity is high. They offer very little in the nutrition department.

When we talk about a ketogenic diet later, it should be understood that we are more interested in limiting these types of carbs and sugars in your diet, rather than taking all carbs away.

Complex Carbohydrates

These carbohydrates are sourced mainly from starchy products such as rice, bran, vegetables, fruit, etc. Complex carbohydrates contain much higher concentrations of soluble and insoluble fiber. They have proven to be an effective weight maintenance tool.

Carbohydrates, on average, contain 4 calories/gram, relatively low in calories considering the carbohydrates you eat are essentially the energy that powers you through the day.

For optimal health, your diet should contain approximately 40-50% of its daily intake of calories from carbohydrates. A diet rich in fruit and vegetables would cover ⅔ of your plate and would be about 800-1000 calories daily.

Fiber and Net Carbohydrates

One of the most important aspects to remember about carbohydrates is that not all are digestible. This is a good thing! Fiber is a non-digestible source of carbohydrates that comes in two main forms, soluble and insoluble.

Fiber has been used for generations to help assist in healthy bowel movement and decrease inflammation. Unfortunately, most people don't get enough. Dietary recommendations for fiber are generally around 30g/day - depending on your weight.

These 30g will not only assist you in maintaining weight and optimizing health, they also lower your net carbs each day. Since fiber is indigestible, each gram you eat lowers your carbohydrate intake.

For example, a Gala apple contains about *22g of carbohydrates* and *5g of fiber*. This 5g of fiber lowers our net carb intake to *17g of carbohydrates*.

This is why it's important to eat foods containing high amounts of fiber whenever possible. A whole food, plant based approach to your diet will ensure you meet your caloric needs without exceeding your carbohydrate allowance.

4.5.6 Using Macronutrients to Determine our Body Composition

We all know that consistent exercise can help us obtain our health and/or fitness goals, but no workout exists that will allow you to outwork your diet. High performance athletes eat scientifically and clinically calculated diets in order to optimize performance. We can use the

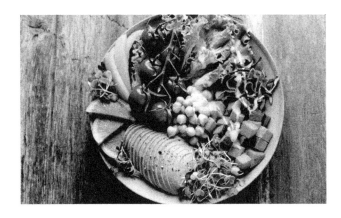

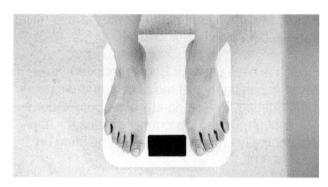

same principles to establish a nutrition program for any specific goal.

4.5.7 Creating a Macronutrient Split That Promotes Weight Loss

Many of us wish to lose weight but few will take the time to regulate the amount of each macronutrient in order to promote weight loss.

To achieve weight loss, your body must be in a state of caloric deficit. This means you eat less calories than your body burns on a daily basis. When your body is in caloric deficit, you may experience fatigue more than normal, which is why it becomes so important to eat a diet that provides the body with the best source of calories.

In order to optimize the amount of weight we lose while in a caloric deficit, we can create a specific macronutrient split. Research[2] has shown that the most effective macronutrient split for weight loss is 40% carbohydrates, 30% protein, and 30% fat.

Not only will this diet help you lose weight, but it's perhaps the easiest macronutrient split to adhere to. Consider a traditional plate of food. This split would look like this: ⅔ plate as vegetables, ⅓ lean protein, and a pinch of fat (used as a cooking oil or to flavor). A recent study found that irrespective of the minor changes in the macronutrient split, accrued time on a consistent diet was the greatest weight loss factor.

What does this mean?

Some people may find eating a diet higher in fat may assist them in losing fat through fat oxidation or ketosis, yet overeating becomes easy on a high fat diet (9k/cal/gram in fat, rather than 4k/cal/gram in carbohydrates).

Finding a macronutrient split that is easy to adhere to and balances the nutrients you will obtain becomes the most important aspect for successful weight loss.

4.5.8 What About Gaining Muscle? What is the Optimal Macronutrient Split?

If your goal is to gain muscle, then you need to follow a very different approach to nutrition. From a fundamental level, if your goal is to put on clean muscle weight, you need to be in a slight caloric surplus from high protein foods.

A caloric surplus occurs when you ingest more calories than you burn on a daily basis. This caloric surplus ensures that your body always has nutrients to source for energy and recovery of soft tissue. And remember gaining muscle is not as simple as just gaining muscle.

Exercise puts stress on joints, tendons, ligaments, and internal systems. Your diet must be balanced to cater to all the demands of exercise. A high protein diet has been shown to promote the greatest effects on muscle protein synthesis, the precursor to muscle recovery.

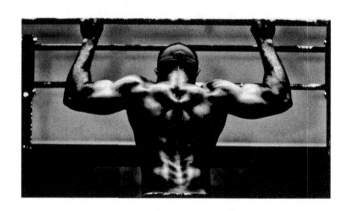

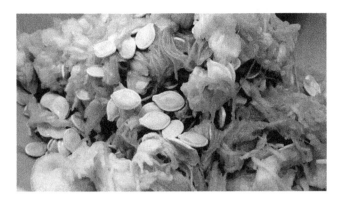

A macronutrient split perfect for your muscle building goals is high in protein, low in fat, and sourced with complex carbohydrates, which are often rich in fiber and health promoting. Complex carbohydrates are commonly found in whole plant foods and, therefore, are also often high in vitamins and minerals.

To build muscle, you should maintain a macronutrient split of 40% carbohydrates, 40% protein, and 20% fat.

All carbohydrates should be sourced from high fiber-yielding plant sources such as vegetables and fruit. A diet that is high in fiber has been shown to assist in weight loss as well as weight maintenance.

Will protein shakes help me gain muscle?

Yes, protein shakes can help you build muscle. Protein shakes are a great way to consume low calorie, high protein sources that digest at a rapid rate. Keep in mind that many protein shakes are based off whey proteins, derived from milk.

For a clean plant-based source try a protein shake that contains hemp, pea or pumpkin seed concentrates (these contain the highest amino acid spectrums).

The rationale behind ingesting protein as a shake/whey form is to consume fast absorbing protein in an effort to stimulate muscle protein synthesis. Once muscle protein synthesis has

been stimulated, amino acids then go to work in repairing muscle tissue.

If my goal is to gain muscle, why eat carbohydrates?

Carbohydrates do not help in any way to induce muscle protein synthesis or hypertrophy, so why eat so many? Carbohydrates are a source of fuel for muscles and internal systems. Muscle contractions are fueled by glycogen, a metabolised sugar from glucose found in carbohydrates.

This is the reason you hear of distance runners "carb loading" prior to a race - they want to create a carbohydrate surplus in the muscle so that they have more energy to draw from during a long run.

We can use a similar principle on a smaller scale to provide the muscle with energy for each workout. Without an adequate amount of carbohydrates in your diet, you will struggle to recover for the following workouts and may feel fatigued earlier in each working set.

4.5.9 Insulin Issues

The next important point to consider when creating a macronutrient split is your insulin resistance. Insulin, made by the pancreas, allows your body to use sugar (glucose) from carbohydrates in the food that you eat for energy or to store glucose for future use - generally in the liver or muscle cells.[38]

On a fundamental level, insulin helps keeps your blood sugar level from getting too high

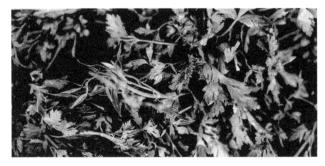

(hyperglycemia) or too low (hypoglycemia) - both of which can be harmful.

The issue arises when our body becomes incapable of regulating insulin. This poor regulation of insulin can lead to diabetes. To create a macronutrient split for your goal, it is important to have a basic understanding of your personal insulin sensitivity.

Take eating a plate of pasta, for example. Considering this food is very high in carbohydrates, 10 minutes following the meal, do you feel energized and ready to tackle a workout or do you feel sluggish and ready to nap?

Most pastas are made with refined white flour, and turn quickly into a sugar source in your body. This is why you feel tired after eating them. However, there are pastas made with non-gluten, high protein grains like quinoa which would not cause your insulin levels to spike.

The added fiber and protein in these traditional pasta substitutes can also help you to feel satiated, and contribute to your gut health as well.

In some cases, you may need that quick energy, but on a daily basis, eating a plate of pasta every night will cause you to gain weight, lose energy, and feel rather blah.

If you are ready to take on a workout, chances are your body excels at handling insulin, and you may thrive on a high carbohydrate diet. If you fall into the second category (as many people

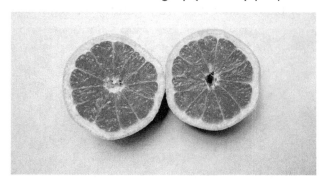

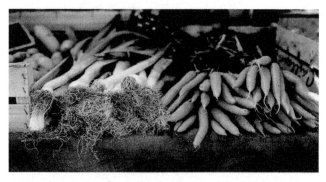

do), you may want to monitor the amount of carbohydrates you have on a daily basis and be conscious about when you consume them.

Pasta is a good example of a food that promotes a strong insulin response, but many other foods have also been shown to promote insulin. For example, a recent study found that consuming red meat and refined grains promoted the greatest spike in insulin - these are foods to stay away from.[39]

To teach your body how to regulate insulin, you should ingest foods that are low on the glycemic index. This index ranks foods on a scale from 1 to 100 based on their effect on blood-sugar levels. Foods that are low on the glycemic index are vegetables, low-fat dairy, and grapefruit.

With this information in mind, insulin response may be beneficial at certain times. In the world of strength and bodybuilding, an insulin response can be used in order to accelerate muscle protein synthesis and stimulate hypertrophy (increase in cell size).

This is why it is common for bodybuilders and powerlifters to consume fruit or high carbohydrate meals with their post workout protein blends. It should be noted that this insulin response, on a daily basis, can be harmful to the body's natural insulin cycle.

4.5.10 Benefits of Minimizing Carbs and Increasing Plant Based Proteins

Our body needs carbohydrates; they are an important source of energy. When we eat more

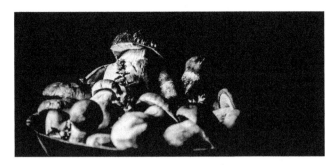

carbs than required, our body starts storing them in the form of fat. However, if we limit the intake of carbs, our body is less likely to store them as fat.

According to a study by Harvard University, a low carb diet helps people lose weight faster and maintain it better than a low fat diet.[40]

People on a high protein and low carbohydrate diet achieved impressive weight loss. Hence, it was considered a safe and effective way to lose weight.[41]

When the body starts burning fat instead of carbs for fuel, it is called ketosis. This phenomenon can take place at any time of day when there is low energy intake. Our body burns ketones as a source of energy, and this has many benefits, including increased energy levels, reduced appetite, and gradual weight loss.

The results are even better if the protein intake is adequately increased while reducing the carb intake.

Studies have shown that people on a low carb diet have more REM sleep in comparison to people with mixed diets.[42]

This sleep type is critical for your body to recover and build muscle after a long day.

REM sleep can also help to boost your immune system to keep you healthy.

Carbohydrates are broken down into sugars (glucose) to fulfill body's energy requirements. This results in an increased blood glucose level. Low carb diet helps you regulate your blood glucose level and reduce HbA1c levels. The foremost cause of type 2 diabetes is a disturbed metabolization of carbohydrates.

If you want to lower your blood sugar level and control type 2 diabetes, you should consider a shift to a low carb diet.[43] This also limits excessive insulin production, preventing several other diseases including heart disease, cancer and obesity.[44]

A 2012 study found that people on a high protein and low carb diet were at a lower risk of metabolic and cardiac conditions.

This study showed that participants experienced a significant increase in high density lipoprotein cholesterol (HDL) and a decrease in triglycerides. However, there was an overall decrease in cholesterol and low density lipoprotein (bad cholesterol).[45]

Those who eat low carbohydrate diets, high in vegetable sources of protein, have a 30 percent lower risk of developing heart diseases.[46]

Bacteria in the oral cavity multiply in the presence of dietary carbohydrates, so having a diet high in carbs can be a haven for bacterial growth. This can result in gum diseases and tooth decay. These periodontal diseases could increase your risk of dementia, heart disease, rheumatoid arthritis, and diabetes.[47]

Lowering carbohydrates in your diet helps lower hypertension, reducing the risk of heart disease. A low carb diet can also be naturally low in lactose and gluten. As a result, people suffering

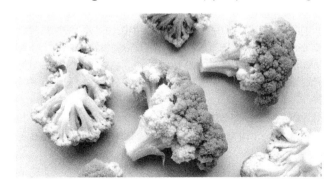

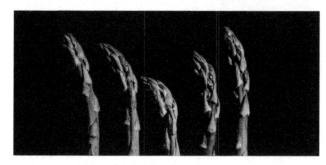

from allergies and gastrointestinal symptoms may observe an improvement in their symptoms.

Some patients dealing with schizophrenia have experienced progress in their health when they shifted to a low carb diet.

A low carb diet has also helped in improving polycystic ovary syndrome and gastroesophageal reflux disorder. As per the experiments conducted on mice, it was observed that mice on a low carb dosage had stunted tumor growth.

It was therefore concluded that a diet lower in carbohydrates and adequately high in proteins prevents cancer by slowing down tumor growth.

Cancer cells feed on high levels of glucose. A low carb diet reduces carbohydrates, which in turn reduces glucose levels. Therefore, cancer cells can be depleted of their energy by keeping to the low carb diet.

According to a study, excess carbs increase the risk of cognitive disorders.[48] By eating a low carb diet, you can significantly improve your cognitive abilities. This diet is now being used to cure Parkinson's and Alzheimer's disease.

High protein intake and high intensity exercise prevents muscle loss and increases fat loss while on a low-calorie diet. This also significantly increases lean muscle mass.

If you want effective results, you should consider eating more protein, along with some strength exercises. This will not only help you retain muscle mass, but improve your overall health.[49]

It is suggested that by following a low carb diet, you add an average of ten years to your life expectancy. Research conducted on mice by scientists at The University of California showed that mice on a low carb diet had a 13% increase in their life expectancy.

It also had several other surprising effects such as improved memory, better coordination, increased strength and slow tumor growth. In this case, many of the things we're looking at aren't much different from human. . .at a fundamental level, humans follow similar changes and experience a decrease in overall function of organs during aging.

This study indicates that a ketogenic diet can have a major impact on life and health span without major weight loss or restriction of intake. It also opens a new avenue for possible dietary interventions that have an impact on aging." said Jon Ramsey from the University of California, Davis.[50]

4.6 Principle One: Eat Clean

Approximately 95% of diets fail according to North Dakota State University.[51] That has as much to do with your mindset and approach to dieting as it does with the *actual* food you consume.

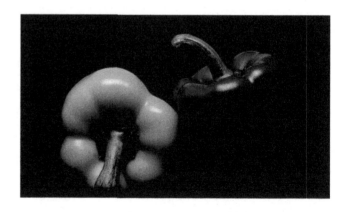

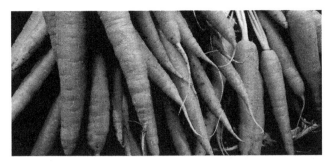

Most diets focus on eliminating specific ingredients or even entire food groups. When that doesn't work, the average person's response is to try even harder at cutting out that ingredient or food.

Yet psychologists say that this focus on simply eliminating food and "trying harder" is one of the key reasons that most diets don't work.[52,53]

Instead, you can benefit from understanding what psychologists call a habit replacement loop. Instead of just trying to cut out a bad habit, whether it's eating junk food or biting your nails, you simply replace it with a new and more positive habit.

Habits can be difficult to change because our minds prefer inertia. Inertia refers to your tendency to want to keep doing the same thing and stick to the same lifestyle patterns.

To put that into simpler terms, researchers at Colorado State University say that you're more likely to succeed by maximizing your health benefits without feeling like you're restricting your choices.[54,55]

If you want to create sustainable change and improve your health and wellness, don't just give up an unhealthy food or a bad mealtime habit. You've got to replace it with something healthier if you want to see lasting results.

For example, if you're trying to reduce your sugar intake, don't just ban all refined sugar in your diet. Find low carb snacks to enjoy whenever you have a craving. This breaks the habit loop and helps you stick to your goals.

Plus, low carb snacks that are high in healthy fats or healthy protein help stabilize and reduce blood sugar better than high-carb, low-protein/low-fat snacks.

If you have trouble giving up potato chips or pizza and fear that you may turn back to your unhealthy diet, it is suggested to follow simple and healthy alternatives, and you will move away from temptations gradually.

Replace potato chips with veggie chips, candy with frozen grapes or berries and soda with water. Also, try making some veggie pizza bites, banana pancakes, and other healthier food replacements. This will help you maintain a sustainable diet routine.

It's All about What You *Can* Eat, Not What You Can't

"Successful people are simply those with successful habits." – Brian Tracy, personal development guru

Remember that you chose to pick up this book and reflect on what it would be like to improve your own health and happiness. If someone offers you food that you know will thwart your weight loss effort, don't think or say, "I CAN'T eat that."

Our language is very powerful, even the language we choose when we talk to ourselves silently, or write in a private journal. Saying that you *can't* eat something is not the whole truth.

You CAN eat it, in fact. No one wired your jaw shut. But you CHOOSE not to eat it. In fact,

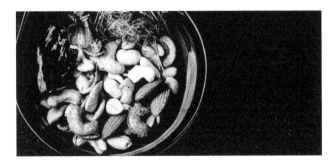

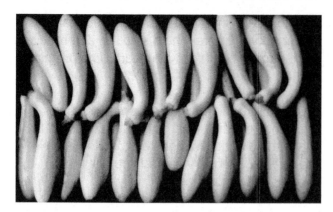

if it thwarts your ultimate goal and creates frustration for you, *the absolute truth is you DON'T WANT to eat it.*

See the difference?

Own your power in this awesome decision you're making for the sake of your vitality and health. We are the master, not the victim, of our own decisions.

Hearing the words "I can't" throughout the day, whether spoken to us by someone else or said internally, is discouraging, demotivating, and disempowering.

A mindset that focuses on what you *can* eat will make the transition infinitely easier since most of us really hate feeling disempowered. Indeed, this is one of the big downsides of the deprivation mindset so pervasive in the dieting world.

The "I can't" mentality also implies you want it, but that some external force has prevented you from being able to eat it. Again, this is not entirely the case, since you are still in the driver's seat. In the beginning, it may be the honest truth that you want the familiar comfort food that you've decided to avoid or cut back on.

If this is the case, go ahead and tell yourself and tell others that you want it - be honest. *And*, you also deserve to hear yourself say why you choose to have less of it or want to avoid it altogether at this moment.

Think of it this way: Every time Cheryl says no to a tempting morning doughnut, she is saying yes to something else simultaneously.

There are two sides to this coin: *no* to hopping onto a blood sugar rollercoaster for the rest of today, and *yes* to starting her day off right with a more satisfying breakfast that gives an energy boost to her morning that really lasts. See the difference?

Focus on what is possible, what new realizations and insights will occur, and all that you have to learn and explore. You are boldly setting out to see for yourself what a whole food, plant-based lifestyle has to offer and how to make it uniquely work for you.

This is an opportunity to put on your mad scientist lab coat and experiment to see what makes your body feel and perform best.

There are so many whole, plant-based foods out there to savor and enjoy, and enhanced vitality and energy and well-being are worth the pursuit.

Why Diets & Deprivation Don't Work

News outlets routinely highlight the latest study suggesting that diets don't work. Anyone who has tried one can attest to this fact. You lose a little, gain it back – and then some.

Current research indicates that willpower is a finite resource. In studies where participants are left alone in a room with a cookie after performing mentally demanding tasks, people who tackled harder questions were less able to

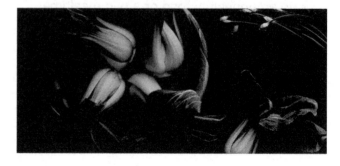

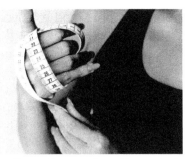

resist the cookie than the others who attempted to answer easy questions.

Translated to a dieting scenario, an individual's willpower to deprive themselves for the sake of their diet will decrease as the stressors and demands in his or her life increase. We can thank science for pointing out the obvious. Who among us hasn't reached for a pint of cookies and cream ice cream when we've had a really stressful week, when otherwise it would have no power over us.

People often find it more challenging to muster the willpower to deprive themselves of foods they want or crave when they are already tired, low energy, stressed, anxious, depressed, or otherwise upset.

For you, the word "diet" may be synonymous with deprivation. A crash diet approach is popular, yet this short-term and sudden effort to lose weight or shift health indicators often involves sacrifices that you never intend to maintain long-term.

As a dieter, you may even see results in the short term, but they rarely last for long. It is all too easy to return to your pre-diet eating and lifestyle habits. This can leave you even worse off than when you started the diet.

Deprivation and extreme calorie deficits can actually signal your body to respond as if it were in a famine. Your body begins to anticipate a long stretch of time before food will be available again. Your metabolism slows, and your body may even begin to break down muscle in its quest to survive the perceived famine and to mobilize fuel.

This is not the path to optimal health. Don't forget that your heart is comprised of muscle, too, and we all want our hearts to be as strong as possible!

Crash diets and fad diets often instruct individuals to cut out entire food groups with little explanation and minimal support to help them find realistic and healthy substitutes. It is also quite routine for the average crash dieter to develop guilt and shame when it comes to their deprivation strategies.

This is a truly harmful situation, both physically and psychologically. If you have had any history with crash or fad diets, you have felt their effects firsthand, and you know the damage an omnipresent sense of deprivation can do.

Instead, our approach here is refreshingly different. We teach you to:

- Learn the power of whole nutrient-dense foods
- Appreciate the benefits of these foods for your short and long-term health
- Understand the risks associated with the Standard American Diet
- Make gradual changes to your eating habits to avoid overwhelm
- Add in more of the good stuff, and skip the worrying about do and don't lists or judging yourself for falling off track at a meal

We want you to think "*Fall down seven times, get up eight*" (Japanese proverb). Not "*No pain, no gain.*" Got it?

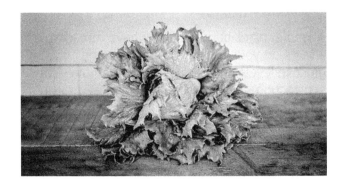

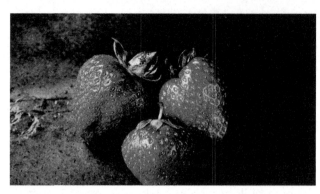

Choose Simple Plant-Based Whole Foods, and Supplement Food with Food

Studies have shown that a plant-based diet provides essential proteins, carbohydrates, fats, minerals, and vitamins. A whole plant-based diet helps prevent some of these diseases: heart disease, high blood pressure, and type 2 diabetes.

Incorporate more plant-based meals into your day and eat less meat. Animal protein has been linked to increased inflammation, while many fruits and vegetables contain antioxidants and plant compounds that help reduce inflammation.

That may be why studies of patients who suffer from inflammatory diseases, such as arthritis,[56] often see inflammation drop once patients move to a vegan diet.

When considering different plant-based foods, get as close as you can to how Mother

Nature intended it. If possible, always choose the whole food version of your food. Shifting to a vegetarian menu does not mean going for processed vegan meals, but eating a whole food, plant-based diet.

A whole, plant-based diet will have remarkable effects on your health, improving blood glucose levels, increasing mental and physical satisfaction, lowering inflammation, and raising energy levels.

Take fruit as an example. While juice cleanses and detoxes claim to be healthy, extracting juice from the whole food robs you of the fiber and plant compounds found in the fruit's skin and core.

Since fiber helps reduce blood sugar spikes, removing this fiber, but keeping all the sugar in the juice can dramatically accelerate how quickly your blood glucose levels rise.

These foods are full of natural soluble and insoluble fibers that help with digestion and reduce constipation. There are more than a dozen recipes we will discuss in chapter five that you can consider for a delicious whole plant-based meal.

The same is true with grains. Whole grains preserve all of the nutrients, while refined grains strip away the germ layer, which is where biotin and many other critical vitamins are stored. Plus, the extra fiber and protein in the whole grain help stabilize your blood sugar better than refined grains. Whenever possible, go for whole foods.[57]

Going From Processed Foods to Whole Foods

"I've long been a dedicated student of food labels, and it's really quite shocking that some breakfast cereals are much saltier than salty snacks. And some pasta sauces have much more added sugar than ice cream toppings." – David Katz, MD, MPH,

Another important part of replacing bad food habits with good ones involves going from a highly processed diet to a more natural one.

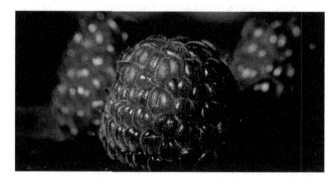

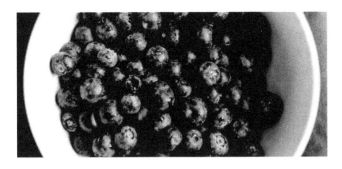

Remember that modern day food environment of ours with the 24/7 availability of food anytime and anywhere? The *processed* aspect of highly processed food products enables this food environment along with the omnipresence of eating opportunities and their seemingly endless shelf life.[58]

The cheap and easy way to recognize a processed food is to ask yourself: will I find this food occurring in this same condition out in nature? For example, there is no such thing as a Froot Loops or Hot Pockets tree.

You will not find the Bologna Barn at your local farm with little Bolognas grazing in the pasture. Joking aside, this becomes a surprisingly accurate shorthand for identifying processed versus whole foods.

By contrast, whole, plant-based foods are recognizable out in nature: even children can point out an apple tree, pull a carrot from the ground, or identify beans growing on a bush or vine.

The processing of our food occurs along a spectrum. Returning to the mythical Froot Loop tree for a moment, this well-known breakfast cereal is an example of a *highly processed food*.

You have to read its ingredient label pretty closely and decipher the long-winded names of many manufactured additives in order to understand the raw materials required to make a single box of Froot Loops.

So, what about applesauce? Using our shorthand test, you know you can walk onto a farm and find apples, but it won't look like applesauce. That's because store-bought applesauce is *lightly processed*: it still retains a lot of what it has in its original state, but it has been ground up, which is one method of processing.

You can still imagine how it was made from whole, fresh apples, though. If the ingredients label only has one ingredient, apples, then you have your answer: the only raw material required to make that jar of applesauce was apples.

The more highly processed a food, the more likely it was stripped of nutrients – such as vitamins, fiber, and minerals – and the more likely it was packaged with unnecessary and sometimes unhealthy additions.

Packaged food companies often include additives such as sugar, salt, artificial colorings and flavors, and certain unhealthy fats to extend shelf life and/or enhance appearance and flavor of the food product, not to benefit our health.

The closer you can get to food in its whole and intact form, the more you benefit from high quality nutrition, and the more you avoid unhealthy additives.

Going From Animal Foods to Plant Foods

"It's not just about taking off the pounds; it really is about improving the quality of the fuel your body runs on." – David Katz, MD, MPH, FACPM, FACP, Director of Yale University's Prevention Research Center

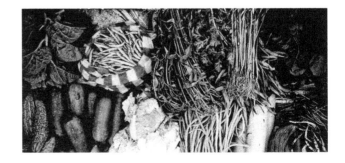

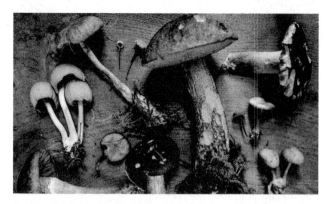

Animal foods and plant foods are exactly what they sound like. Animal foods are derived from an animal, and plant foods originate from a plant. Animal foods include milk, cheese, all dairy, meats, processed meats like bologna and sausage, fish, and eggs.

Plant foods include fruits, vegetables, legumes, grains, herbs and spices, sea vegetables like nori, kombu and dulse, fungi (mushrooms), nuts, and seeds.

Phytonutrients are chemicals unique to plants that benefit our health in many ways – there are thousands of them, many of which are still being studied.

Phytonutrients are a relatively new and exciting frontier in nutrition science research. Despite the hype surrounding the latest food to be deemed a *superfood*, the discovery of a new phytonutrient is often responsible for these labels.

In the monumental 20-year China Study and book by the same name published in 2005, Dr. T. Colin Campbell found that rates of a variety of cancers correlated with the introduction and increasing volume of animal-based foods in the diets of numerous populations in China.[59]

While animal-based foods often possess more concentrated protein by weight, plant-based foods outperform them as fiber-rich (animal foods have none), cholesterol-free (plant foods have none), and nutrient-dense (more vitamins, minerals, and phytonutrients per calorie) choices.

In fact, dark leafy greens always top the list of most calorically efficient foods, evaluated in terms of the nutrients we get in return compared to the overall weight of the food.

Animal foods are so damaging to your health and the environment, we've compiled a list of 128 different scientific studies elaborating on the disease they cause, and the mayhem to our planet that they induce. Instead of putting them all here for you to read, you can go to Addendum I, and reference them to educate yourself further.

Throughout this transition, we will encourage and show you how to make more and more food choices from the plant world.

Replace Processed and Artificial Foods

Processed food is often very high in refined sugars and high fructose corn syrup. This can be seriously detrimental to your health, loading you down with empty calories, having severe negative effects on your metabolism, leading to insulin resistance, and other problems with abnormal organ fat accumulation and high triglyceride levels.

This leads to a high risk of heart disease, obesity, diabetes, and cancer.

Processed meat is the worst choice you can make for any meal. This includes hot dogs, deli meat, and beef jerky options. Many processed meats are produced by a method to last for long periods, and typically they are consumed in "healthy" lunch options.

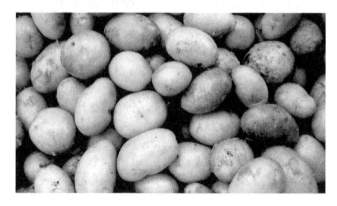

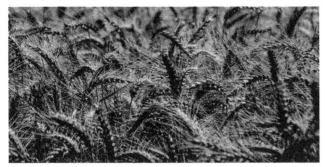

Processed meats should not be considered healthy, even if they are organic.

Processed foods have been specifically tailored and manufactured to be as appealing as possible. We naturally gravitate towards salty, sweet and fatty foods, as our bodies know they should be high in nutrients and energy.

Food manufacturers compete with each other. Making their foods tastier is one way to do this. Sugar and junk foods activate the same brain areas as drugs like cocaine, so be mindful at how powerful your taste buds are. This means most foods we consume are so 'rewarding' to the body, affecting thought patterns and behavior, that they lead to massive overconsumption, which messes with your energy balance regulation mechanisms, which leads to excessive weight gain.

All processed foods are high in additives, chemicals, and food dyes that may trigger your body to release hormones and compounds that cause swelling and inflammation.

For example, researchers have found that polysorbate-80, a common food additive, was linked to gut inflammation.[60]

Eating artificial foods like breakfast cereals on a regular basis is not a very healthy choice. These foods have been processed, and many of the added ingredients are not the best for your health, even though it appears that they are.

Also, cereals tend to be loaded with added sugar as a way to make them taste better.

Replace Fried Foods

Fried food is often very high in salt, and a high sodium diet leads to fluid retention, high blood pressure, and higher risks of stroke, heart disease, and kidney disease. High blood pressure makes your heart's job a lot harder and can damage blood vessels and the heart muscle.

The trans fats often found in fried foods can wreak havoc with your digestive tract, slow down your digestion, and cause you to swell up. You are more prone to obesity if you over consume fried foods.

Continued consumption of these foods can lead to atherosclerosis. Researchers from the Mount Sinai School of Medicine found that people who reduced fried foods from their diet experienced reduced inflammation.[61]

Fast food restaurants are known for providing fried food options using various types of oils, but usually the hydrogenation process in frying foods leads to increased trans fats.

Trans fats lower good cholesterol (HDL) levels and raise bad cholesterol (LDL) levels, increasing your chance of heart disease. Hydrogenated oils are especially unhealthy when they are reused, which occurs in a number of restaurants. Oil breaks down more and more with each frying, changing their composition and making the food absorb more trans fats.

Another fried food issue is a chemical, acrylamide, that forms in food cooked at a high temperature, especially fried food. Acrylamide has been shown to cause cancer in animals.

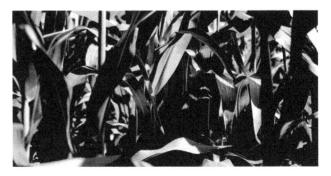

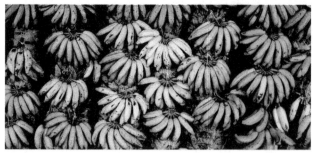

French fries, potato chips, hash browns, and other fried foods are high in this neurotoxin.

Switch Alcohol for Something Better

The next time you pick up another glass of beer, wine, or liquor, keep in mind that it is a toxin not beneficial for your health. The process of breaking down this toxic and addictive substance releases toxic by-products that damage liver cells, cause inflammation, and weaken the immune system.

Heavy drinking can lead to a variety of liver problems such as steatosis, fibrosis, and alcoholic hepatitis or cirrhosis.

Alcohol impairs gut and liver functioning, causing persistent inflammation. It also increases the blood sugar level, and its prolonged consumption can lead to other complications, including heart issues like an irregular heartbeat, high blood pressure, pancreatitis and heightened stroke risk.

Alcohol can change mood and behavior and change the way the brain works. It can even change looks, by messing with the brain's communication pathways.

Overconsuming alcohol weakens your immune system, making you much more susceptible to disease. Chronic drinkers are much more likely to contract pneumonia, tuberculosis, and other diseases than moderate consumers. It even contributes to a higher cancer risk.

Since most of us drink to be social, try going to a clean juice bar, ordering tonic water, or telling friends you can't drink because you're training for a marathon. You may just inspire them to pass on that round of beer or cocktails, and join you!

Replace: Alcohol, Meat, Fish, Dairy, Gluten, Soy, Processed, Artificial, or Fried Food

Some of the most common ingredients in modern food are also the major underlying causes of inflammatory symptoms. Avoid these nine major culprits:

Replace Meat

The World Health Organization has stated that processed meat is a "carcinogen," increasing your risk of colon and rectal cancer by 18%. It is rich in inflammatory saturated fats and omega-6.

It not only results in making us sick but can also cause excessive weight gain.[62] Vegan diets are also linked with generally higher metabolic rates (around 16% faster compared to meat-eaters).

By limiting your intake of meat, you can expect to lose weight, reduce inflammation and enjoy a lower risk of developing cancer, diabetes, and many heart diseases.

Meat processing often adds many toxins and additives to the finished product. One example is 'pink slime', or "lean finely textured beef (LFTB)."

This is where fatty leftover meat is heated and spun to remove excess fat, and then is sprayed with ammonia gas to kill any bacteria.

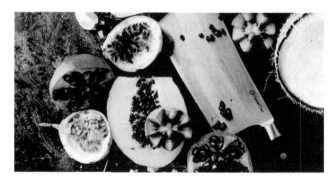

Red meat often has added hormones which can increase breast cancer risk.

Researchers believe that hormones and hormone-like compounds attach to hormone receptors on tumors, and so increase cancer risk.

Charring meat increases the toxin called nitrosamines which can lead to an increased risk of stomach cancer. Nitrosamine precursors are also found in cured or smoked meats such as bacon and sausage. The iron content in red meat is also a nitrosamine precursor.

This iron content in meat can also raise the levels of iron in the brain, which could increase Alzheimer's disease risk. Excess iron in the brain can cause the fatty tissue that coats the nerve fibers, myelin, to be destroyed, causing disrupted brain communication.

Carnitine, a compound found in red meat, has been found to cause atherosclerosis, leading to increased risk of cardiovascular disease.

Because animals are being fed corn and soy with high omega-6 oil content, processed meat can disrupt your omega-6 to omega-3 ratio. Maintaining this ratio is important in minimizing your diabetes, cardiovascular disease, depression, Alzheimer's, cancer, and rheumatoid arthritis risk.

A higher omega-6 to omega-3 fatty acid ratio suggests increased inflammation in your body, which is why it is important to decrease omega-6 fatty acids.

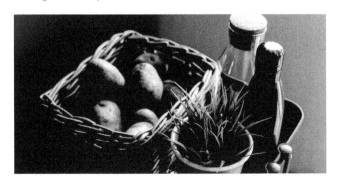

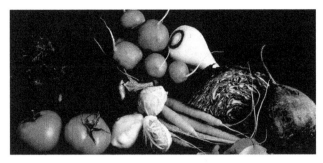

High levels of phosphates in your blood has been linked with increased cardiovascular disease risk, calcium deposit, hardening of the arteries, and poor bone health.

Eleven different phosphate salts are allowed to be added to red meat and chicken to help bind more water, making the meat juicier after it has been frozen and reheated.[63]

The industry itself says this is to "enhance the moisture absorbance, color, and flavor of the meat and reduce product shrinkage".

Phosphate additives have been linked to possible increased levels of Campylobacter bacteria in chicken exudates. Chicken exudate is the fluid that seeps out of poultry carcasses and has often been found full of Campylobacter bacteria in high numbers.

This increases food poisoning risk considerably. Campylobacter can leave people paralyzed.

Our body is in a constant state of attack due to the leftover antibiotics and hormones present in most all meats. Overexposure to antibiotics makes you more likely to develop resistance. For example, vancomycin, a drug that is often a "last defense" in fighting staphylococcus bacteria induced pneumonia and blood infections, is losing much of its potency now because many cattle farmers in years past would give antibiotics as a way to prevent cattle from dying, which improved profit for farmers.

This antibiotic consumption increases your risk of succumbing to infections and superbugs.

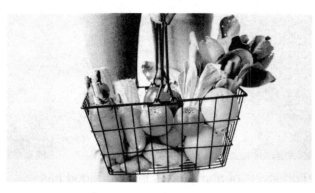

Replace Fish

People quite often include fish in their healthy diet choices assuming that nothing could possibly go wrong with this option, based on its reputation for being heart healthy.

Fish is considered a type of meat and has some disadvantages too. The protein level in fish is so high, it can be very harmful, as the body fights to excrete the extreme levels it cannot handle.

This has been linked to osteoporosis and kidney stones, because it leaches calcium from the body to cleanse itself.

Fish like tilapia and many others have high levels of omega-6 fats, causing chronic inflammation and other related diseases.

Fish is often wrongly recommended for its omega-3 fatty acid content, but there are much better, plant-based sources, including flax seeds, walnuts and pumpkin.

Fish, such as tilapia, do contain omega-3, but the ratio to omega-6 is very poor and is actually detrimental to health. It also contributes to arthritis, heart disease, asthma, and autoimmune and allergy issues.

Because of the inflammatory response it can cause, fish consumption can contribute to heart, lung and joint damage and can also harm the digestive tract, skin and blood vessels.

Fish is often contaminated with toxic chemicals such as arsenic, lead and mercury (a neurotoxin associated with birth defects, seizures, cerebral palsy, and more), and even traces of other substances, such as industrial-strength fire retardant, that can cause cancer and other problems.

Of all foods, fish is most likely to make you ill from bacterial contamination. The flesh of the fish can contain as much as nine million times the chemical residue as that found in the water in which they live. This is because they concentrate the industrial and municipal contaminants dumped in their environment.

Much of the seafood we eat are bottom feeding animals, and therefore collect feces, pesticides, bacteria and parasites. The water our fish live in is so polluted, you would be revolted at the thought of drinking it. But you're ingesting all this pollution every time you eat fish.

Issues like cancer, fetal damage, poor behavioral development, nervous system disorders, memory loss, and more have been linked to pesticides, PCBs (polychlorinated biphenyls), dioxins, cadmium, lead, arsenic, chromium, insecticides like toxaphene, and substances that are radioactive, like strontium 90.

Farmed fish are even fed dye to make the flesh artificially pink, and they are fed high levels of antibiotics, more per pound than any other food animal.

You can replace fish with plants that contain high levels of Omega 3 fatty acids and proteins, like hemp seed or plant oils.

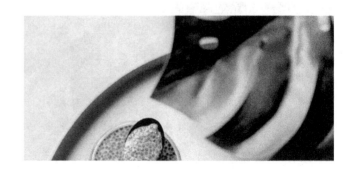

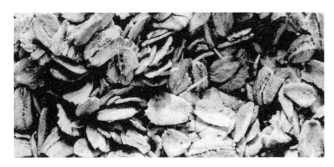

Replace Dairy

Dairy is one of the most inflammatory food groups. It is a common allergen and can easily initiate inflammatory reactions through the release of histamines. It contains varying amounts of lactose (the sugar in milk), which slows down weight loss.

It also speeds up the process of aging and leads to poor skin health.

Sticking to a dairy-free diet can save you from this while lowering the risk of prostate, testicular, breast and colon cancer and chronic digestive problems.

Dairy is often lauded as a prime ingredient in a healthy diet, due to its high calcium content. But this calcium is not as beneficial as it seems. In reality, milk (especially pasteurized milk) can actually be detrimental to bone health.

Milk has an acidifying effect on the body's pH, as all animal products do, which causes the body to pull calcium, a wonderful acid neutralizer, from the body, primarily the bones. After neutralizing the body's pH, this calcium is lost via the urine, so your body is actually depleted of calcium through dairy consumption.

This loss can affect your bones, teeth, muscle function, the regulation of nerve signals, your heartbeat, and blood clotting processes. To increase your calcium intake naturally, turn to foods such as almond milk, oats, chickpeas and dark leafy greens.

We know that all mammals consume specially formulated milk for the species, including humans, and cow's milk is a perfect food - for a calf. On average, cow's milk contains three times the protein in human milk, and the proteins contained in it are specific to the species.

This protein mismatch can cause metabolic disturbances leading to bone health issues.

The high casein content in milk may cause a raised risk of prostate cancer and other cancers, especially hormone related cancers. Hormones in milk may even contribute to unhealthy early puberty in young girls. It has been suggested that a variant of beta-casein, A1 beta-casein, may cause type 1 diabetes in children that are genetically vulnerable.

All animal products promote aging for the whole body, dairy included, due to its links to many diseases and issues, such as obesity, chronic inflammation, and hyperinsulinemia, a condition where the insulin in the blood is higher than normal.

On top of all that, dairy can be very bad for your skin health. As your body's largest organ, your skin is a pretty good gauge of the overall health of your body. Your skin tries to get rid of toxins your body can't handle, so it is important to pay attention to it.

Skin breakouts are often the first sign of digestive distress, and dairy can easily trigger redness, blotchy skin, acne, eczema, or poor general skin health. When you cut dairy from

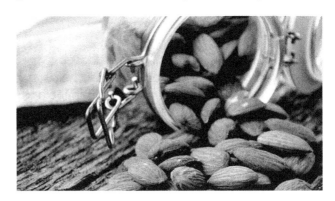

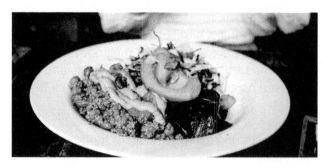

your diet, you can expect to see improvements in your skin within just a few days.

Dairy can also cause major gut damage and is a major contributor to gut illnesses regardless of your age. This leaves you prone to autoimmune diseases, digestive issues, IBS (irritable bowel syndrome), bloating, diarrhea, and constipation. It can also can also cause worsening of conditions such as Crohn's disease.

There are many dairy replacements now, ranging from macadamia, almond, and hemp milk to non-dairy cheese. Be adventurous and see what plant-based non-dairy items you can find to replace your cheese habit.

Replace Gluten

Gluten is at the top of the list of inflammation-inducing foods. Gluten is a protein that is found in many grain products, and it can lead to gut irritation and inflammation for many adults.

Wheat alone also contains a number of other gut irritants that can cause major problems for your general digestion and nutrient absorption.

Many people are sensitive to gluten and cannot tolerate even small amounts of it.

Avoiding gluten supports not only reduced inflammation and weight loss, but also helps in better digestion, exposure to more vitamins and antioxidants, and increased energy levels.

It certainly does not help that most wheat is commonly drenched in glyphosate (aka RoundUp) while it is growing.

Gut inflammation is a phrase used to describe intestinal permeability. It can lead to an issue known as leaky gut. This is a key factor for the development of autoimmune diseases.

The gut generally lets nutrients into your bloodstream from your food, while not allowing non-beneficial particles through.

A combination of inflammation, gluten's effect on the protein zonulin (which causes loosening of the cells in the gut), and wheat's effect on gut permeability means your gut may allow viruses, bacteria, molecules such as dust, and other particles through its lining, directly into your bloodstream.

Instead of thinking going gluten-free restricts your food horizons, imagine that it expands your food possibilities.

In fact, going gluten-free lets you swap traditional refined carbohydrate meals, such as white bread, for more nutrient-dense foods. For example, swapping wheat flour for quinoa flour delivers more fiber, protein, and antioxidants, which in turn can help reduce inflammation, level out your blood glucose levels, and reduce sugar cravings.

Replace Soy

There are many reasons why you should refrain from consuming soy. It can cause digestive problems like bloating, constipation, and irritable bowel syndrome. The fatty acids soy contains are mainly Omega-6 polyunsaturated fats. Too

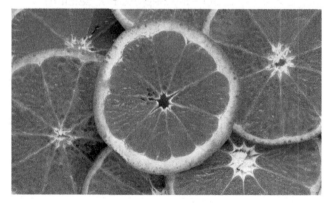

many Omega-6 fatty acids can contribute to inflammation.

Soy also contains high levels of phytates, an anti-nutrient which inhibits the absorption of minerals such as calcium, magnesium, manganese, copper, iron and zinc. High phytate consumption can cause iron and zinc deficiencies.

Lectins are a protein found in everything you eat, but soy contains particularly high amounts of a specific lectin called agglutinin. It can tear holes in the lining of your gut, causing irritation, diarrhea and vomiting, allergies, and other issues like leaky gut syndrome.

Agglutinins can also lead to an intestinal overgrowth of E. coli, as it feeds it. Lectins will disrupt your energy expenditure and hunger signals, known as your leptin sensitivity, and this will trick your brain into thinking it's hungry when it's not. This could also lead to insulin resistance.

Aside from lectins and phytates, soy contains toxins called protease inhibitors, or trypsin inhibitors. These block enzymes that are needed to digest certain proteins and can cause other issues too.

Soy has been known to increase estrogen levels, which can cause lowered testosterone levels. This throws your hormones out of whack, and can, in men, lower libido, increase fat accumulation, lower energy levels and stamina, and cause other health problems. For women, this imbalance can disrupt periods, mess with fertility levels, and increase the risk of breast cancer.[64]

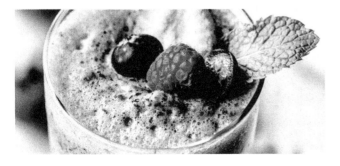

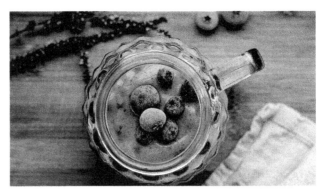

Soy formula can have similar devastating effects on babies throughout their lives. A study has shown that babies on soy based formula had blood estrogen levels 13,000 to 22,000 times higher than the normal estrogen concentration levels.

Soy can contribute to thyroid dysfunction due to its high levels of goitrogens, specifically soy isoflavone genistein.

Compounds that inhibit the thyroid's ability to utilize iodine correctly, goitrogen over consumption can lead to hypothyroid problems, and the thyroid gland may even form a goiter, a swelling or enlargement, to make up for the inadequate hormone production.

Soy also contains calcium carbonate, increasing the risk of heart disease, and has been compared with cow's milk, sharing some inflammatory properties.[65]

You can find many soy alternatives, just be cognizant that soy is lurking in many processed and packaged foods, so you may have to be vigilant for awhile as you switch from a bad habit to a better one.

Smoothies Make an Ideal Breakfast for Nutritional Optimization

Dietitians say that breakfast is the most important meal of the day.[66] Many people have trouble making healthy choices in the morning, as they get their children ready for school or rush off on their morning commute.

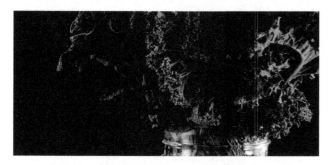

A breakfast smoothie delivers a quick, easy-to-digest dose of protein, fiber, vitamins and minerals in a portable format. By incorporating plant-based whole foods, research shows that a healthy breakfast can promote a healthy metabolism, improve weight loss, and sustain energy.[67]

Developing a habit of consuming healthy smoothies on a daily basis is a worthwhile use of your time, but "healthy" ingredients means adding no sugar at all to your shakes.

Consuming the daily recommended proportion of fruits and vegetables can be challenging; however, smoothies help you to meet your body's nutritional requirements quickly.

To start your day off right and establish a baseline of wellness that helps you keep sugar cravings and blood sugar levels under control, don't forget the basic principles and research that we've outlined so far. Follow these tips when creating a delicious smoothie:

- Add a source of fiber, such as dark leafy greens. Fiber reduces blood sugar spikes.
- Avoid consuming fruit juice (high in sugar, low in fiber) and aim for low-glycemic fruit[68] like cherries and grapefruit. As a bonus, grapefruit can help lower your blood sugar.[69]
- Add a source of healthy fat to help reduce your blood sugar. Try avocado. Not only is it rich in plant-based essential fats, but it also adds a rich and creamy texture to your smoothie.
- Add a source of lean, plant-based protein, such as hemp hearts or flax. Protein in every meal stabilizes blood sugar.

- Top it off with a plant-based milk, such as almond milk. Dairy spikes blood sugar and is also linked to inflammation.

Search online and you'll find a variety of diet smoothie recipes that will not only help you lose weight, but also detox your body. Making smoothies using vegetables like kale or spinach along with berries and unsweetened coconut milk and ice can help you lose weight in a healthy way. These contain a good amount of fiber ensuring improved ingestion.

If you don't have time to make a smoothie from scratch, there are many pre-made mixes that you can simply blend with non-dairy milk and ice cubes, so be sure to look for these in your health food aisle at the grocery store.

Smoothies have many health and beauty benefits including glowing and fresh skin, healthier hair, stronger immunity, long-term energy, improved mental ability, and a calmer and better mood. And the best part is, you can have smoothies at any meal!

4.7 Principle Two: Eat Consistently

"Food is the most intimate thing you can buy... Unlike clothes and shoes that dress the outside, food goes into your body and builds who you become." – Ani Phyo, cookbook author, speaker, and raw foods expert

Do you struggle to make healthy choices? Do you feel overwhelmed by the growing number of healthy products at the grocery store, so

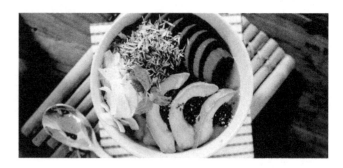

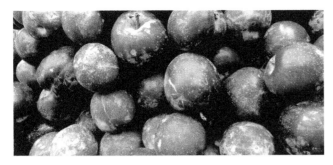

much so that you feel overwhelmed in making a healthy decision?

You are experiencing what psychologists and behavioral analysts refer to as the "paradox of choice."[70] The more choices you need to make, the harder it is for you to make a decision, and the less likely it is that you'll make the right choice.

It's really hard to keep your macro ratios and nutrient intake consistent each week unless you're eating a consistent diet. Unless you're consistent in what you eat, it's also extremely difficult to figure out how certain foods make you feel and to continually optimize your diet.

Eating consistently each week and making small tweaks over time is the crucial key to finding a nutritional profile that meets your personal needs.

Moreover, buying consistent and simple meals (with nothing extra) saves you some money too. While planning your week's meals, you should be keeping your fitness goals in mind, and they should match with your eating patterns as well.

If you have ever set out to lose weight in the past and that involved diligently counting calories or worrying about portion sizes, then you are in for a real treat. As if the high nutrient density of whole plant-based foods wasn't great enough, they bring another advantage to the table: low calorie density.

It typically takes a greater volume of plant foods to arrive at 100 calories than with animal foods. Compare 207 calories in one 4-ounce serving of beef sirloin steak with 40 calories in one 4-ounce serving of broccoli, for example. The fiber in broccoli also contributes to feeling more full or satisfied, whereas the steak has zero fiber.

By enhancing the quality of your food, you increase your intake of *micronutrients* – vitamins, minerals, and phytonutrients.[71]

Why are micronutrients so important?
We all know that we need enough of the macronutrients – carbohydrates, proteins, and fats – for our bodies to carry out all the amazing functions they perform on a daily basis.

But, did you know that micronutrients often act as *cofactors* in those very functions?

A cofactor is a substance that plays a supporting role but is absolutely necessary for that function to occur.

It may not get the fancy title or the media spotlight, but we need it just as much as the leading actor for the show to go on.

Micronutrients are the underestimated, underappreciated little guys who keep the machine humming.

While the amount of vitamins and minerals we need and absorb from our food is typically very small compared to macronutrients (hence "macro" and "micro"), we still very much rely on their presence throughout the body.

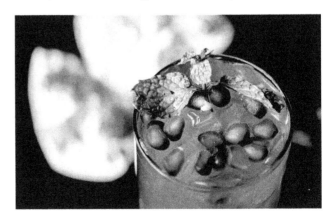

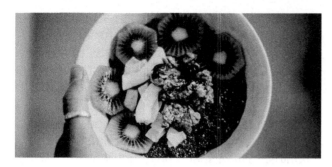

Deficiencies in some of the most important vitamins and minerals can also interfere with processes and dangerously impede certain functions altogether.

A whole, plant-based approach to eating ensures a higher micronutrient intake than any plate of food possible on the average S.A.D. diet because you are eating directly from the source.

Take dairy milk: we celebrate cow's milk for its high calcium content, yet have we ever stopped to consider how or why so much calcium ends up in the milk to begin with? The calcium is not inherent to cow's milk per se. Instead, the cow's intake of calcium-rich greens and other plants causes the cow's milk to contain calcium.

Why not go directly to the source of your calcium, skipping the unnecessary saturated fat, cholesterol, and hormones?

Vegetables, nuts, and seeds are among the most calcium-rich foods we can eat. Despite claims to the contrary, an increasing body of research suggests that the bioavailability (or, the ease with which our body absorbs calcium from this source) of calcium from plant foods is just as high, if not higher in some cases, than from dairy.

Bok choy, kale, sesame seeds, watercress, kidney beans, almonds, and figs are just a few excellent plant-based sources.

We encourage you to take this opportunity to re-examine your food choices in terms of quality, not quantity.

Even though the average crash diet involves a serious reduction in calories and portion sizing, and even though leaders in the food industry and government frequently prescribe an "exercise more, eat-less approach" to losing weight, we instead urge you to identify foods that offer your body the highest quality of nutrition possible.

If you are new to choosing whole, plant-based foods, your choices are likely to have lower calorie density and higher nutrient density than ever before, and you won't have to fret over portion sizes.

Supplement food with food: While we will talk more about supplementation in its own chapter, there are two key things you should know.

Most people, regardless of whether they eat animals or plants, are deficient in many key nutrients due to degrading soil quality and other factors; a fantastic way to ensure that you get all the nutrients on a very consistent basis is to add them in powdered or pill form, but to make sure that those powders *are* simple powdered plants (like ginger, nopal cactus, etc.) with relatively little processing

Every day, 70 million Americans suffer from digestive issues, estimates the American Nutrition Associatio   n.[72] And according to a study in the *Journal of Gastroenterology and Hepatology*,[73] nearly a third of adults experience indigestion with it ranking as the #1 digestive complaint in the entire country.

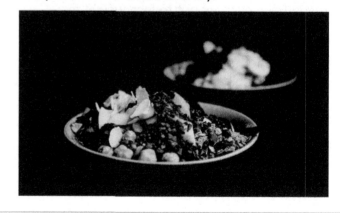

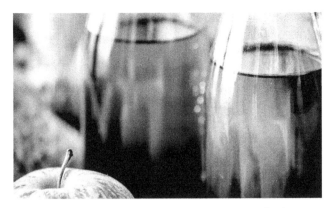

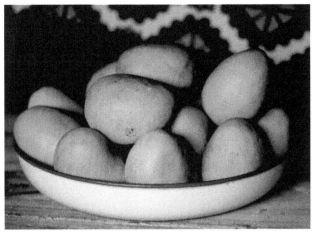

Not only does poor digestion leave you feeling crampy, bloated and uncomfortable, it also could mean that you're not getting all of the nutrition out of your meals. Calorie for calorie, you're getting less out of every bite, and you're starving your cells of energy.

There are several key ways to improve digestion. First, ensure your gut is well-populated with beneficial bacteria. Scientists currently estimate[74] that there are approximately 1,000,000,000,000,000 (10 to the 14th power) of such bacteria cells lining your gut right now. That's more bacteria cells than cells in your entire body.

Probiotics

Many gastroenterologists recommend probiotics because of their health benefits, enhancing the intestine's barrier function and fighting pathogenic bacteria. Studies have demonstrated that probiotics are effective in preventing disorders like ulcerative colitis, colon cancer, inflammatory bowel diseases, gastric ulcers, and diarrhea.

By incorporating more probiotics in your diet, you improve your digestion, absorb more nutrients from the food you eat, and even strengthen your immune system.[75]

Plant-based, whole food probiotics include sauerkraut and apple cider vinegar. You can find them in most health food stores.

Probiotics are found in yogurt, pickles, some kinds of cheese, and it is very healthy to consume these products.[76,77] You can also take probiotic supplements, which are a quick and convenient way to send millions of microbes to your gut. When shopping for a probiotic supplement, look for one that contains live, active cultures contained in an enteric-coated capsule.

These coated capsules help the microbes survive your stomach acid better so they can reach your gut. Check the ingredients label, too. Some brands, especially cheap generic probiotic supplements, contain sugar, dairy, gluten or soy.

Enzymes

Digestive enzymes help restore wellness in the gastrointestinal (GI) tract. The three main enzymes that help in the digestion of protein, carbohydrates, and lipids are amylase, protease and lipase. Foods like papaya, mango (contains amylase for starch digestion) and honey (containing protease, amylase, and sucrase which help in the digestion of both carbohydrate and proteins) are good for optimizing digestive health.

While your body has natural levels of these enzymes, eating an unbalanced diet can deplete these.

If you've only recently begun moving towards a healthier, whole foods diet, you may want to jumpstart your digestion with an enzyme

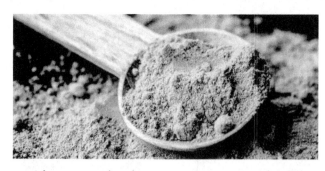

supplement. Take these supplements with each meal to rev up your metabolism.

Ginger

Studies have shown that ginger can be used to avoid seasickness and nausea after chemotherapy. It can also lessen arthritis because of its anti-inflammatory properties. And it helps to decrease the effects of diabetes, inflammatory bowel disease, colitis, migraines, and asthma. Ginger tea can also be used to improve digestive juices and help in weight loss.[78]

In one study, taking ginger helped speed up digestion by four minutes.[79] In another, taking 1.2 grams of ginger in the form of a ginger powder supplement improved digestion by 50%.[80] It's no wonder that naturopaths and doctors often recommend ginger for chronic indigestion.

And here's a bonus, if you are trying to reduce whole-body inflammation and control your blood sugar, studies have shown taking 2 grams of ginger powder every day can lower your blood sugar by 12%.[81]

Turmeric

Turmeric has been used for thousands of years as a spice, but lately, researchers have been exploring what it can do for your health. Curcumin, an active compound in the spice, stimulates the production of bile in your digestive tract,[82] which helps your body break down food[83] and improves digestion. It has also been successfully used to manage symptoms of indigestion, such as bloating and gas.

According to additional studies, turmeric is expected to help fight against many infections and even some cancers.[84,85,86,87]

In addition to being a digestion aid, turmeric is also a potent anti-inflammatory compound. In fact, it can be just as effective as some prescription anti-inflammatory drugs,[88] and it may help reduce Western diet-related chronic diseases linked with inflammation like heart disease,[89] cancer,[90] and obesity.[91]

Turmeric is available as a tincture, fluid extract, or powder-based capsule. If you are taking a standardized powder capsule, adults typically take 400-600 mg three times a day.[92] If you're taking a 1:1 extract, dosages vary from 30-90 drops daily. And if you're consuming a 1:2 tincture, dosages range from 15-30 drops four times daily.

Fiber

Add more high fiber foods to your diet. This includes dark green leafy vegetables and fiber supplements like psyllium husks.

Approximately 97% of adults don't get the recommended minimum daily amount of fiber.[93] In fact, most people only eat approximately 15 grams of fiber every day, even though we should be eating roughly 25 grams every day.

Eating more fiber helps move your food through your digestive tract more efficiently.[94] Fiber also helps moderate blood sugar levels[95] and works in sync with probiotic supplements to feed

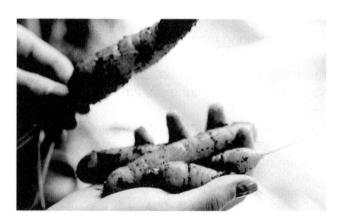

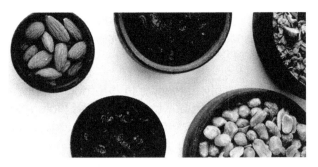

beneficial bacteria and help your gut microbes to flourish.[96]

There are two types of fiber that you'll want to include in your diet.[97]

Soluble fiber helps with blood sugar levels and improves the efficiency of your probiotics. Examples include nuts, seeds, and psyllium. This form of fiber is healthier for your cholesterol levels and can help to regulate your cholesterol levels.

Insoluble fiber aids in digestion and is what you will find in many leafy vegetables and whole grains.

4.8 Principle Three: Abundant Water, Not Sugar

Water is the perfect beverage to appease thirst and rehydrate the body.

Your body is approximately 60 percent water.[98] It might seem plain and boring, but water is key to all areas of life, and it's the health and beauty secret that doctors swear by. For example, drinking more water and keeping your brain well-hydrated can help you to be more focused,[99] think faster,[100] and feel happier.[101,102]

It also maintains body temperature and protects against many ailments like constipation, kidney stones, heartburn, gastritis, migraines, ulcers, cardiovascular disorders, rheumatoid arthritis, and osteoporosis.

Water boosts your metabolism and helps to increase productivity, giving a healthier look and improving digestion, making you happier and more energetic. Water also supports and nourishes your digestive system.[103]

Fiber absorbs water, which increases fiber's ability to move food through your stomach and intestines. Water also helps flush food through your body and circulate bile and other enzymes that break down your food.

Water is an excellent way of burning calories, and it helps in weight loss. As associate professor Amanda Salis, from The University of Sydney told the Huffington Post, "The research is showing that plain water consumption -- not salted water or diet soft drinks -- does cause a small but significant increase in energy expenditure or the number of kilojoules that your body burns."

And finally, not drinking enough water can increase your blood sugar levels. Because your blood is mostly water, dehydration causes sugar levels to become more and more concentrated.[104] Your body loses water, but the sugar stays behind in your blood. This is why people with diabetes are cautioned to stay hydrated, and chronic dehydration is a common symptom of diabetes.

Despite all these incredible benefits of drinking more water, nearly 75 percent of adults are chronically dehydrated.[105] Chronic dehydration can lead to prolonged inflammation, low vitality, and chronic high blood sugar.

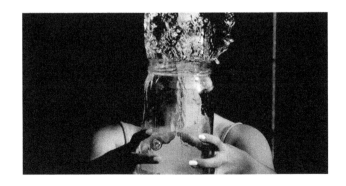

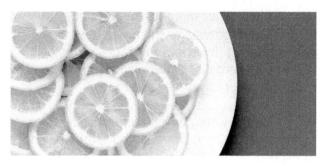

Stay hydrated by drinking at least eight glasses of pure, clean, filtered water every day. Remember, plain is best.

Caffeinated beverages, fruit juice, and sweetened drinks may only serve to dehydrate you even more, and sugary drinks increase your blood sugar levels, as well as amp up your levels of cytokines, which boost inflammation.[106]

To remind yourself to stay hydrated, keep a water bottle with you at all times and fill it up any time you stand up to go somewhere. You can also consider using a notepad or an app to track your water usage. You may be surprised by how little you drink.

Sugar: A Special Case

"My advice is to give up stevia, aspartame, sucralose, sugar alcohols like xylitol and malitol, and all of the other heavily used and marketed sweeteners unless you want to slow down your metabolism, gain weight, and become an addict." **-- Mark Hyman, MD, functional medicine physician and best-selling author of several books including** *The Blood Sugar Solution*

If you are like millions of Americans, you have a sugar addiction. That's not an overstatement. Recent studies have found that sugar has the same effect on the brain as cocaine. One study didn't mince words when describing the effects of this single food substance:

"Animal data has shown significant overlap between the consumption of added sugars and drug-like effects, including bingeing, craving,

tolerance, withdrawal, cross-sensitisation, cross-tolerance, cross-dependence, reward, and opioid effects."[107]

Sugar is incredibly pervasive in our food supply. Its unique appeal to our tastebuds and biological reward systems makes it impossible to ignore. Moderation in all things, sure, but there really ought to be an exception for sugar.

If you have ever tried to stop eating added sugar and found it difficult, you are not alone. It is not all in your head. The neurotransmitters that are activated in your brain every time you eat a single ounce of the stuff are setting you on a trail to full-blown addiction.

If you think you can weasel your way around this problem with sugar alternatives – not so fast.

Unfortunately, the growing list of sugar substitutes and alternatives available nowadays does not solve the problem, as Dr. Hyman explains. Many of today's sugar alternatives are 10-100 times sweeter than cane sugar, so we quickly run the risk of overdoing it with stronger stuff than good old cane sugar.

We are wired to seek out a sweet taste thanks to an evolutionary process. However, refined and added sugars oversaturate our taste buds without the fiber, vitamins, and minerals that nature normally packs into natural sources of sweetness such as fresh fruit or a subtly sweet yam or beet. If we just ate sugar as nature intended, we'd probably be fine, but American

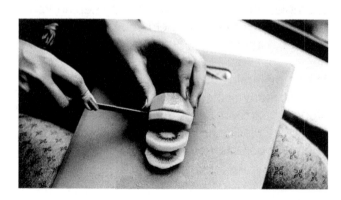

sugar consumption is the highest in the world at 126 grams a day.[108]

Many people sign up for a daylong roller coaster ride without even knowing it, simply because of their sugar consumption. The rollercoaster ride starts when they wake up in the morning with low blood sugar.

After a highly sweetened coffee drink loaded with hidden sugars, maybe paired with a sweetened morning pastry or cereal, their blood sugar levels skyrocket. Not much later, their blood sugar levels drop as steeply and sharply as they skyrocketed, bringing a craving for instant energy.

Their bodies are literally fiending for their next "hit" which they believe can only be gotten from more sugar. And so the rollercoaster continues.

A spike in blood sugar triggers the release of insulin, the hormone that regulates blood sugar and stimulates hunger. Insulin also prompts the conversion and storage of sugar into fat.

Sure, insulin transports much of the starches and sugars we consume into muscles for energy storage, but only when our stores are low and we are actively working hard like during intense exercise.

For the majority of the day, the body doesn't know what to do with a continuous stream of sugar, so the body does what it does best – it stores energy as fat to protect us from famine and hard times.

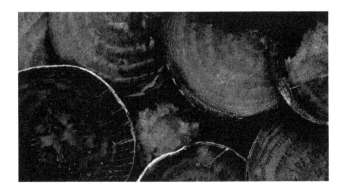

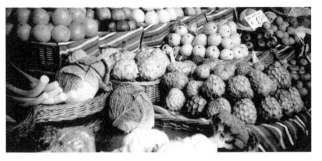

Insulin activates hunger signals, so it is no help that blood sugar spikes and consequent insulin rises also lead to sudden hunger pangs, at least some of which have more to do with imbalances in our diet and insulin response than an actual need for more food.

Sugar, and the simple carbohydrates that break down quickly to become sugars once we eat them, are not the whole story, but they are a big part of it.

Unfortunately, the growing list of sugar substitutes and alternatives available nowadays does not solve the problem, as Dr. Hyman explains. Since many of today's sugar alternatives are 10-100 times sweeter than cane sugar, we quickly run the risk of overdoing it on even stronger stuff than good old cane sugar.

We are wired to seek out a sweet taste thanks to an evolutionary process. However, refined and added sugars oversaturate our taste buds without the fiber, vitamins, and minerals that nature normally packs into natural sources of sweetness such as fresh fruit or a subtly sweet yam or beet.

If we just ate sugar as nature intended, we'd probably be fine, but American sugar consumption is the highest in the world at 126 grams a day.[109,110]

Many people sign up for a daylong roller coaster ride without even knowing it, simply because of their sugar consumption. The rollercoaster ride starts when they wake up in the morning with low blood sugar. After a highly sweetened coffee drink loaded with hidden sugars, maybe paired

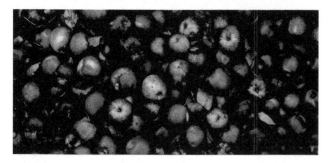

with a sweetened morning pastry or cereal, their blood sugar levels skyrocket.

Not much later, their blood sugar levels drop as steeply and sharply as they skyrocketed, bringing a craving for instant energy. Their bodies are literally fiending for their next "hit" which they believe can only be gotten from more sugar. And so the rollercoaster continues.

A spike in blood sugar triggers the release of insulin, the hormone that regulates blood sugar and stimulates hunger. Insulin also prompts the conversion and storage of sugar into fat.

Sure, insulin transports much of the starches and sugars we consume into muscles for energy storage, but only when our stores are low and we are actively working hard like during intense exercise.

Sugar, and the simple carbohydrates that break down quickly to become sugars once we eat them, are not the whole story, but they are a big part of it.

Remember that insulin activates hunger signals, so it is no help that blood sugar spikes, and consequent insulin spikes also lead to sudden hunger sensations. Some of this has more to do with imbalances in our diet and insulin response and less to do with genuine hunger and a need for calories.

Whole grains, legumes, vegetables, soda, and pastries – each of these has different kinds of carbohydrates, of which varying amounts break down and become blood glucose, or blood sugar, through the course of digestion.

Clearly, our body requires a reliable supply of glucose, and steady blood sugar levels power many critical systems in our body – in fact, the brain alone consumes up to one-fifth of our blood glucose. The determining factor in sugar regulation is then to consume whole, raw foods that are loaded with healthful nutrients, vitamins, and energy.

4.9 Principle Four: Replace the Carbs

Minimize Carbohydrates, Limit Fruit Intake, Supplement with Daily Nopal Cactus

According to the U.S. Centers for Disease Control and Prevention, the average adult gets nearly half of their daily calories from carbs like fruit and added sugar, with protein comprising 15-16% of their calories and fat rounding out the rest.[111]

This creates a protein-carbohydrate-fat ratio of approximately 15-50-35. But if you want to bring down your blood sugar and stabilize it, this ratio is out of sync. Researchers[112,113] are finding that we need to eat fewer carbs and eat more healthy proteins and fats if we want to manage the current sugar crisis.

Minimizing carbohydrate intake means cutting down our intake of cereals, bread, and potatoes. But it's not just restricted to these. You also need to avoid fruit juices, also a high glycemic food.

According to a study by Harvard University, people who consumed 2-3 servings of fruit juice

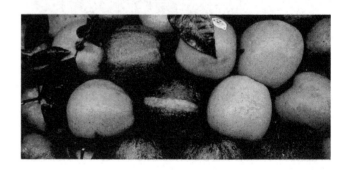

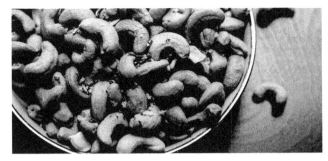

a day had a 31 percent higher risk of developing type 2 diabetes. Because it is stripped of all fiber, fruit juice is also very different from fruit itself.[114]

Common high-glycemic fruits include:[115]
- Bananas
- Pineapples
- Watermelons

If you want to experience optimal health by minimizing inflammation, minimize carbohydrates, especially from fruit and other foods that are high on glycemic index.

In one study, bringing down carbs and increasing proteins and fats to the ratio of 30-40-30 (proteins-carbs-fats) reduced blood sugar by 40%.

In another study, simply adding a minimum of five grams of healthy protein or fat also helped the body naturally manage blood sugar.

Opuntia ficus-indica (nopal cactus) is a common ingredient in several Mexican dishes.

The nopal cactus contains fiber and pectin, lowering blood glucose by decreasing the concentration of sugar in the intestine and stomach and has been used traditionally in the treatment of dyspnea, ulcer, glaucoma, wounds, liver conditions, and fatigue.

Studies have suggested that a daily consumption can be beneficial to our cardiovascular health as it reduces bad cholesterol and we suggest adding it to your diet as a powder in a capsule, so you can get it in your system every single day.

Prioritize Healthy Fats and Proteins So You Feel Fuller

Proteins are very important for cell building and tissue repairing. Protein is thermogenic, meaning it helps you burn calories. Fats found in avocados, pistachios, walnuts, cashew nuts, almonds, and olive oil help to fight obesity and lower bad cholesterol. However, you must eat healthy fats in moderation, as they are high in calories per gram of fat.

If you consume the right amount of proteins with appropriate healthy fats and reduce your carbohydrate intake at the same time, you can observe a miraculous stabilization of your blood glucose level.[116]

Prioritize fat first, protein second, and carbs last in all your meals.

Because fat has an average of nine calories per gram whereas carbs have four, prioritizing fat helps you feel fuller and satisfied, thus leading you to crave less carbs.

Omega-3 fatty acids can also reduce inflammation as well as a lower the risk of chronic diseases like heart disease.[117]

4.10 Principle Five: Regularly Abstain from Eating

Ancient cultures understood that fasting allows our body the much needed time and space to digest, rest, and reset myriad biological and psychological functions.

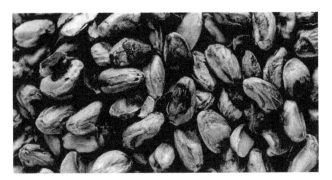

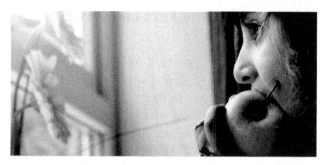

When we fast, we are better able to absorb nutrients, get rid of toxic build up, and free our bodies to fight disease, restore tissues, and even to think more clearly.

In Chapter 12 we talk at length about the different types of intermittent fasting, so that you can choose a fasting plan that works for you. Once you've tried it a few times, you'll be pleasantly surprised with how new and refreshed you feel after a fast.

4.11 From Mindless Eating to Mindful Eating

"Eat, drink and be mindful." – Susan Albers, Psy.D., eating psychology expert

With 20% of meals being eaten in cars (figures may have increased since 2008), more and more foods are designed specifically to be eaten on the go with one hand. Have you ever experienced looking down on your plate and realizing that you've eaten something without remembering it? This phenomenon is caused by our contemporary "on-the-go" food environment.

Eating more mindfully, connecting with the signals your body sends, and noticing how and when your body responds to what, can provide both motivation and results in your quest to enhance your vitality and lose weight.

Do this at your next meal: chew a single bite of food at least 50 times before swallowing. You will likely need to focus and count to be sure you chewed at least 50 times.

This is challenging and eye-opening for most people who try it. You may notice tastes and textures you never before noticed in a familiar food, or you may realize your current chewing habits are a small fraction of the 50 times you do in this exercise.

Depending on what you are eating, you may also notice that your food tastes sweeter than ever before: we have enzymes in our saliva that begin to digest complex carbohydrates into their sweeter-tasting building blocks right away as we chew.

If you swallow your bites whole or after only a couple chews, you may never experience this sweet taste. This process has evolved in alignment with our biological needs, too. It facilitates absorption of key nutrients at the very first step of our digestive tract, our mouth.

Whatever you notice, it will open your eyes to a process that usually occurs under the radar and outside of our awareness, although it is a process that happens many, many times throughout the day.

Maybe you'll notice the taste of your food more often. Maybe you'll slow down in ways that enhance your body's nutrient absorption and give your body more time to realize you are full, to avoid overeating and for digestive discomfort.

Maybe you'll notice undesirable side effects for the first time from one of the foods in your daily routine. The journey of mindful eating is always evolving and is different for each of us. There is no "wrong" place to be on this path.

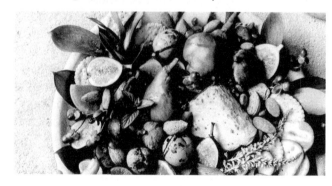

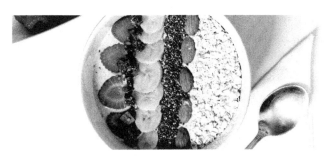

It is a continuous practice of noticing, optimizing, re-calibrating, and experimenting.

Another way to approach mindfulness in your meals is to notice the environment and the company you keep at mealtimes. You are sure to notice some habits and routines that already work well for you, and perhaps some others that don't support your health and wellness goals.

Do you eat differently at different times of day? Do you make different choices after a restful night of sleep or a stressful work day? Do you order differently when you're out with a crowd of friends versus a business meeting versus a family dinner when you know your kids are watching?

Think of the two healthiest friends or loved ones in your life: how often do you eat with them? Do you know whether your food choices, the pace of eating, or anything else is different when you eat with them versus other people in your life?

Are you aware of anyone who might be a negative influence on your eating habits, someone with whom you behave differently when it comes to how much you eat or what you decide to order when dining out, or who judges you or makes you uncomfortable about your food choices?

Eating with others is an irreplaceable social element of cultures around the world. Eating with others can also be very distracting if we are currently making efforts to observe and change our eating habits in any way.

Taking a completely private, undistracted, solo meal on your own once a day, week, or month might help you on this path.

Talking openly with your friends and family about what you're up to and how they can support you on your journey to a healthier life may also really help. Simply engaging with these questions and answering them for yourself may lead you to insights and the next step all on their own.

4.12 Foods to Optimize Energy Levels

Feeling tired and lethargic in the middle of the day? Most people will go straight for a warm cup of coffee, yet this cup of coffee can become a bad habit and does not solve the problem.

Unfortunately, caffeine sourced from coffee in no way provides the body with calories for energy. Instead, it induces a stress response in the body that elevates your senses and makes you feel like you have more energy.

Instead of grabbing a cup of coffee, you should pay close attention to your diet and see if there is any way in which you can promote sustained energy all day long.

We now understand that our body's main source of fuel is carbohydrates, yet eating carbohydrates all day long can play a negative role in terms of insulin sensitivity in the long term.

A balanced macronutrient split throughout the day is vitally important. Traditional North American diets have us eating high carbohydrate breakfasts, which will promote energy for a couple hours but are not optimal for sustained energy all day long.

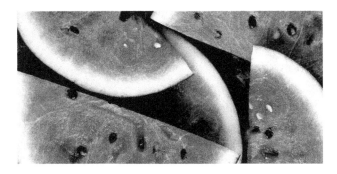

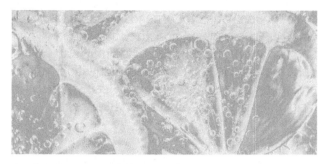

Finding sustained energy the entire day comes down to splitting your meals throughout the day. Your first meal should have a focus on lower carbohydrates, higher protein, and higher fat.

Lower carbohydrates will induce a lower insulin response; more protein will help replenish amino acid stores after sleeping. Higher fat (with more calories) may provide you with sustained energy for a longer duration.

As the day progresses, you should lower your fat intake and raise carbohydrates. Especially if you exercise in the evening, you will want the meal before and after your workout to have a decent amount of carbohydrates to fuel performance.

Keep in mind, this process is not an exact science. You will need to cater the macronutrient splits depending on the specific meal and how you feel throughout the day.

As a general overview, you can use the following split to determine your meals. Don't over complicate it. For optimal results, always try to have a source of complex carbohydrates rich in fiber and lean protein sources in each meal.

Meal #1: 50% protein, 30% fat, 20% carbohydrates
Meal #2: 40% protein, 15% fat, 35% carbohydrates
Meal #3: 30% protein, 20% fat, 40% carbohydrates

4.12.1 The Role of Micronutrients in Weight Loss and Overall Health

Macronutrients are the building blocks of the human body. Yes, macronutrients are where we source many of our calories and without them we could not determine our goal or build our body, but micronutrients are the little guys that do all the background work.

Micronutrients are substantial chemical elements that are needed in trace amounts to promote immune health, blood regulation, growth, and normal tissue development and function.

Micronutrients are vitamins and minerals that are found in everyday foods we eat such as vitamin B, C, D, and minerals like magnesium and iron.

All of these vitamins and minerals become important to the overall success in our respective health and fitness goals.

You will struggle to thrive with a diet that does not have a normal amount of micronutrients. You may experience regular fatigue, mood swings, headache, and much more.

In order to obtain all the essential vitamins and minerals in your diet, it is crucially important to eat a balanced diet.

A diet that is too high in protein will see a lack of vitamins and minerals important to immune health and hydration.

A diet that is too high in fat will see a lack of essential vitamins sourced from fruits and vegetables.

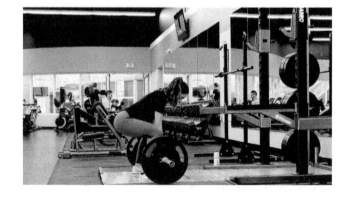

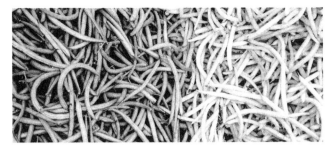

To maintain adequate amounts of micronutrient values, it is important to eat a diet rich in vegetables, fruit, high fiber carbohydrates, lean proteins, and unsaturated fats.

The argument for macronutrients is one that strongly promotes a plant-based nutrient profile. Diets that are heavy in meat lack strong micronutrient profiles and thus have a greater chance for immune dysfunction and lack of tissue development.

A diet rich in fruit, vegetables, nuts, beans, and seeds displays the greatest spectrums of all micronutrients, macronutrients, and amino acids.

What Does Science Say About Macronutrient Splits?

Finding the best macronutrient split for your goal can be difficult and time consuming. That's why we consulted research-based science to help determine which macronutrient profiles are best for specific goals.[118]

4.12.2 Weight Loss and High Fiber

The argument for high protein is extensive, yet there is emerging evidence to show that losing weight on a high fiber diet may be just as effective and much safer for your internal systems.

Fiber is an indigestible source of carbohydrates that is found in soluble and insoluble variations. It is found readily in natural plant based sources such as beans, whole grains, fruit, vegetables, and nuts/seeds. The benefits of nuts/seeds go exceedingly further than most people understand.

Not only do nuts/seeds demonstrate a near perfect macronutrient profile, they are high in fiber and readily sourced with essential vitamins and minerals - they should be a staple in your diet.

High fiber diets have been used to treat and reverse obesity and obesity caused illnesses and have been shown to be the most effective method at maintaining weight loss.

4.12.3 Strength and High Carbohydrates

When it comes to strength and bodybuilding, protein has always been the main nutrient in the discussion. Research[4] has shown, however, that when it comes to pure strength, power and endurance, carbohydrate consumption is king. Let's get one thing clear though, this isn't an excuse to indulge in white flour, candy and cakes. The *kind* of carbs you consume for strength and energy are essential.

Carbs are so effective at creating energy due to glycogen availability in the muscle. Muscles that have a higher glycogen availability have a greater ability to resynthesize ATP (Adenosine Triphosphate) and therefore can induce a greater effect on strength and performance.

If your goal is total energy output, such as cycling, sprinting, or strength training, your diet should include high consumption of fruit, vegetables, whole grains and other complex carbohydrates. This will not only provide you with greater energy for your workouts, but also high fiber and moderate amounts of intra-workout amino acids to draw from.

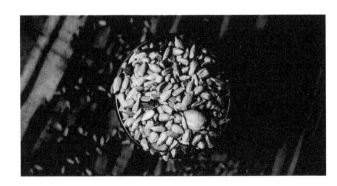

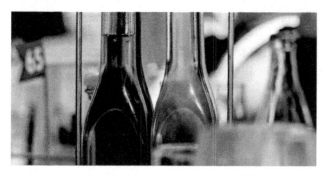

4.12.4 Weight Gain and High Fat

Fat is by no means the enemy in your life. You need to have an adequate amount of fat in your diet in order to have proper immune function and normal growth, yet you should take time to consume good sources of fat and avoid those that have been shown to promote weight gain.

A diet that maintains a fat macronutrient split lower than 30% and is rich in saturated and unsaturated fats from plant sources such as almonds, avocados and olive oil should be considered when avoiding weight gain. Keep in mind, as stated above that of all three macronutrients, fat contains the highest amount of calories per gram (9k/cal/gram).

Irrespective of the type of fat, when consumed in high amounts, fat has been shown to promote weight gain. Due to its high amount of calories per gram, it is very easy to overeat and difficult to achieve a ketogenic effect (like many people attempt). It is much safer, and easier to maintain lower fat intakes from clean, plant-based unsaturated sources.

4.13 Adapting This Diet for Your Life

New diet regimes are difficult and progress can be slow. If dieting was easy, everyone would be fit and healthy. With a fast food restaurant on every corner, it can be quite difficult to stay on a new meal plan or adhere to your macronutrient split for your goal.

Here are three tips to adapting your lifestyle to a new diet regime.

4.13.1 Set Action Based Goals

Many people struggle to stay on a new health/ fitness regime because they do not create goals that have action items. Let's use an example to describe how action items can assist with your goal.

Example #1
Joe wants to use a macronutrient split to put on muscle and lose weight. After a month or so of trying various splits, he found that 40% carbs, 30% protein, and 30% fat worked best for him.

Simple action items can enable Joe to succeed in his specific goal. In order to achieve this macronutrient split Joe will need to eat a good amount of whole foods from various sources. Here are some action items Joe could use to achieve his goal.

- eat 4 servings of fruit and vegetables daily
- replace morning bagel with handful of almonds
- consume protein shake after each workout
- limit fast food to 1x/week

Although these actions seem small and insignificant, when enacted consistently and daily over the span of a year, they become new habits and will promote success.

4.13.2 Monitor Progress

This is done in order to ensure progress is constant - which is exactly what you need for any goal. Not seeing objective progress is

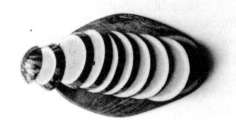

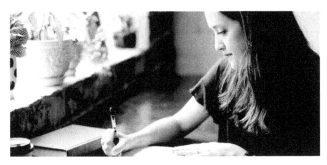

the largest determinant for most people who attempt new lifestyle changes. Monitoring your progress insures that you see ongoing results.

Progress can be monitored in a few simple, yet effective ways.

1. Weekly weigh in
Most people weigh themselves every morning, which is not necessarily a bad thing, but with long-term goals, we can move to a weekly weigh in so we don't obsess over weight every day.

2. If you exercise, Write down your weights, reps and sets
Working out really is a science - that's why we have kinesiologist and exercise physiologists planning complex exercise routines for Olympic athletes. Take advantage of progress markers by writing down your weight, reps, and sets for each workout.

3. Keep a diary
Starting a new health and fitness routine can be difficult and taxing. Taking time to unwind and write down some simple notes about your day can be a great way to track progress without it feeling like work. Two to three months into the new year, you can go back and read about all the challenges you overcame boosting your confidence and seeing objective results at work.

4. Be Patient
Patience is the greatest weapon when it comes to health and fitness. The stars you see in the magazine with toned and sculpted bodies worked for months, if not years, to achieve their figures. The process you are getting into will take time and dedication.

Be patient with your goal and consider that progress is progress, no matter how insignificant.

4.13.3 Finding Your Balance

Macronutrient profiles are a tricky subject. The values are always open to constructive criticism, but we cannot deny the research that backs specific values and their success.

If your goal is to build muscle, you need a diet that is high in macronutrients sourced from carbohydrates and protein, while a goal catered towards weight loss should see lower carbohydrates, low fat, and high protein.

You should not forget to consider the effect each choice you make will have on your insulin response. After all, not keeping an eye on this could lead to diabetes and obesity caused illnesses.

The macronutrient value comes down to your specific goal and adherence to the values. From lower risks of heart disease to cancer prevention, controlling your macronutrient values and eating a whole food diet can have lasting benefits. Staying on track requires careful attention to detail, tracking each day and watching the results come in.

Consistent work yields consistent progress. Find your split and work to your goal.

4.14 Ketogenic vs Low Carb Diets

A ketogenic diet (also known as keto) is a low carb diet, but, low carb does not necessarily

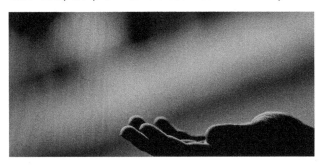

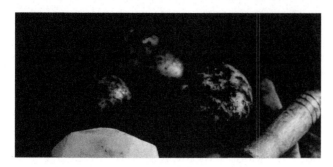

mean ketogenic! The difference is how low carb you go.

The recipes and advice in this book may induce ketogenesis, but as long as you aim for healthy carbs which make up about 20% of your total calories, you'll succeed at almost anything you do.[119]

In such a case that you are training for a marathon or expending lots of energy in athleticism, then by all means – up your carbs. Just try to keep them complex. For example, eat more sweet potatoes rather than white flour or carbs that cause an insulin spike and dump.

All this advice and the recipes we share at the end of the book will be useful when applied to any diet plan, including a low carb diet or a ketogenic one.

Our aim is for you to be consuming plant-based and low-carb foods, as this offers the best results from our perspective.

The difference between keto and low carb is basically that one is low carb, and the other is lower carb. Low carb diets generally range between 50 to 150 grams of carbs per day, whereas the keto diet aims for 20 to 100 grams per day, but it generally is below 50 grams daily, with a ratio of 75% fat, 5% carbohydrates and 20% protein.

If you go above the level suitable for your body, you will no longer be in ketosis (this occurs when your body uses fat as its primary energy source) and burning fat as fuel. You can stick to one or the other, or you can vary your carb intake to cycle in and out of ketosis.

Either way, lowering your carb intake will be very beneficial for your health, in helping you lose weight, improve your cognitive function, and reduce your risk of heart disease, cancer, and type 2 diabetes.

4.14.1 What is a Plant-Based Ketogenic Diet? How Does it Work?

Before jumping directly to the definition of plant-based ketogenic diet, first, let's have a look at the definitions of both "plant-based" and "ketogenic diet" separately. A plant-based diet requires eliminating all types of animal products from your diet.

A ketogenic diet is a high-fat, low carb diet with an adequate consumption of protein. With the diets compared, they typically are considered to be opposites of each other.

You must be wondering, if they are opposites, how come they can work together and benefit your health? Well, a two-word answer - "opposites attract". It's easier than you think to follow a ketogenic diet plan using plant-based foods.

It is true that the biggest issue you might face while shifting to this diet would be getting "enough" protein, as plant-based diets contain low amounts of proteins, and a ketogenic diet narrows the option further.

But don't worry, your body does not need loads of protein on a regular basis. The required amount varies for every person and is easily achieved if you choose the right foods.

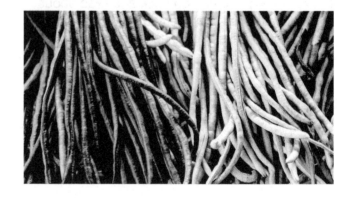

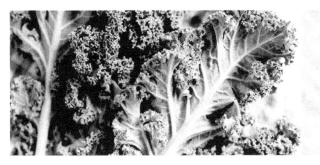

Also, keep this in mind, the most important rule for a plant-based, ketogenic diet is not much different than any other ketogenic diet – eating the right amount of fats and proteins and reducing the carbohydrate intake to almost 50 grams a day.

4.14.2 Types: Standard, Targeted, and Cyclic Ketogenic Diet

There are three primary types of a ketogenic diet.

1. Standard Ketogenic Diet (SKD)
2. Targeted Ketogenic Diet (TKD)
3. Cyclic Ketogenic Diet (CKD)

We will be discussing each of these in detail so that you can decide which one is best for you and your health.

4.14.3 Standard Ketogenic Diet (SKD)

This is the basic version of a ketogenic diet. It works best for fat loss, people who are not physically active or who have insulin resistance. If your performance is not affected by the carbohydrate restriction, then SKD is a good choice. It is a high-fat low carb diet with medium-protein content.

This diet will put you in a state of ketosis; when deprived of carbohydrates the body mainly depends on fats for energy. Fats are broken down mostly by the liver to form fatty acids and glycerol. Fatty acids are further broken down to acetoacetate (acetone body), and the process is called ketogenesis.

Athletes, bodybuilders, marathon runners and obese people are groups of people who can benefit from the standard ketogenic diet. It also helps people suffering from different diseases like Parkinson's disease, type 2 diabetes, autism, celiac disease, and cancer.

4.14.4 Targeted Ketogenic Diet (TKD)

The targeted ketogenic diet requires consuming carbohydrates specifically around workout times. This is mainly to refill the glycogen storage to prevent loss of muscle mass and sustain exercise for a long time.

TKD helps to maintain exercise performance and enables glycogen synthesis without inhibiting ketosis for a longer period.

In TKD, we consume carbohydrates for a specific purpose. If the proper amount is consumed then it helps to fuel the body in optimal ways, especially when you are active. This is known as 'macro timing,' specific timing for introduction of carbohydrates to your targeted keto diet.

Although it varies with individuals, usually between 25-50g of carbohydrates are introduced to your body 30 minutes before being physically active.

The main form of carbs in the TKD is sugar (glucose), because it is digested easily and enters quickly into the blood. Cyclists and Sprinters usually follow a TKD as a way to get immediate energy for races.

4.14.5 Cyclical Ketogenic Diet (CKD)

This is recognized as the "most advanced" form of ketogenic diet. If you are an advanced bodybuilder and do intense workouts throughout the week, you might think that your performance is lacking on SKD or TKD.

It's time to consider CKD and see if that helps bring your performance up to par.

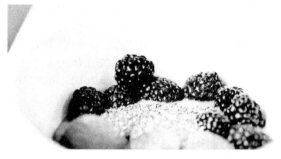

CKD focuses on cycling "high carb," "low carb" and "no carb" days throughout the week. Having no carbs at all is very difficult to achieve, which is why the CKD is for experienced and dedicated athletes. Also, high water consumption is required during the cyclic ketogenic diet.

The main goal of CKD is to temporarily switch out of ketosis to deplete muscle glycogen. For challenging workouts, there are high carb days, and after that, you continue cycling through "low carb" and "no carb" days.

Manage your carb load and nutrient intake according to your lean body mass and physical activity levels. It is not recommended for beginner or intermediate athletes, but again, you make the decision in your diet.

It is very important for you to find out which ketogenic diet is right for you according to your health and physical activity levels. Consider giving each a try if you are unsure which is best for you, but consider starting with the SKD if you need a baseline.

4.14.6 Common Plant-Based Ketogenic and Low Carb Foods

A plant-based ketogenic diet is much more than consuming shakes with coconut milk, protein powder, and ice. You should not be afraid of exploring new options, consuming new vegetables or the same ones in a different, but delightful way. Do not forget the food you eat must meet the nutritional requirements of a vegan ketogenic diet. Below is a list of low carb vegetables:

- Spinach
- Swiss chard
- Kale
- Lettuce
- Garlic
- Green beans
- Cucumber
- Asparagus
- Red and white cabbage
- Cauliflower
- Onions
- Broccoli
- Bell peppers
- Tomatoes
- Eggplants
- Summer and winter squash
- Mushrooms
- Celery
- Parsley
- Zucchini
- Snow Peas

Mostly, fruits should be avoided, but you can have avocados and berries because of their low carb and low sugar content. Nuts have high fat, appropriate protein, and low carbs. Consider these options:

- Macadamia nuts
- Pecans
- Brazil nuts
- Hazelnuts
- Walnuts
- Almonds
- Coconut meat
- Pine nuts

Along with these, you can also consume coconut oil or olive oil, boiled kidney beans, pumpkin seeds, and nut-based butter. Some of the foods you should avoid while on this diet plan

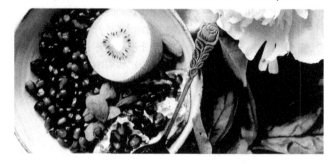

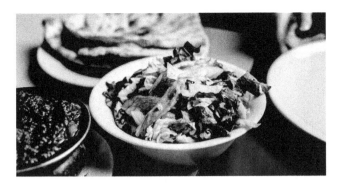

include yams, parsnips, and yucca. Fortunately, yams are seasonal in most places in the U.S., and parsnips and yucca are not commonly consumed.

4.14.7 Ketosis Cycling

As mentioned above, ketosis cycling works by alternating high-carb and low carb days to shed body fat and build muscle. This is more like a hormonal strategy; when carbohydrates enter the body, they are broken down into sugars (glucose), and insulin is released to help clear the blood of excess sugar.

On the low carb days, the insulin levels remain low. Hence, glucose is not taken up by cells, and stored fats are used as a source of energy. During high-carb days, the insulin levels raises, and the empty muscles restocks with glycogen and other nutrients.

Carbohydrates are the body's source of energy, but when there is a shortage of glycogen, the body starts relying on fats for its fuel source. Ketogenic cycling helps the body to use fats stored in muscle and dietary fats as its basic source of energy. By limiting your carb intake on the low carb days, your energy requirements are fulfilled by protein and fats.

Gradually, your body will get used to fat as an energy source. You may experience the 'metabolic switch' period initially, also known as 'brain fog.' It is when your body begins to create certain enzymes needed for the keto diet and it is a way for your body to adapt to this new energy source.

Ketosis cycling offers many benefits other than just building muscles or losing weight. It allows you to learn more about your body, and you feel physically and mentally empowered. If you consume too many carbs, your body becomes resistant to leptin (the satiety hormone).

This means it is unable to identify when you are full. This will cause the body to feel hungry frequently, which can lead to overeating. However, ketosis cycling helps to keep leptin levels regulated in a nice way.

In addition to regulating leptin levels, a keto diet can help to improve signs of autism and migraines. According to a recent study, 18 out of 30 children suffering from autism showed signs of improvement by following a cyclic ketogenic diet for six months.[120]

Another study of two sisters reported that while they were following ketogenic cycling for weight loss, their migraine headaches vanished during the four-week ketosis cycle.

The first couple of days are designed to get your body into ketosis, often resulting in drowsiness and muscle fatigue. When you have finally achieved ketosis, your body gains some equilibrium.

However, if you are not strong enough and start with ketosis cycling immediately and then stop and eat carbohydrates, your body exits ketosis and the fatigue phase repeats.

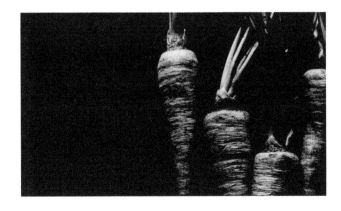

4.14.8 Ketosis Health Implications and Therapeutic Potential

Ketosis promises fast and easy weight loss because it reduces food cravings and reduces the amount of calories you consume each day.

Other than weight loss, it has several health benefits including fighting cancer, improving mental focus, preventing heart-related disease, decreasing inflammation, improving energy, better sleep, improved fertility, increased endurance, and reduced metabolic syndrome.

Metabolic syndrome is a collection of health conditions that increases your risk of premature death. You have metabolic syndrome if you have at least three of the following conditions:

- Hypertension
- High cholesterol
- Abdominal obesity
- Type 2 diabetes

The keto diet has been used since the 1920s to treat children with epilepsy. Even today, under the direction of a pediatrician, a keto diet can be helpful in reducing and eliminating the effects of epilepsy disorder.

4.14.9 Health Benefits of a Plant-Based Diet

There was a time when an unhealthy life was caused by malnutrition. Now, however, it is due to the shift to processed foods and more animal-based foods that have resulted in too much food, which is the cause of several chronic diseases.

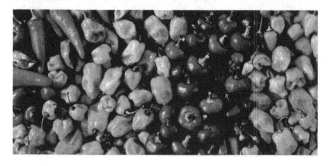

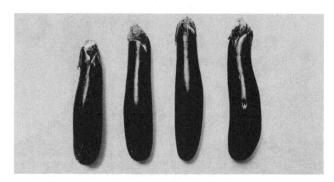

With a plant-based diet, you have a lower risk of diabetes, obesity and high blood pressure. Moreover, a vegan diet helps increase your intake of some of the most important vitamins and minerals needed for health.

You have a better chance at lowering your blood pressure levels, since this diet typically is low in sodium and higher in potassium and fiber.

In addition, research on blood pressure levels among adults found that people on a vegan diet have a lower systolic and diastolic blood pressure[121] because their meals are lower in saturated fats and contain almost no cholesterol.

Health authorities may now be leaning to plant-based diets even for mothers. From the Medical Association of Pediatrics to the American Academy of Pediatrics, all medical associations now favor a vegan diet during pregnancy.

A plant-based diet not only provides the expectant mother with the required nutrients, but also helps to avoid morning sickness, constipation, hemorrhoids and many other side effects.

4.15 Frequently Asked Questions

4.15.1 Can I eat this way if I'm just cooking for one? For my whole family? For my children?

Whole food, plant-based meals are every bit as scalable, upward and downward, as any other way to eat.

The actual cooking isn't all that different, so this lifestyle is fortunately relevant for both individuals and families.

People can actually "catch" habits from each other as if they were a contagious cold. In other words, we influence our peers and social networks with our eating and lifestyle habits, and similarly, we are influenced by the people with whom we spend the most time.

Your pursuit of a healthier life will positively influence others, sometimes in ways you cannot possibly imagine.

Use this fact to your advantage and make your transition a social one. The popularity of this eating approach is rapidly growing, and you are never alone on this journey.

Finding a community during this transition is a great way to line up support for yourself and make new friends. Online recipes, social media groups and platforms, and cookbooks and magazines are all easy to find nowadays and there are many that cater to whole, plant-based foods.

4.15.2 What if I can't imagine life without cheese?

If you can't imagine life without cheese, then don't. There are a variety of nut-based homemade cheese recipes as well as a rapidly growing market of plant-based, non-dairy cheese substitute products available at grocery stores and larger big-box stores like Target, Walmart, and Costco.

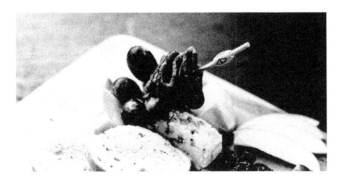

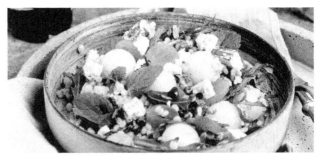

What makes dairy cheese so popular? It often has a complex, savory flavor, often called the fifth flavor (after sweet, salty, sour, and bitter), or *umami*. Parmesan cheese has a particularly high score in terms of umami flavor, but it shares that score with another food group, seaweed.

Specifically, kombu is one type of seaweed that contains high amounts of an amino acid called glutamate. Kombu is the foundation for Japanese stock soup, which then becomes the base ingredient for a variety of traditional dishes. When our taste receptors detect the presence of glutamate in foods, that is the umami taste.

This is really good news, and seaweed is only one example, as many plant-based foods boast a strong umami flavor owing to their high glutamate content, such as fermented foods (kimchi, or fermented Korean vegetables, and balsamic vinegar for instance), tomatoes, shiitake and porcini mushrooms, spices like cumin and smoked paprika, and so on.

It is natural to crave the tastes we grew up with. It is natural for your taste buds to adjust to new flavors, too, and it is easy to trick your taste buds to enjoy new flavors that are similar to the old favorites.

Lastly, the anticipation is often worse than the reality. That goes for many, many things. Remember, you don't have to make all these changes today. And when you are ready to make them, they may not be as difficult as you fear.

4.16 Change is a Process

"You're off to Great Places! Today is your day! Your mountain is waiting, so… get on your way!"
– Dr. Seuss, *Oh, The Places You'll Go!*

You've made it this far. You are ready and committed to creating a healthier life for yourself.

If you lightly skimmed this chapter, skipped over several pages, and/or read it half-heartedly while doing other things, you may have trouble remembering anything from these pages at all, wondering what value you really obtained.

If this happened to you during your first read, start over from the beginning and give it another try – we bet you'll surprise yourself and create something valuable from your experience. Let this chapter be the beginning of a powerful story of transformation into the next best version of yourself.

Remember, habit change is a process, and there may be moments when old and familiar habits are pretty tempting. There may even be moments that feel like a step backward. That's all just part of the process. You didn't learn to ride a bike without ever taking a fall.

You didn't learn to play an instrument without ever playing one wrong note. Pick yourself back up wherever you are. Start riding again.

More energy, vitality, and well-being await you.

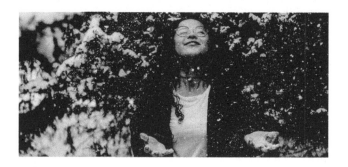

5.0 Intermittent Fasting: The Secret to Ultimate Health and Simple Weight Loss

You are what you eat, as well as *when* you eat.

When people are searching for ways to manage their weight, burn fat, and stabilize their blood sugar, they often focus on specific foods or diets.

While those factors are key in reaching optimal health, it's also important to focus on the timing of your meals. In this area, intermittent fasting can unlock your health goals and help you achieve new levels of health, wellness, and energy.

Intermittent fasting is an easy and quick way to make a simple habit change that impacts your weight and your waistline. Anyone can try it, starting at the end of your next meal. If you're looking to improve your health, burn more fat and lose more weight, fasting could be the strategy that finally gets you the results you need!

5.1 What is Intermittent Fasting?

Fasting is not *just* abstaining from eating.

Fasting for religious and spiritual reasons and health and longevity has been common among people across the world for ages. Plato and Hippocrates are considered the earliest founders of fasting to improve health.

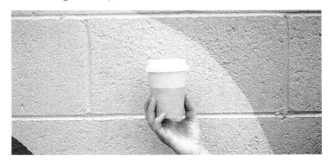

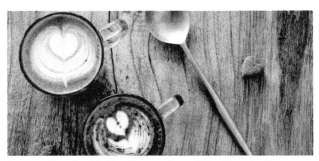

According to Philip Paracelsus "Fasting is the greatest remedy – the physician within".

Fasting poses the same challenge for the brain as regular exercise, but it may have some benefits to your health as well. Intermittent fasting has been gaining popularity in recent years, and now it has made its way to the fitness scene.

Intermittent fasting is an eating schedule rather than a diet. It doesn't require changes in your diet; rather, it is an eating pattern with set feeding periods and fasting periods. Parts of the day or week are divided into feasting and fasting windows depending on the pattern you follow. It is a decision where you choose to skip certain meals of the day on purpose, all to better your health.

It is the easiest way to lose weight, increase energy, reduce insulin resistance, lower risk of type 2 diabetes, reduce stress, protect your heart, and prevent cancer and Alzheimer's disease.

5.2 What are the Benefits of Intermittent Fasting?

The benefits of intermittent fasting are well documented. It improves your metabolism, aids

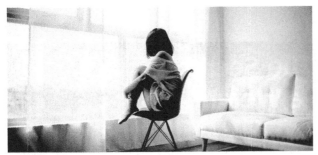

in weight management, and drastically reduces obesity.

In a massive study published in the *International Journal of Obesity*,[122] researchers measured how intermittent fasting affected blood sugar, insulin sensitivity, inflammation and weight loss in overweight women.

They monitored the women over a period of six months and found improvements in all areas. These results were present even when the actual amount of calories were the same and only the timing of meals was changed.

Another study noted how intermittent fasting stabilized blood sugar and helped improve sugar metabolism, which helped boost general wellness and even improved brain health. And speaking of brain health, studies report that intermittent fasting may help reduce your risk of depression, Alzheimer's, Parkinson's, stroke and more.[123]

If you're still not convinced, the research on intermittent fasting is quite comprehensive:

- *American Journal of Clinical Nutrition*: Intermittent fasting improved insulin levels significantly (insulin is important for managing your blood sugar) and helped people burn fat.[124]
- *International Journal of Obesity*: Fasting just a couple days a week helped people lose weight.[125]
- Multiple studies: Intermittent fasting increases your metabolism by up to 14%.[126]
- *Translational Research* journal: In just a few weeks, intermittent fasting sig-

nificantly stabilized people's blood sugar, reduced their blood sugar by up to 6%, and helped them lose up to 8% of their weight and up to 7% of their waist size.[127]

It's dramatically clear that intermittent fasting as a lifestyle habit can help you shed the pounds, burn fat and feel healthier.

"For individuals to sustain healthy lifestyle changes, we must make the healthy choice the easy choice," says Dr. Scott Young in a research report recently published in the *Permanente Journal*.[128] In other words, if you want to make intermittent fasting a way of life and truly change your lifestyle habits, you have to make it easy for you to follow this fasting program.

5.3 Whole Day Fasting and Time-Restricted Fasting

Intermittent fasting can be divided into two popular categories: whole day fasting and time-restricted feeding. Whole day fasting or alternate day fasting is a type of fasting that involves fasting for a complete 24 hours, followed by a 24-hour feeding period.

The feeding period is the usual pattern of eating and does not give you the ok to splurge on ice cream and fattening foods. In time-restricted feeding, food is allowed in only a certain number of hours, fasting for the rest of the hours.

In previous chapters, we went into depth on plant-based, ketogenic diets. Let's learn how we can combine a plant-based keto diet with

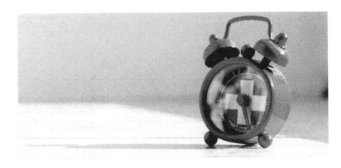

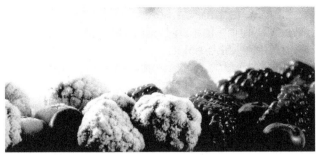

intermittent fasting methods. These two types of eating are highly complimentary and can enhance the benefits of each if combined correctly.

The combination of a plant-based keto diet and intermittent fasting is ideal for those who are already on a plant-based keto diet. You just need to be mindful of your fasting window and eat the required calories during your feeding window, keeping the plant-based keto diet in mind to keep your body in ketosis.

Sounds pretty easy, right?

If you aim for ketosis, intermittent fasting will help you get there quicker and more efficiently. Moreover, with a keto diet, intermittent fasting becomes more feasible as the body is already adapted to fasting.

Both these diets not only go together well but also complement each other. Starting intermittent fasting along with plant-based keto will help you avoid the common side effects of keto diet like the keto flu. The keto diet will make your fasting window very comfortable, and it can be a nice transition into a new lifestyle.

In the beginning, intermittent fasting may be uncomfortable, but with time, your body will get used to it; and if you use a plant-based keto diet along with intermittent fasting, you may not even feel very hungry during the fasting periods.

To successfully achieve all the benefits, make sure you eat enough plant-based foods and be sure to hit your caloric goals. Let's discuss some of the popular intermittent fasting methods in more detail.

5.4 Leangains (The 16/8 Method)

Leangains is a type of intermittent fasting founded by Martin Berkhan, a nutritional consultant. The 16:8 protocol is very easy to follow. You simply fast for a period of 16 hours a day and adjust your calories in the remaining 8 hours. This is by far the easiest method to start with, as the body is in fasting for at least eight hours from the time you go to bed from the time you wake up.[129]

The time of day that you are not fasting, you can eat as you normally would. You can adjust your fasting times to your daily routine. Most people find it easier to fast at night (after dinner) and then skip breakfast, so their first meal of the day is around lunch or early afternoon.

While on the 16:8 protocol, the protein intake remains moderately high. On workout days, fat intake is considerably lower as compared to non-exercise days. This also depends on your age, sex, body fat, and activity levels.

The workout days can be started with a medium-sized meal of veggies, and it's usually best to work out within three hours of this meal.

On non-exercise days, you should have a lower calorie intake. It is better to eat vegetables as the first meal of the day. The last meal of the day before fasting should preferably contain a slow digesting protein. This will maintain a feeling of fullness, ensuring that your body has plenty amino acids during the 16 hour fast.

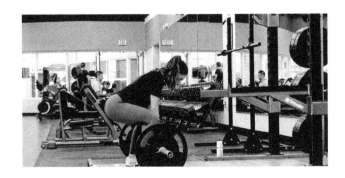

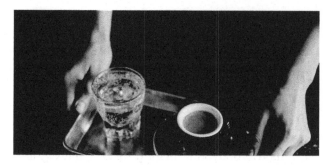

While on the 16:8 protocol, do not overeat. If you are fasting using this method, it does not mean you can eat all sorts of unhealthy foods in that 8-hour stretch and increase your calorie intake so that it lasts until your next feeding. Although it is better to avoid all foods during fasting, coffee, water, and sugar free gum can be taken as they have an extremely low calorie count.

Once you start with the leangain protocol, you will notice the benefits immediately. It increases the rate of fat loss and prevents you from craving unhealthy food. It suppresses hunger, making you feel more satisfied after a meal. It also helps you to differentiate between when you are really hungry, and when you are just craving something to chew on for flavor or to fill an emotional need.

After fasting for 16 hours, and you finally have your first meal, you will be more sensitive to insulin. Therefore, your insulin levels will fluctuate less and be more stable following your feeding.

5.5 Eat - Stop - Eat (Fasting for 24 Hours Once or Twice Every Week)

Brad Pilon initiated this type of intermittent fasting, and most people can follow it when first starting. Eat-stop-eat was the result of the graduate research thesis he did at the University of Guelph, Canada.

How does it work?

It's simple: fast for 24 hours once or twice a week. During the 24-hour long fast, also referred as "24 break from eating," you do not consume any food. However, some calorie-free beverages are ok to drink.

Following this way of fasting, your muscular strength is maintained, so don't worry if you are looking to increase muscle mass. It is preferable to start your fast after dinner, around 7 p.m.

You sleep all night, and when you wake up, you will be more than halfway through your 24 hour fast. You need to drink plenty of water on this protocol.

After completing the 24 hours, you should break your fast by eating some of your favorite vegetables same as you would if you were not fasting. Have some healthy vegetables as your first meal after the fast and chew slowly so you don't suddenly burden your digestive system, as it has been resting for a while.

You should never break the fast just because you're hungry. This will help you to have stronger self-control to deal with your hunger cravings. You should learn to restrain yourself from breaking the fast unless you have achieved the 24 hours.

During the fast, your empty stomach might start making funny noises; this doesn't require you to break the fast or start panicking. Instead, satisfy your stomach with water.

Practice this for at least 2 to 3 months, and you'll experience all the amazing benefits of fasting. Your first fast will be the hardest, but

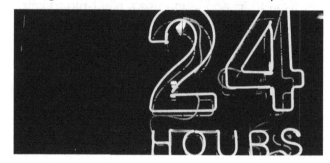

after the sixth one, you'll get completely used to it and hopefully will enjoy it.

Like Leangain fasting, the eat-stop-eat method has its benefits, including fat loss, regulation of hunger hormones, better memory and concentration, better insulin sensitivity, and a lowered risk of diabetes.

5.6 The Warrior Diet

Warrior dieting means sticking to a form of fasting during the day, eating small amounts of raw fruits and vegetables for 20 hours, and then eating one large meal at night. Ori Hofmekler started it in 2001. The fasting phase is more like restricting your calories to nearly zero, or at zero. You can eat some raw fruits or vegetables, fresh juice, or a small amount of protein and lots of water. This is to stimulate fat burning and boost your energy.

Managing your calories during that "one large meal" is also very crucial for a successful warrior diet.[130]

The four-hour eating phase is at night to help promote calmness, relax digestion, and allow the body to use the nutrients for repair and growth. It may also help the body to produce hormones and burn fat as well.

While fasting on the warrior diet, you should drink at least 8 glasses of water per day. You can also supplement water with nutrients by adding lemon, mint, and cucumber. This helps to naturally flavor your water and it is a good way to boost nutrient intake as well.

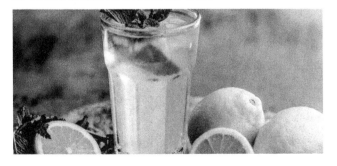

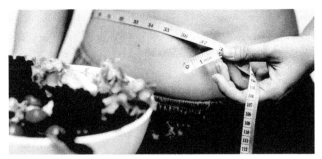

5.7 Alternate-Day Fasting (Fasting Every Other Day)

Alternate day fasting means that you fast every other day and, while fasting, you simply restrict your calories to 25% of your daily calorie intake. Let's say you have determined that you require about 1800 calories a day to lose weight. Then on the fasting days, you will have to limit this intake to 450 calories. So, you do not completely cut off food while fasting, but you restrict it severely.

You will need to keep carbs low and protein intake moderate in order to meet your body's needs. On the day when you are not fasting, you can have anything you want, but don't use this as an excuse to overdo it.

There is no definite rule about what you should eat or drink while fasting, so long as your daily calorie intake does not exceed the required amount. As mentioned earlier, it is always better to drink low-calorie or calorie-free drinks on fasting days, such as water, green tea or unsweetened coffee and tea.

As your calorie intake is strictly limited, try to eat nutritious, high-protein foods and low-calorie vegetables. These will help you feel full and can help you to succeed in your fasting. Vegetable soups are another good option while fasting, as they help you controlling your hunger and reducing your meal intake.[131] Some other low-calorie meal choices include:

- Grilled vegetables
- Kale soup
- Avocado hummus

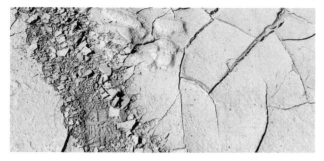

- Berry & almond smoothie
- Pumpkin muffin bites
- Roasted vegetable salad

Studies have shown that alternate day fasting is very effective for weight loss in average weight or obese adults.[132] In addition, alternate day fasting helps reduce inflammatory markers in obese individuals, along with reducing harmful belly fat.[133] If combined with exercise, this method may help you lose a lot more fat than you would have lost with exercise only.[134] If weight loss is your primary goal, consider this an effective method.

Alternate day fasting also lowers the risk factors for type 2 diabetes among overweight and obese individuals. Studies have also shown that alternate day fasting can benefit heart health and reduce the risk of cardiovascular disease.[135] It reduces hypertension, LDL levels, waist circumference and lowers blood triglycerides.

Other studies conducted on animals have shown that both long-term and short-term fasting increase autophagy, a procedure in which old and worn out cells are degraded and recycled.[136] Both are, therefore, helpful in delaying aging and reducing the risk of tumors, helping to decrease your risk of certain cancers, heart disease, neurodegeneration, and infections.

If you are following this diet just for weight loss, then you have the tools here to achieve it, as long as you stick with your eating plan.

5.8 Fat Fasting

Fat fasting is eating around 1200 calories a day, with more than 80% of your calories coming from fat sources alone. You can break these 1200 calories into 4 or 5 meals a day according to your activity levels and schedule.

Usually, fat fasting is done for 2-4 days at a time and never recommended for more than five days. Going over five days may cause you to lose muscle mass, something that you'd probably not be pleased with.

This is often suggested to those who are already keto-adapted. When you fast, your ketone level will increase because energy is coming from fat (termed lipolysis). This is the mechanism of the breakdown of fats, involving hydrolysis of triglycerides into glycerol and fatty acids. The longer you're fat fasting, the more of these free fatty acids will be released.

Lipolysis cannot occur if there is a substantial amount of glucose present. However, you do not need to worry about excess carbs converting into glucose, as 80% of your calories are coming from fats. But why is it so important?

Fatty acids create small ketone bodies and use them as fuel.

At first, you are more likely to feel hungry. But as soon as your body starts adjusting to this way of eating, your hunger will decrease.

This is because you will have your meals at regular intervals with high amounts of fat, which improves the satiety levels. Although most people get used to 2-3 meals per day along with some coffee, some also find 1-3 meals convenient and satisfactory. More than four

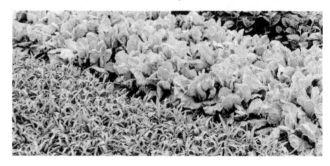

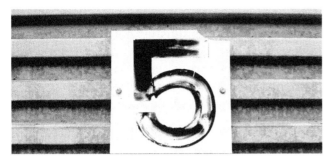

meals a day is likely to make you think about food all the time, and you'll feel hungrier.

It is completely normal if your calorie count or fat percentage fluctuates a little at the start. Sometimes you end up eating 75% of your calories from fat or might over consume some 200 calories. But this is normal, and you shouldn't worry about it. If you try to focus on the rules of this diet when eating, you may find it easier to adjust.

Some preferred foods while fat fasting are:

- Avocados
- Nuts
- Mushrooms
- Dark chocolate
- Coffee with coconut milk

The most important benefit of ketogenic induced fat-fasting is that it increases your body's capacity to use fats as fuel. This way, your body starts selecting ketones over glucose.

As a result of lower levels of glucose, there is a reduction in insulin levels, which enables more lipolysis. The fundamental use of the fat fasting diet is to help people with metabolic disorders. Fat fasting can help those with metabolic issues lose weight, burn fat, and improve insulin sensitivity following a feeding.

5.9 Only Eating When You're Hungry

Some people might find it difficult to control their hunger. This can make it difficult to lose weight. You may think you need far more calories than you truly require. You can control your appetite by finding out when you are *actually* hungry.

Let's look at hunger more closely.

It is neither the urge to eat when you are sad or bored, nor is it something that you feel when you walk past a restaurant. Hunger is a physical feeling that builds up gradually throughout your day. It serves a vital function in human life. It occurs when your stomach requires food. Some of the healthy signals of hunger include:

- Gnawing in the stomach
- Difficulty concentrating
- Headache
- Feeling faint
- Irritability
- Lightheadedness

It's better to eat only when you are hungry rather than following a time-based eating schedule. Unrequired snacks will hinder your weight loss. What's the point in eating a meal when you are not hungry and skipping a meal when you are? Eat until you feel full, but dig deep to find out what feeling full truly means.

Your stomach usually doesn't register the full capacity of food you put in it until a whole 20 minutes after your last bite. Consider this when you are eating, and stop before you feel "full."

They are many people with success stories using intermittent fasting. However, you should keep one thing in mind: these intermittent fasting methods are not for everyone.

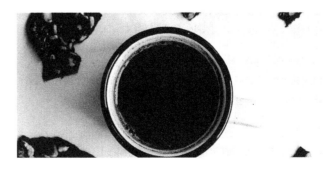

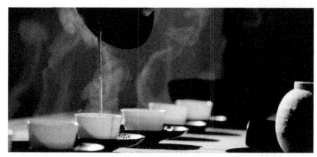

Specific methods are geared for differing health goals, and some people respond better to a particular fasting plan. Only do what works best for you.

5.10 Three Ways to Make Intermittent Fasting Much Easier

You can support your health goals during a fast with several key supplements and dietary choices. These add-ons, while not essential for enjoying the benefits of intermittent fasting, can help make intermittent fasting a lot easier by eliminating food cravings.

5.10.1 Drink Abundant Amounts of Tea

Hydration helps you to control appetite and cravings, which is beneficial when doing intermittent fasting. In fact, many people think that they're hungry when in fact they're thirsty, warns a report in the *American Dietician* journal.[137]

If one reason you're doing intermittent fasting is to lose weight and stabilize your blood sugar, take note: According to doctors, becoming dehydrated can spike your cravings for sugar and junk food.[138]

Staying hydrated also boosts your metabolism, further enhancing the results of your fast. In one study, drinking 500 ml of water increased people's metabolism by an incredible 24%.[139] Drinking fluids can even boost metabolism down on the cellular level.[140]

Staying hydrated is also essential for healthy digestion, according to research in the Nutrition Review journal.[141] It moves digestive fluids through your system, flushes out waste and toxins, and helps deliver the nutrients from your food to different parts of your body. All of these elements are critical when you're shrinking your meals to a narrow window. Your body needs more support to digest and move that food in a quicker period of time.

Besides drinking water, consider herbal teas. Their flavors can encourage you to drink more water. They can also bring their own distinct health benefits. Herbal teas like ginger tea, peppermint tea, chamomile tea and cinnamon tea have all been shown to help you improve waste elimination and boost digestion.[142]

5.10.2 Utilize Branch Chained Amino Acids (BCAAs)

BCAAs is a powdered supplement full of healthy amino acids with multiple health benefits.[143] Research shows that this supplement can help reduce fatigue, reduce hunger and improve how much fat you burn, which can speed up the beneficial results of your fasting. Studies also show it may help lower your blood sugar and even influence the production of ketone bodies, the chemicals your body produces when you're on a fast.[144]

BCAAs are especially popular among those who are on an intermittent fast. For example, some people worry that extended periods of fasting can cause a breakdown of muscle, especially if you partake in exercise. BCAAs help prevent muscle breakdown so that you maintain healthy lean muscle no matter how long you're fasting.[145]

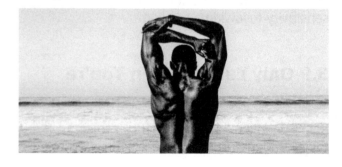

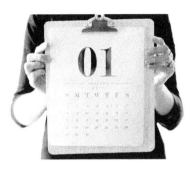

Women should take approximately 5 grams of BCAAs a day while men usually take approximately 15 grams.

5.10.3 Use Medium Chain Triglycerides (MCTs)

Eating fewer carbs and more healthy fats moderates your blood sugar and helps you maintain a healthier weight. MCTs, which is naturally found in coconut oil, is one type of healthy fat. You can also find MCT oil supplements.

MCT can be beneficial for intermittent fasting in several key ways. First, it helps control your appetite and reduces cravings. This can make it easier to stick to your fasting plan and avoid the temptation to break your fast too early, thus robbing you of the benefits of a true fast.

Second, MCT can help stabilize your blood sugar. In a study published in the journal *Diabetes*, they found that it could help moderate your blood sugar-and-insulin response, which is a key factor in diabetes risks.[146]

Third, it can provide a boost of energy that can sustain you through your fast. A side benefit is that it may lead to a reduction in body fat. You see, when you're fasting, your body uses fatty acids instead of sugar as energy. By taking MCT oil, you encourage your body to continue to use fat as an energy source instead of sugar and carbohydrates.

While you can find MCTs in coconut fat, eating enough coconut fat to get the amount of MCTs you need can be difficult. Instead, a concentrated MCT oil can help you hit your intake goals. While every supplement varies in its dosage, studies suggest taking 1-3 tablespoons of MCT oil supplements a day.

With these added nutritional supports, you can fast with greater success.

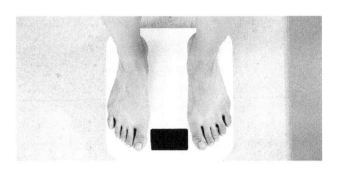

6.0 Mental Health and Nutrition

"I'm not faking being sick, I'm faking being well."
– Facebook meme

It is completely normal to feel anger, frustration sadness, and even rage at some point in our lives, but depression affects far more people than it needs to.

Our modern society has normalized depression, and far too many doctors and health "experts" ignore the fact that food is inextricably linked to how well we feel. Our mental health and happiness simply cannot thrive on the S.A.D. diet.

In this chapter we'll be discussing how food affects your mental health and what you can do to feed your brain foods that will help it thrive.

6.1 Your Brain On Food

Your brain is like a rare, collectible car. If you give it anything other than premium fuel, it's going to break down.

Our high sugar, inflammation promoting diet in the West causes oxidative damage to brain cells, allows free radicals to run wild within a closed space, and depletes our ability to feel happy.

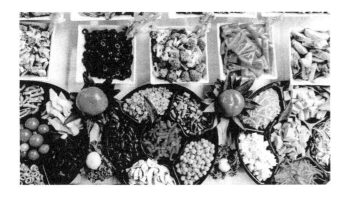

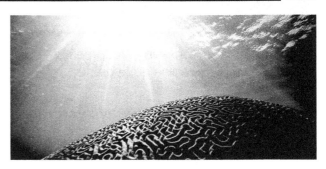

Many people have heard of a commonly noted brain chemical – serotonin, yet few people are aware that 95% of serotonin is produced in your gastrointestinal tract.

Why is what you eat so important?

The gastrointestinal tract is lined with hundreds of millions of neurons, that don't just make it possible for you to digest your food, but which also regulate your emotional state.[147]

6.2 Nutritional Deficiencies and Mental Health

6.2.1 How does nutrition influence mental health?

Many nutrient deficiencies threaten your mental health[148] because the correct functioning of your mind and emotions is very complex.

Your mood is an intricate dance between functions in your brain, nerves, hormones, and gastrointestinal tract.

At a cellular level, there's a symphony of many different vitamins, minerals and amino acids[149] that all must work together to keep you on top of your mental game. If any one of these

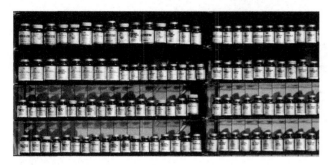

essential elements is missing, your mental health can start to decline quite quickly.

6.2.2 Eating well isn't always enough.

Even though you might think you eat well and live a healthy lifestyle, it's still possible that you're not getting all the nutrients you need for optimum health.

This is because our modern lives are stressful and it's common to skip meals or eat on the run. Convenience foods are often nutritionally poor[150] because they've been heavily processed.

Even foods that you think of as healthy, such as home cooked meals, can be lacking the nutrient density[151] you need to live your healthiest life. This is because they've been grown in depleted soils or fertilized with chemicals that don't contain the full range of necessary nutrients. It's virtually impossible to tell just from looking at your plate whether your food is nutritionally rich or not.

6.3 Supplements are key to Overcoming Nutrient Deficiencies.

With supplements, you get a controlled dose of the nutrients you need. If it's a good supplement, it will be delivered primarily from plant food sources, which are easy for your body to digest and utilize. Taking a supplement gives you added assurance that you're getting the nutrients you need, even if your food isn't providing them.

6.3.1 Nutrient deficiency and stress can perpetuate each other.

It can quickly become a perpetuating cycle when your sleep is disturbed or your stress levels are out of control and you just can't regain your balance. Living with sleeplessness or excess stress can put even more strain on your body, and it starts to burn through nutrients faster than ever in an effort to heal.

By using up vital nutrients to try to counter the stress it's under, your body becomes even more depleted. Your symptoms may worsen at this point, and it begins a cycle of compounding symptoms and nutrient deficiencies. To reverse this and head back towards health, it's necessary to interrupt the cycle through boosting nutrition and breaking the pattern of your symptoms.

6.3.2 Lifestyle choices are an essential factor in mental health.

It's important to address your lifestyle if you have mental health issues. Look at the things you find stressful and ask yourself if you can let go of any of them. Make a plan to move away from stressful circumstances and towards things that relax you.

Reach out to your support network and ask for help when you need it. If you feel that you don't have the support network you need, look for ways to create this. Even if you don't have friends or family on your side, you can seek help from professionals.

Make sure you have a doctor you feel comfortable with, whom you trust and can speak

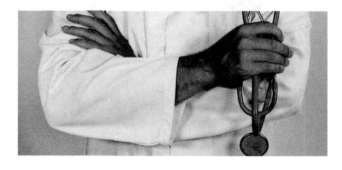

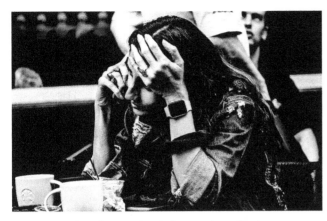

with openly. If you don't have this, find a new doctor. Make it your first step towards improving your wellbeing. Your doctor can have a big influence over whether or not you get the right help, so this is really important.

6.3.3 Common Nutrient Deficiencies Associated with Mental Illness

Magnesium

Magnesium deficiency is common in virtually every mental health imbalance. This includes depression, anxiety[152], stress, personality disorders, and attention disorders. This mineral is essential because it's involved in energy production. The energy your body produces powers all of your cells and therefore every function that maintains life and health.

Another vital role magnesium plays in your body is in forming proteins. Proteins are the building blocks of all life; they make up your bones, muscles, brain, and internal organs. You need to be able to make proteins effectively in order to maintain your mental health.

Magnesium is deficient in many people's diets and it gets depleted by factors such as alcohol, oral contraceptives, diuretics and excessive sweating. The recommended daily allowance for magnesium is 200-300mg.

Foods that contain magnesium[153] in high amounts include:

- Almonds
- Cashews
- Brewer's yeast
- Brazil nuts
- Pecans
- Walnuts

Any dose over 150 mg[154] elemental magnesium should be enough to top up your magnesium stores because your diet will be providing the rest.

Zinc

Zinc is in every body cell! This amazing nutrient is not needed in very large amounts, but it's absolutely essential for hundreds of different processes in your body. Zinc deficiency is associated with depression, aggressive behaviors, attention disorders, and learning difficulties[155].

Zinc is heavily involved in signaling and message systems within your body. When it's time to make your happy hormone, serotonin, or your sleep hormone, melatonin, you need zinc to send the message and facilitate the process. If zinc isn't there in adequate quantity, levels of these important hormones will decline. That's when you start to see symptoms.

Every aspect of your mood and energy are regulated[156] closely by hormones and nerve signals, and zinc is always involved. Without it you have trouble sleeping, your mood is

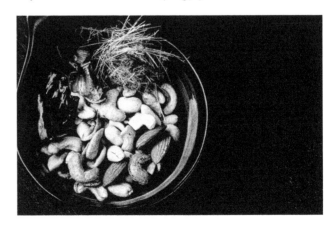

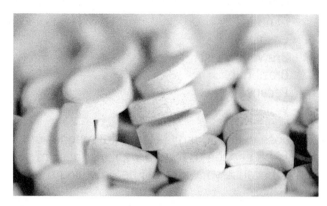

unstable, you have trouble concentrating or learning. In fact, your entire personality can be affected.

A lot of people in the United States are marginally deficient in zinc, receiving about half of the amount they need daily. The recommended daily allowance is only 15 mg, and most people consume only 7-8mg of this important mineral. So when it comes to supplementing, look for a formula that gives you at least 7 mg of zinc daily.

There are many different states that can cause zinc deficiency[157,158]. If you suffer digestive issues, it's likely you have reduced zinc absorption, so even if you're getting enough in your diet, it's possible your body can't digest it. Liquid formulas and zinc in the form of chelates can help to counter this. But ultimately, healing your gut is going to give you back your health in the most profound way.

Eating a diet that's too high in calcium or iron can disturb your zinc absorption because these nutrients compete for the same digestive channel. Alcohol consumption can prevent proper zinc absorption and so can a diet that's excessively high in fiber.

Plant sources of zinc include pumpkin seeds, pecans, Brazil nuts, almonds, walnuts, peanuts, split peas, rye, oats, and Lima beans.

B Vitamins

B vitamins are included here as a group because of the way they work together synergistically. They need to be in balance to give you optimum health benefits. There are specific B vitamins that are more strongly associated with mental health, but when you take them in supplement form, it's best to choose a formula that contains the full spectrum of B vitamins.

B vitamins work on the most basic functions in the body[159]. They're essential for making energy, hormones, and neurotransmitters. These then direct the activities of all the organs and systems that work together to keep you healthy.

Digestion, sleep, energy, and mood are all coordinated by the hormones and chemical signals that are produced using B vitamins.

Vitamin B6[160] is one of the most important vitamins with regards to brain function. It's involved in brain chemistry at a very fundamental level because your body needs it to make hormones.

This includes serotonin, melatonin, and all the other molecules that regulate mood, energy, and sleep. Vitamin B6 is very commonly deficient in people who have depression, especially in women who are taking the oral contraceptive pill. It's useful to supplement it in the range of 50-100 mg daily.

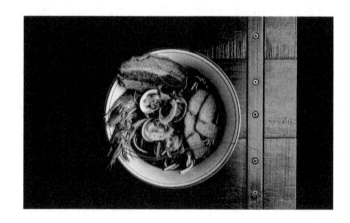

Vitamin B9[161] is also called folic acid. Its deficiency is common in psychiatric patients and in certain cases, folic acid supplementation can bring about surprising improvements in mental function. It's a mild antidepressant and works especially well when depression is accompanied by mental fog - trouble concentrating, difficulty in thinking clearly, and a general sense of confusion.

Vitamin B9 needs to always be supplemented in combination with vitamin B12 because B9 supplementation can mask B12 deficiency. 400mcg daily is enough folic acid to reverse a deficiency.

Vitamin B12[162] works with vitamin B9 in many body processes, including the making of nerve covers, which are essential for good signaling between the brain and the rest of the body. B12 also works on energy production and the collection of hormones and transmitters in the brain that regulate sleep and mood.

One of the first symptoms of B12 deficiency is in the nervous system, where you experience numbness, tingling or a burning sensation, often accompanied by impaired mental function.

B12 deficiency is often mistaken for Alzheimer's disease,[163] especially in older people. The recommended daily dosage range of 100-2,000mcg is broad because vitamin B12 is largely non-toxic, so there's no disadvantage to taking higher doses. It ensures that even if you have a very low absorption rate, you'll still receive the minimum dose you need of around 2-3mcg.

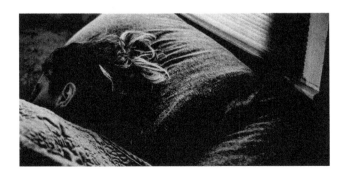

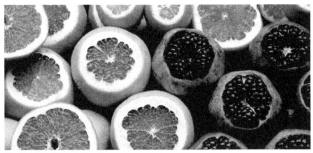

Tyrosine

This amino acid is a stimulating antidepressant, useful for fatigue and mental exhaustion. It improves concentration and mental clarity, making it appropriate for Alzheimer's, attention deficit, stress, adrenal fatigue and depression.

Tyrosine[164] can be supplemented in the range of 500-1,000mg daily. It's often used in combination with tryptophan. Tyrosine is taken in the morning to stimulate and energize, then tryptophan is taken in the evening to tranquilize.

Tryptophan

This amino acid is tranquilizing and calming, helpful for stress, anxiety and tension. It improves sleep quality and duration, making it easier to fall asleep as well as ensuring that sleep is deeply rejuvenating. Tryptophan increases your body's production of serotonin so it's good for all mood disorders. Supplement with a daily dose of 100-200mg.

Tryptophan[165] works in a similar way to SSRI antidepressants, so some people who are taking these types of antidepressants find the combination too potent and need to be careful when taking both. Starting with a very low dose of tryptophan will give you an indication of whether you're likely to have a negative reaction to the combination.

If you have any doubt at all, stop taking the tryptophan and talk to your health professional. Some people find that they can take both at the same time and see great improvement in their symptoms.

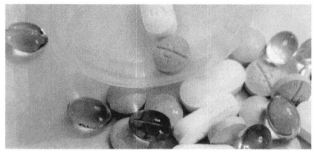

In certain cases, it's possible to use tryptophan to replace pharmaceutical antidepressants, but this should always be supervised by a health professional.

Omega-3 Fatty Acids

Sometimes called vitamin F, the Omega-3 essential fatty acids are found in every cell in your body, in the cell membrane, also called the wall of the cell. The cell wall plays some very important roles in your mental health. It's the interface for messages between different parts of your body.

So when it's working well, your cells can receive instructions from your brain and nerves. And when it's not working well, these instructions can get confused. If this happens, your cells begin to make the wrong hormones and chemicals. This can affect your mood, your energy levels, and your mental acuity.

Omega-3 fatty acid deficiency[166] is associated with mood disorders, attention disorders, personality disorders and mental fatigue. It's often deficient because people don't get enough of it in their diets. Unless you live near the ocean and eat a lot of oily fish, it's unlikely that you get enough Omega-3 from your food.

While most people take fish oils to supplement their Omega-3 levels, there are also vegan options available that extract the Omega-3 oil from algae.

The advantage of this is that it can be grown on land, where it doesn't affect fish stocks. Fish also carries the risk of contamination from ocean pollutants such as plastics, heavy metals and even radioactivity.

Algae-extracted Omega-3 oils don't carry this same risk because they're grown in a controlled environment.

The oil from algae is just as effective as the oil from fish. Daily supplementation of Omega-3 oils needs to be in the range of 3,000-5,000mg to positively impact mental health.

6.4 Common Symptoms of Mental Illness

6.4.1 General Fatigue

When your body is struggling to make enough energy, you become generally fatigued. This often feels like a heavy, aching sensation in your muscles. It can also show up as lethargy or a lack of motivation.

Physical feelings of fatigue are often closely linked to mental exhaustion because your brain and your muscles use the same method of energy production. When this system is under-functioning, it affects all parts of your body.

Sometimes fatigue follows a pattern of energy surges and slumps throughout the day. A classic sign of stress and adrenal exhaustion[167] is the need to fall asleep early in the evening, unable to stay awake. This is followed by waking in the small hours of the morning, usually between 2am – 4am.

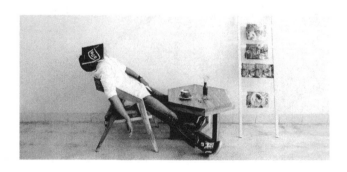

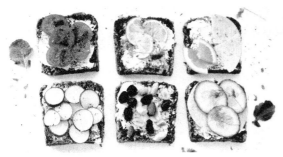

You lie awake for an hour or more, sometimes not getting back to sleep at all. Then when it's time to get up you feel tired and have trouble waking up properly. If you have this pattern of fatigue, then treating your adrenal glands is essential.

Another common sequence of fatigue is caused by extreme blood sugar levels. If you find yourself craving sugar, and your energy levels swing wildly through the day, it's likely your blood sugar levels are not well controlled.

Often there's a slump after lunch, around 2pm, when you suddenly feel like you could fall asleep. Cravings for sugar and caffeine kick in around this time. Blood sugar levels can affect mood as well as energy, as the two are closely linked.

If you have this pattern of fatigue, you need to focus on eating low GI (glycemic index) foods. Also try eating small meals more often, five or six throughout the day, rather than one or two large meals. This will even out the supply of sugar and energy to your body.

6.4.2 Poor Memory and Lack of Focus

There's a broad range of cognitive symptoms that go along with mental health conditions[168]. It can be a subtle lack of focus and poor short-term memory. Or it can be expressed as confusion, attention deficit, slow learning, poor concentration and hyperactivity.

These symptoms relate to energy production and hormonal and chemical balances in your brain. Energy production is key to brain function because the brain is one of the most demanding organs in the body for energy.

It's also one of the organs that is first to be ignored when there's not enough to go around. This is because the process of digesting food is more essential for your survival than whether or not you can learn to use a new computer program.

Energy is also required for making the hormones and chemicals that control your brain function. These can be thought of as the master hormones, because they dictate the behavior of other systems in your body.

They give instructions to your digestive system, your immune system and your reproductive system, influencing your mood and health hugely.

So you really need to be generating a lot of energy to maintain mental health. When your body is functioning optimally, it makes plenty of energy to feed your brain as well as your muscles and digestive organs.

Your thinking is clearer and you can focus more sharply on the tasks you apply yourself to. Your memory improves, with a longer attention span and better learning ability.

6.4.3 A Heightened Stress Response

One of the earliest signs of mental illness can be an increased sensitivity to stressful situations. Ongoing stress[169] can also lead to mental illness because it depletes your body of vital nutrients

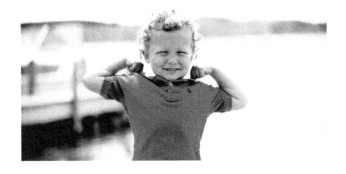

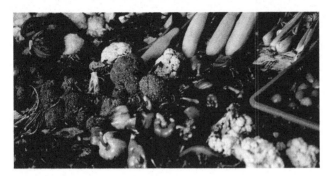

as well as creating a pattern of behavior that normalizes stress and anxiety states.

It takes a certain amount of strength and resilience to respond to stress well. In addition to manufacturing stress hormones, your body also has to break them down and remove them from your bloodstream.

Your body also has to counter the effects these hormones have because they're inflammatory and can damage body organs and systems.

All these chemical processes require nutrients. So, you become depleted if you're constantly facing stressful circumstances as these nutrients get used up in the cycle of making and breaking down stress hormones.

The cycle can perpetuate itself as you become gradually weaker and more depleted, which makes you more vulnerable to stress. The more you overreact, the more depleted you become, and so on.

Stress hormones also shut down your digestive system because they're intended to strengthen your muscles and brain in case you need to run away or think yourself out of a dangerous situation. This compounds the problem with nutrient deficiency because you're no longer able to absorb nutrients optimally.

You can end this downward cycle and start making your way back towards good health by boosting your nutritional status. The nutrients we've been talking about that feed into energy production, relaxation, and sleep are essential

in this process. Once your nutrition improves, you're better able to respond appropriately to stress and you can reverse the cycle.

6.4.4 Irritability and Aggression

When you're deficient in key nutrients for energy and hormone production, your body struggles to maintain normal, healthy patterns of thought and behavior.

The effect can be profound in some people as their entire personality seems to change. Someone who has always been rational and gentle can become irritated and aggressive, and it can be difficult to see your loved one in this new version of themselves.

It's frustrating for the person suffering the personality change because they usually don't understand why they feel the way they do. And they still feel guilt and remorse if they hurt people. It can be heart breaking and even scary for friends and family to watch someone they care about set on a path of self-destruction.

Irritability and aggression[170] are often due to imbalances in hormones and neurotransmitters. While pharmacy medication is effective a lot of the time, there are cases where it simply doesn't give the desired outcome.[171]

And sometimes it leaves the patient with unwanted side effects, such as weight gain, impaired mental function and addiction.

Nutritional therapies can be very effective and they have the advantage of being non-addictive.

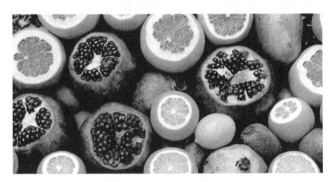

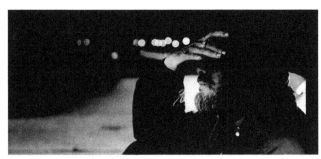

They can also be used in conjunction with pharmacy medicines.

6.5 Body Systems Involved in Mental Illness

It's easy to think that mental health is all about brain function. There are thousands of people who have been duped by psychiatry into thinking that their brain is simply broken.

Is it any surprise that Americans are some of the most medicated people in the world, with almost a quarter of the popular on some type of pain med or anti-depressant?

Could it have anything to do with the S.A.D. diet? At this point, you already know. The answer is a resounding YES!

Some call this the Americanization of mental illness.[172] The American Psychiatric Institute has come up with ever more interesting terms for mental illness, all while practically ignoring nutritional deficiencies, and failing to effectively treat depression for more than a decade now.[173]

However, there are intricate connections between your brain and different parts of your body, and therefore, this will become the "new frontier" of psychiatric science.[174]

Nutritional therapies must address the entire system to be effective. Brain chemistry is influenced by reproductive hormones, digestive activities, immune responses and stress responses to name just a few of the major players.

6.5.1 The Gut-Brain Connection

"Digestion is the seat of health," is a classic naturopathic adage that means if you have a healthy gut the rest of your body will follow. This is because proper nutrient absorption is absolutely essential for well-being.

When this foundational process is working well, it ensures that every cell in your body is nourished. This includes the structures in your brain such as nerve cells, hormones, chemicals and neurotransmitters.

Recent discoveries about the gut[175] have added another level of understanding to this concept as the importance of the gut bacteria has been revealed. Your gut and its resident bacterial population have a huge influence over brain function.

This control is exerted through chemical and nervous messages that are sent through your bloodstream and your nerves from your gut to your brain. This is known as the gut-brain connection, or the gut-brain axis.

A thorough treatment plan for improving mental health needs to include remedies for your gut because mental health and digestive health are elaborately connected. In addition to the nutrients already discussed, glutamine and probiotics are specific nutrients for gut health.

6.5.2 The Brain-Adrenal Connection

Your adrenal glands are responsible for manufacturing stress hormones, including

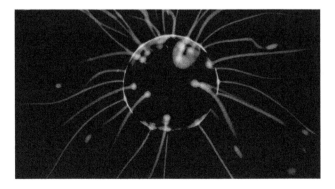

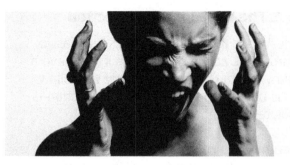

cortisol and epinephrine. They receive the message to make these hormones from your brain. These instructions are sent and received through hormone signals as well as nerve signals.

Stress hormones in turn are active in your brain and the loop is closed between your brain and your adrenals. This is known as the brain-adrenal connection, or the hypothalamic-pituitary-adrenal axis[176] (HPA axis).

Stress and anxiety states come about because of the interaction between the brain and the adrenals. You can try this out by thinking of something scary or stressful. You should feel an instant rush of epinephrine, which is released from your adrenals in response to instructions from your brain.

It usually gives you a noticeable sensation of tension in your gut and an alert, edgy feeling. This is your brain-adrenal axis in action.

Treatment for stress, anxiety and irritability needs to include nutrients that nourish and support your adrenals. In addition to the other nutrients already mentioned, vitamin C and the herb Rehmannia are specific for adrenal replenishment.

6.5.3 The Nervous System

Your nervous system includes your brain and your nerves. Your brain[177] is the obvious organ involved in mental health but nerves are also essential for good mood and energy balance. Your nerves come out of your brain, go down your spine, and spread out at various points to cover virtually every part of your body.

Nerves have the hugely important task of sending and receiving messages between your brain and all your other organs. So your hormone balance, mood, energy, digestion, immunity, all are affected by how well your nerves can transmit messages.

To keep your brain and nerves functioning at their optimum, vitamin E and calcium can be added to the list of nutrients you can take daily to protect your mental health. By nourishing these important organs, you give your brain the opportunity to function optimally. This can prevent and even reverse the conditions that can threaten your mental wellbeing.

6.6 Summary: Nutrients are Vital to a Happy Mental State

There are certain key nutrients that are commonly deficient in people with mental health issues. This has been shown in many studies, and nutritional therapy is a legitimate and effective way to get relief.

Conditions that can be helped by nutritional treatment include stress, depression, anxiety, obsessive-compulsive disorder, schizophrenia, bipolar disorder and Alzheimer's disease, to name just a few.

Serious and chronic mental health conditions should always include treatment from a qualified physician. And if you have any doubts at all about the effectiveness of your nutritional therapy, see a professional.

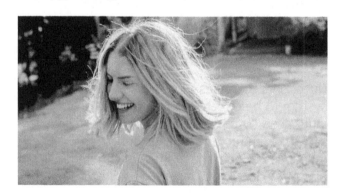

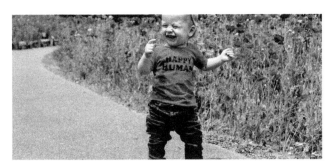

Make adjustments to your diet and use high-quality vegan supplements. This combination will give you the nutrient boost you need to start making the elements necessary for optimum mental health. This includes energy, hormones, neurotransmitters and other bioactive chemicals.

Treat your whole body, not just your brain. Include nutrients for your digestion, adrenal glands and nerves. This is especially relevant if you have symptoms in other parts of your body apart from your mental function.

Focus on the following nutrients for optimum mental health:

- Magnesium
- Zinc
- B vitamins
- Tyrosine
- Tryptophan
- Omega-3 essential fatty acids
- Glutamine
- Probiotics
- Vitamin C
- Rehmannia herb
- Vitamin E
- Calcium

7.0 Your Guide to Ultimate Gut Health

The father of medicine, Hippocrates, said, "All disease begins in the gut." The gut is also known as the second brain.

Just how smart is this second brain? Think about that immediate sinking feeling in the pit of your stomach the last time you opened your credit card bill following a holiday spending spree. You are stressed out, and your gut *immediately* knows it.[178]

Between your brain and gut there are millions of neural connections, like an information superhighway. This superhighway evolved over time to protect us. It was created as a signaling system to let us know if we ate something containing bad bacteria, but also to alert us to danger.

These neurons transit information about how we feel for a very good reason, but the food we eat can interfere with that signaling system, causing a host of diseases, including depression.

Ultimate gut health will lead to your ultimate health.

Let's learn more about why and how.

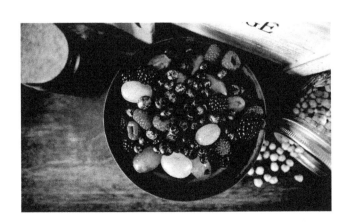

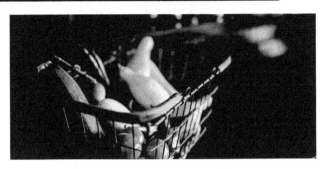

7.1 What Makes a Healthy Gut?

The digestion process is vitally important to health. Your intestines are wrapped in a rich supply of nerves and blood vessels[179] so that they can respond with great sensitivity to their environment.

This includes nerve signals from other parts of your body and your brain, as well as physical and chemical signals from the food you eat.

Your intestinal wall, also called the gut wall, is made up of a layer of cells that act as a barrier between your blood vessels and the contents of your gut. These cells make a liquid coating for themselves called mucus[180], which serves as an extra layer of protection against disease-causing bacteria, fungi, and viruses.

A whole ecosystem of microbes lives within this mucus layer, called the microbiota[181]. This collection of beneficial bacteria and fungi help with nutrient absorption and crowd out any species that might make you unwell.

Digestion is complicated. Your nerves, blood vessels, gut wall, mucus, and microbiota all work together to digest your food. There are thousands of messages being relayed every second[182] between the different parts of this intricate system. But when you look at the end

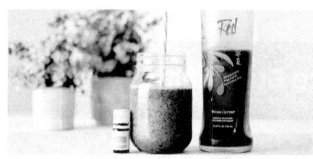

goals, the overview is actually quite simple: digestion serves to absorb nutrients and remove waste.

You need nutrients to feed your body – your muscles, nerves, internal organs, and brain all need constant nourishment to continue functioning well. And you need metabolic waste removed, because once your body has used the nutrients from your food, there are residues left over that can't be recycled. They need to be taken out of your body in feces.

A healthy gut works tirelessly[183] to absorb nutrients and remove waste, keeping your body nourished and energized. It usually goes unnoticed and it's only when you have digestive symptoms that you become aware of it. If it's not functioning optimally, you can experience gas, bloating, cramping, pain, diarrhea, constipation, and many other uncomfortable sensations.

Your gut becomes unhealthy because one or more parts of the system is not operating properly. It could be your nerves, blood vessels, gut wall, mucus, or microbiota that first lose their optimum function. Often, other structures will follow soon after if the dysfunction isn't corrected. This is because all the components that make up your gut need to act in symphony for good digestion.

A gut that's not working well can also create a range of symptoms in other parts of your body[184]. It's not always obvious that there's a connection between your gut and your other health concerns, but it often follows that when you heal your gut, your other issues improve greatly.

7.2 Why is Gut Health Important?

Gut health is a vital process to health because proper digestion of food is essential to survival. It's possible that you could be eating all the right foods but not absorbing their nutrients.

Certain minerals such as iron are known for their low absorption rate, and even if you're really healthy, you'll only get about 10% iron absorption[185] from your food. So you can imagine, if your gut isn't healthy, the amount of iron you absorb from your food could be really low. This could leave you iron deficient even if you're eating plenty of iron-rich foods.

The waste removal function of your digestion is also essential to health. Your body is constantly dumping unwanted substances into your gut. Once there, they're bound into a solid lump that becomes feces and gets expelled.

The dumping, binding, and removing processes can be disturbed in the same ways that nutrient absorption is. If this happens, toxic byproducts can build up in your body and upset your health.

The barrier function[186] of the microbiota, mucus and gut wall is also a key part of staying healthy. The barrier stops things from entering your bloodstream and therefore the rest of your body. It keeps out bacteria, fungi, and other particles that can cause inflammation and disease.

When this barrier function breaks down, it's called leaky gut[187], or increased intestinal

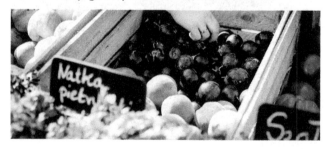

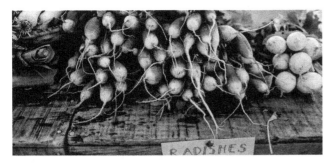

permeability. This condition is thought to cause an immune response in your body that leads to autoimmune diseases such as psoriasis, rheumatoid arthritis, multiple sclerosis, inflammatory bowel, and celiac.

Your gut is so intimately involved in your body's processes that it affects other systems apart from your digestion. It has a close connection to your brain and nerves, which is known as the gut-brain connection, or the gut-brain axis[188]. It also has a relationship with your adrenal glands and your immune system.[189]

The gut-brain axis refers to the way that your gut and your brain communicate with each other and influence each other. The connection goes both ways. Your brain tells your gut when and how to digest food, but it also gives it instructions to make hormones and immune cells.

Your gut tells your brain when it's time to feel hungry or satiated. It also generates inflammatory or anti-inflammatory chemicals, which affect your brain function.

Your gut is heavily involved in your immune system responses. Around 80% of all your immune cells are located in your gut, and your gut microbiota is at the center of much of this. Interestingly, gut microbes control immune responses in other parts of your body[190] as well as your intestines.

Your gut microbes give instructions to your immune cells[191] on how they should mature and what sorts of cells they should attack. If this messaging gets confused, your immune cells can miss disease causing bacteria and start to focus on destroying your body's own cells. This is the beginning of possible autoimmune illness.

Put simply, autoimmune illness is when your immune system receives the wrong instructions about what it should consider a threat. Instead of attacking only things that could cause disease, it attacks your body's own cells. This leads to inflammation and illness.

Depending on which body part your immune system acts against, you could have symptoms in virtually any system. It could be in your gut but could also show up in your skin, joints, muscles, nerves, brain and internal organs. If it affects your brain, it can show up as mood and personality disorders. Autoimmune conditions are often accompanied by fatigue and pain.

7.3 Symptoms and Conditions Associated with an Unhealthy Gut

As you can see, your gut influences many other body systems and functions. Usually people can tell if there's gut involvement in their illness, because they'll have digestive symptoms along with any other condition.

It does happen that digestive dysfunction can be quite subtle and not always considered a causative factor in disease. But a good health practitioner should pick it up during a thorough consultation if there's anything unusual happening.

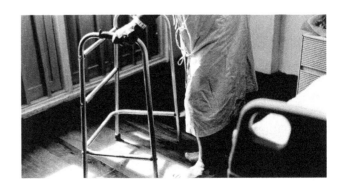

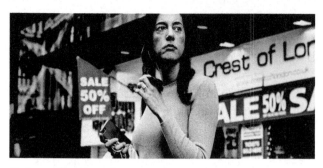

7.3.1 Signs of an unhealthy gut:

- **Gas** – Gas[192] is caused by ineffective digestion, especially of carbohydrates. Food makes its way from your stomach to your small intestine and then through to your large intestine.

  If a lot of undigested carbohydrate particles remain in your gut by the time it reaches your large intestine, the bacteria that live there will break it down and release gas in the process. Gas may be a sign that your stomach acid is under-producing, or that you have an imbalance in your small intestinal microbiota.

- **Bloating** – Bloating[193] can simply be a sign that you've overeaten. But if it happens after every meal, even when you've limited your meal size, it could be an indication that you have an infection or an imbalance in your gut microbiota. It can be caused by an immune response.

  If you can pinpoint a particular food that's causing the bloating, such as lactose or gluten, then it's highly likely your immune system is hyperactive. This goes back to your gut microbes and making sure you have the correct balance of bacteria in your gut to give your immune system the correct instructions.

- **Cramping and pain**[194] – Cramping is associated with your gut wall and involves your nerves. When your natural rhythm of gut wall contractions is disturbed, it can lead to irregular movements which cause cramping and pain. Inflammation in the gut wall also causes cramping and pain.

This is often an indication that your gut microbiota is out of balance, because of the important role it plays in keeping inflammation down.

- **Irregular Bowel Movements** (Irritable Bowel[195]) – Bowel movements are controlled by the nerves that wrap around the intestines. There's an electrical signal that passes form the brain down through the nerves and into the gut. It tells the intestinal muscles to contract, which forces gut contents further along the digestive passage.

  In irritable bowel syndrome, the signals become random, sometimes over-active and sometimes under-active. The gut wall loses its normal rhythm and the gut content pass too quickly or too slowly through the intestines. So by the time they're expelled, they're too soft or too hard, depending on the frequency of the signals.

- Diarrhea[196] – If the nerves around the gut are constantly over-active, the gut wall receives too many stimulating signals and the muscles contract too often. This pushes food through the digestive passage too quickly and it's still undigested by the time it passes out of your body.

  You're not absorbing all the available nutrients from your food if you suffer from ongoing diarrhea. Diarrhea can also be caused by an imbalance in your gut microbiota.

- Constipation[197] – If the nerves around the gut are constantly under-active, the gut wall doesn't receive enough stimulation

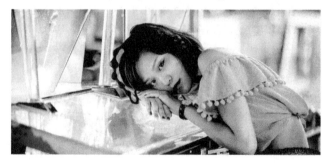

to get food moving through properly. Gut contents remain inside the intestines for too long and the waste removal function is ineffective.

This can lead to a build-up of metabolic waste in your blood and organs. You may have signs of toxicity such as body odor or skin rashes.

7.4 Nervous Symptoms and Conditions Associated with an Unhealthy Gut

- **Depression** – One of the main contributing hormones to maintaining a healthy mood is serotonin. 95% of your body's serotonin is produced in your gut[198], helped by your microbiota.

    If your microbiota is out of balance or weakened, then you won't be able to make enough serotonin to remain happy. Known as the "happy hormone", serotonin deficiency is thought to be the major cause of depression.

- **Stress and Anxiety**[199] – An unhealthy microbe balance can increase anxiety because of the way the gut microbes influence brain chemistry. They alter the balance of mood controlling hormones as well as affecting the brain cells directly.

    There's a tentative link between the barrier function of the gut and mental health. Some studies have shown that particles passing through a leaky gut can cause inflammation in your brain which leads to mood disorders.

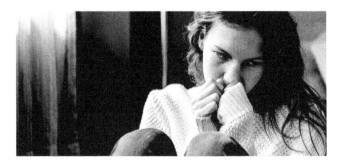

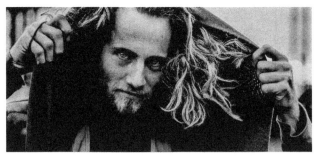

- **Parkinson's** – Parkinson's disease[200] is believed to be an autoimmune condition with increasing evidence pointing towards it starting in the gut. Inflammatory and immune responses can be seen in your gut before any symptoms appear in your nerves. Your microbiota and gut wall are vital for preventing this disease-causing process.

- **Alzheimer's** – Alzheimer's disease[201] is strongly associated with a leaky gut. This is where the barrier function of your microbiota and gut wall breaks down and foreign particles can cross from your intestines into your bloodstream. From here, they cause inflammatory responses throughout your body and specifically in your brain. This eventually leads to Alzheimer's disease.

- **Multiple Sclerosis** – Multiple sclerosis[202] is an inflammatory disorder that aligns strongly with a disturbed gut-brain axis and a dysfunctional immune response. Constipation and underlying irritable bowel syndrome are common among multiple sclerosis patients. As with other gut-brain diseases, the microbiota is pivotal in understanding the cause of the disease.

7.5 Immune Symptoms and Conditions Associated with an Unhealthy Gut

- **Psoriasis** – Psoriasis is categorized as an autoimmune disorder[203], and in this case your skin becomes the target for your overactive immune and inflammatory responses.

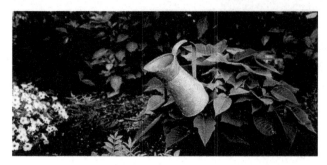

Chronic inflammation exists in the active layer of your skin, and your skin cells respond by reproducing faster and faster. This is what creates the scaly, flaky skin you have if you've got psoriasis.

- **Rheumatoid Arthritis** – Rheumatoid arthritis[204] and psoriatic arthritis follow a very similar disease pattern to psoriasis, except that the inflammation affects your joints instead of, or as well as, your skin.

  It's quite common to have symptoms in both skin and joints. Again, the microbiota and its influence on the immune system are at the root of these conditions.

- **Celiac Disease** – Celiac disease[205] occurs when the autoimmune response is directed towards the gut wall. It's specifically triggered by gluten, which is a protein found in wheat and other grains.

  The wall of the gut becomes inflamed and some of the cells die, resulting in a breakdown of the barrier function. Once the barrier function of the gut is inactive, inflammation spreads from the gut out to other systems in your body. People with celiac disease get symptoms in many different parts of their bodies, not just the gut but also joints, skin, muscles, nerves and brain.

7.6 How Can I Heal My Gut Naturally?

7.6.1 Choose Foods that Feed Your Good Gut Bacteria

The microbial balance in your gut plays a big part in digestion and your nutritional status, but its effect on health is much broader than that. More and more scientific studies are showing that it's intricately connected to virtually every body system[206], through its influence on the nerves, brain, hormones and immune cells.[207]

It makes sense to address your gut health even if your symptoms are showing up in a different part of your body. Sometimes it can be difficult to see the connection between your digestion and your health concerns, but improved digestion will always lead to better health, even if a nutritional boost is the only effect.

Food choices have a huge influence on digestive health because you're not just feeding yourself, you're also feeding your gut microbiota and different foods encourage different bacterial species to grow in your gut. Foods that feed good bacteria are known as prebiotics[208] and foods that contain live populations of good bacteria are called probiotics[209].

Prebiotics are found in the following foods:

- Garlic
- Onion
- Tomatoes
- Leeks
- Asparagus
- Radishes
- Carrots

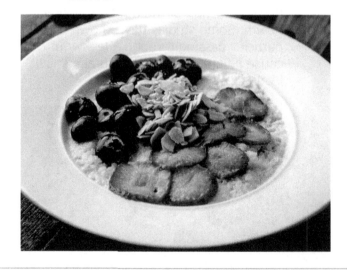

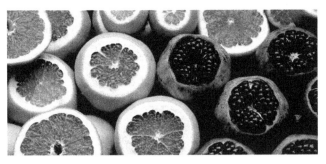

- Bananas
- Apples
- Oats
- Flaxseed (linseed)
- Chia seed

Probiotics are found in the following foods:

- Sauerkraut
- Yogurt
- Miso
- Pickles
- Kimchi
- Kombucha
- Apple cider vinegar
- Soft cheeses
- Green olives

Include at least 5 servings of these foods in your diet daily. Make an effort to switch it up and eat a variety so that you get different nutrients over time. This will lead to a good balance of many different bacterial strains in your gut. Diversity in your gut microbiota helps to keep your digestion strong and protects your gut population from getting out of balance.

7.6.2 Use Our Top 8 Supplements to Support Good Gut Health

The best supplements to support gut health work on your gut function as one of its basic levels. Prebiotics, probiotics, and digestive enzymes support your natural bacterial population to work optimally, while L-glutamine and quercetin help restore the integrity of your gut wall.

Aloe vera and licorice work on supplementing your body's protective mucus layer. And

omega-3 oils work directly on your nerves and the gut-brain connection, as well as directly reducing inflammation in your gut.

1. **Prebiotics** – You can get prebiotics in supplement form. You should always include dietary prebiotics alongside supplements because even the very best prebiotic supplement is no replacement for prebiotics from food. Supplements are made to boost a healthy diet, not replace it.

   Prebiotic supplements are available in powder or capsule form and the powder can be taken as part of a super food smoothie. Prebiotic supplements are often made from inulin, psyllium or flax seed.

2. **Probiotics** – Probiotics in supplement form contain more beneficial bacteria than any food source, so taking a probiotic supplement is a really good idea. Probiotics are usually delivered in powder or capsule form.

   A lot of research has been done on different bacterial strains over the last few years, which has given rise to more variation in commercially available probiotic strains. Some are sold for specific illnesses, for example, *Lactobacillus plantarum* is often used for irritable bowel[210].

   If you're not using a specific strain for a specific illness, look for probiotics that contain multiple strains of beneficial bacteria. Diversity in probiotics is more important than potency.

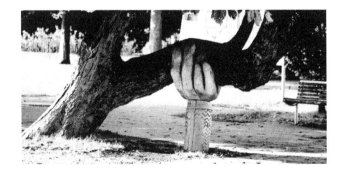

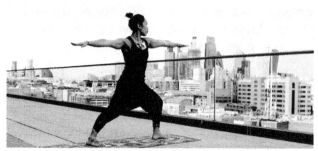

3. **Digestive Enzymes** – Digestive enzymes[211] boost your natural enzyme levels. Enzymes are active in your digestive system helping to break down food and are found in your saliva, stomach and small intestines.

   Sometimes you may be under-producing enzymes so your digestive process is not as effective as it could be. This contributes to digestive symptoms such as bloating and gas. It also disturbs the balance of your microbiota, which can lead on to other illnesses.

   Digestive enzymes can stimulate long term healing of your gut because the increased enzyme activity encourages other parts of your digestion to become more active. You need to take them daily for at least 3 months for them to have an impact on your long term gut health. They usually come in capsule or tablet form.

4. **L-glutamine** – L-glutamine is used by your body to maintain the integrity of your gut wall[212]. It helps to form strong bonds between gut cells, keeping the barrier function intact and ensuring that your gut doesn't become leaky.

   By preventing leaky gut, L-glutamine stops and even reverses inflammation in your body. This also prevents your immune system from overreacting to everything and can go a long way to healing autoimmune conditions at a fundamental level.

5. **Quercetin** – Quercetin acts as an anti-inflammatory[213] at the level of your gut wall. One of the chemicals your body uses when it's creating inflammation is histamine.

Quercetin prevents histamine from being released in your gut by calming the cells that make it. It also contributes to the strength of your gut wall by helping gut cells attach to each other.

Quercetin encourages your body's natural antioxidants to function better and stay longer in your system. It also reduces the potency of some of the immune cells that are overactive in autoimmunity.

6. **Aloe Vera Juice** – Aloe vera is a cooling, soothing herb that acts on your digestive system in a few different ways. It contains its own type of prebiotic that feeds your beneficial bacteria population. It also encourages your regular healthy gut cells to reproduce at a faster rate.

   Aloe vera is really useful if you have a digestive illness that is causing lesions[214], such as ulcers, diverticulitis, inflammatory bowel or colitis.

   Aloe vera also contains a mucilage that can mimic your body's own mucus, adhering to the gut wall and coating the cells with a layer of gelatinous gum. It's very soothing and calming if your gut is suffering inflammation[215] due to under producing this important protective substance.

7. **Licorice Extract** – A deglycyrrhized licorice extract is a powdered form of licorice root that's had the glycyrrhizin removed. While glycyrrhizin isn't really dangerous, it can raise blood pressure if used for a long time, so it's taken out of the powder in order to make licorice safe for everyone.

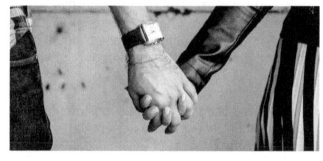

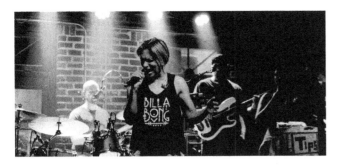

With or without glycyrrhizin, licorice can contribute to your body's own mucus layer and gut wall. It works in a similar way to aloe vera, creating a physical barrier of a soft, mucus-like substance over the lining of the digestive tract. This protects against ulceration and other inflammatory gut conditions[216].

Licorice is soothing and anti-inflammatory in your gut and it's often used as a lightly pressed tablet before meals, where it can help to reduce symptoms of reflux and indigestion.

8. **Omega-3 Fatty Acids** (oils) – Omega-3 oils have traditionally been extracted from fish. But there are now many vegan options for omega-3 supplementation[217]. Fish acquire their omega-3 oil from algae and it's possible to extract it directly from algae, without needing to harvest fish.

   This is good news for depleted fish stocks the world over. And it also eliminates the risk of contamination from polluted oceans because the algae is grown on land in special tanks, away from the ocean environment.

   Omega-3 fatty acids are active on many of the structures involved in your digestion. They act directly on the cells that make up your gut wall, strengthening them and helping them to attach to each other properly. Omega-3s are also active in your nerves and your brain[218], improving the ability of your nerve cells to send and receive messages between your gut and your brain.

These important oils can also influence the functioning of your immune system by reducing inflammation[219], thus preventing overactive immune responses. Omega-3 oils are often used for mood disorders and painful and inflammatory conditions. They can help digestion, skin, joints, immunity, nerve, and brain health.

7.7 Live a Lifestyle that Supports Good Gut Health

It can be difficult to keep up with your commitments to your health when you're crazy busy. Even when you know that home cooked meals and whole foods containing prebiotics and probiotics are better for you, you don't always have the time to spend on preparing these nutritious treats.

If you find yourself eating on the run a lot, it could be affecting your health. You can still choose the healthy option when eating out, but it's likely you'll miss at least some of the foods you're trying to eat. Unless you pick a place that specializes in health-giving foods, there's not much chance you're going to be offered a side serving of sauerkraut with your lunch.

Eating while rushed or stressed is also detrimental to good digestion because you tend to chew and swallow much more quickly. Chewing your food is the first part of digesting it[220], where it gets thoroughly crushed by your teeth and then dissolved slightly by your saliva. If you miss these steps, your stomach and intestines have to work hard to make up for it.

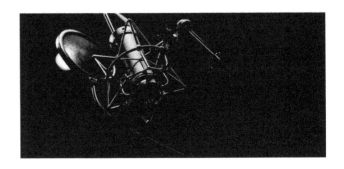

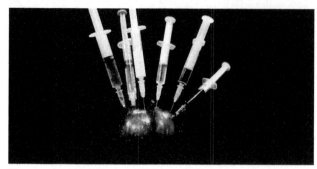

Even more importantly, your body is programmed to shut down digestion during times of stress[221]. The blood vessels that wrap around your intestines, that are so important for good digestion, will have reduced blood flow when you're stressed. That means less oxygen and less nutrients reaching your gut, so it can't function optimally.

If you were faced with a real emergency it would be useful to have the blood diverted away from your digestion and into your muscles and your brain. This is so that you could run away from the threat or think yourself out of the situation. But when you have a lifestyle that stresses you every day without a break, the long term consequence is often digestive illness.

Avoiding stress is the best lifestyle choice you can make for yourself. Stress has been implicated in virtually every illness that can be diagnosed[222], and the evidence is getting stronger with each new study that's done on the topic.

Stress is not just mental and emotional, but can also be physical. Some things that cause physical stress include UV radiation, exposure to toxic chemicals, hidden additives and residues in food, and bad air quality.

Take a moment to analyze your lifestyle and think about what's really important to you. Are you spending time and energy on things you could let go of? Would you really like to do some things for yourself that would help to relieve your stress levels but you don't currently have time?

7.7.1 Here are some quick pointers for living a stress-free lifestyle:

- **Make Time for Relaxation** – Choose a type of relaxation that works for you, something you feel comfortable with. It could be a formal practice such as yoga or meditation, or it could be a pampering day at the spa, or taking time out to catch a movie.

- **Make Time to Eat** – Being relaxed and eating slowly are important for good digestion. Try to sit down while eating and remove distractions as much as possible.

- **Prioritize** – If something really isn't important, don't give it your precious time and energy.

- **Surround Yourself with Positive People** – as much as possible, spend time with people who lift you up and give you a better outlook on life. Try to avoid people who influence you negatively.

- **Exercise** – At least 3 times weekly, getting your heart rate up. This creates an endorphin release that will leave you smiling. It also increases circulation, oxygenating your body and helping with waste removal.

- **Practice Positivity** – There are many ways to brighten your mind, and it's amazing what a difference it can make when you adjust your mental attitude. Try listening to positive affirmations for 10 minutes daily, or learn some cognitive behavioral techniques.

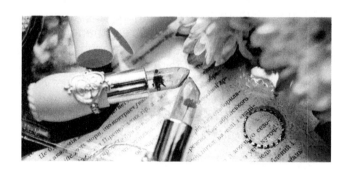

8.0 Vegan Supplementation

"Everyone has to find what is right for them, and it is different for everyone. Eating for me is how you proclaim your beliefs three times a day. That is why all religions have rules about eating. Three times a day, I remind myself that I value life and do not want to cause pain to or kill other living beings. That is why I eat the way I do." – Natalie Portman

Your reason for going vegan may simply be to experience better health. If you're going to eat well, you need to supplement well too. Here's how.

8.1 Best Vegan Whole Food Supplements for Quality, Purity and Effectiveness

8.1.1 How do I know if I need supplements?

It's extremely difficult to maintain the perfect diet and lifestyle. Perhaps you know what you're supposed to be doing, eating only certified organic whole food and living a clean, stress-free life.

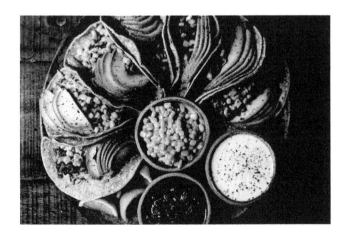

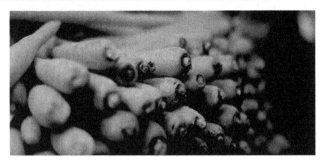

The practicalities of living mean that stress is unavoidable. And insisting on strictly pure food means you're the picky one that ends up hungry whenever you eat out.

Using whole food vegan supplements tops up your nutrient reserves and gives you peace of mind about your long-term health.

Even if you think of yourself as someone who eats well and has generally good health, there are many contributing factors that can lower your nutritional status.

8.1.2 Most Soil Used for Farming is Nutritionally Depleted

Much of your food is grown in soil that's been fed with chemical fertilizers. These fertilizers usually contain nitrogen, phosphorus and potassium. This combination makes crops grow fast, so they're ready for market sooner, but it doesn't add to the nutritional value of the food that's produced.

Unless minerals and trace elements[223] are added to the soil, they gradually diminish. Crops absorb these important nutrients but they're not replaced. So the nutritional value of the food diminishes with the soil[224].

8.1.3 Processing Food Removes or Destroys Nutrients

To create salable convenience food from freshly grown produce, there's usually a lot of processing[225] involved. Foods are cooked, frozen, ground, separated, chemically altered, and even irradiated. Each step in the process reduces the nutritional value of the food. So by the time you're eating it, the health boost you're hoping for could be unrealistic.

For food to contain maximum nutrients, it needs to be fresh and unprocessed. Growing your own produce, or buying from a farmers' market, is the best way to ensure good nutrition from your food. You also need to prepare it with minimal processing[226], eating it raw or lightly cooked to preserve nutrients.

8.1.4 Stress and Digestive Issues Can Stop You from Absorbing Nutrients

Your body is programmed to shut down digestive processes when you're stressed. This is so that all your energy can be directed towards your brain and your muscles, in case you need to think your way out of a dangerous situation, or run away. Continuous, low-level daily stress can leave your digestion weakened[227].

If you have ongoing stress or digestive illness, then it's almost certain you're not absorbing all the available nutrients from your food. Even if you're eating well, much of the goodness will be passing straight through your body, leaving you depleted.

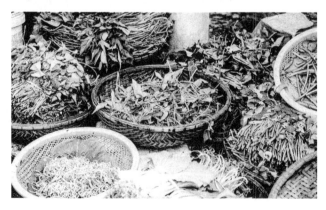

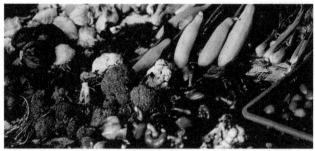

8.1.5 Everyday Chemicals Can Deplete Your Nutrient Stores

Caffeine, alcohol, and other everyday toxins need to be eliminated from your body. This uses up nutrients and energy. Some chemicals also interfere with nutrient absorption, including alcohol[228]. So the bigger your toxic burden is, the more depleted you will be of essential nutrients.

Avoiding the obvious chemicals such as alcohol and caffeine is a great start. But there are many hidden chemicals in your daily life[229] too - in cosmetics, household cleaners, work environments, and of course your food. Detoxifying your choices of personal and work products can contribute towards better nutritional status and improved well-being.

8.2 Signs and Symptoms of Nutrient Deficiency

8.2.1 How Do I Know if I Have Nutrient Depletion?

Nutrient depletion can be obvious at times. If you go to your doctor with fatigue, they'll likely take a blood test. And if you're iron deficient, it'll show up in the test. It's a simple deficiency with a simple solution – take iron supplements. But if you have chronic inflammation, you could get a low iron blood test result when actually your body stores of iron are okay[230].

And if you have fatigue but your blood test comes back normal, the next step isn't always clear. It could be that your blood has plenty of iron in it, but your vital organs don't. Or it could

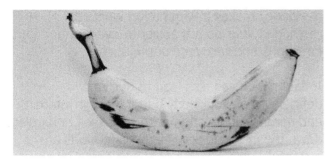

be that your iron levels are okay in both blood and tissues and it's a different nutrient that's low in your body. It could even be a combination of nutrients that's lacking.

8.2.2 Fatigue: A Common Symptom of Nutrient Depletion

Nutrient depletion often shows up as fatigue because making energy requires a complex range of different nutrients and enzymes. If even one of the essential elements is missing, the process will be much less efficient. Energy production in your body uses zinc, iron, magnesium, B complex vitamins, and vitamin C, to name just a few.

Often there are multiple deficiencies[231] because the things that cause depletion usually affect the whole body. For example, if you have weak digestion, you'll be missing out on absorption of a broad range of nutrients which will include all minerals.

Not all deficiencies will show up in a blood test because sometimes it's your tissues and organs that are lacking, rather than your blood.

Your body has systems that move nutrients from your digestion to your blood to your organs, keeping your blood levels balanced and your organs nourished.

These systems don't always work effectively, especially if you're unwell. So blood tests don't always give you accurate information about your nutritional status.

8.2.3 Anxiety and Mood Disorders are Strongly Associated with Nutrient Imbalance

Stress, anxiety, and depression can contribute to nutrient deficiency. But they can also be caused by nutrient deficiency[232]. It can easily become a perpetuating cycle.

Your low mood triggers your digestion to shut down and you stop absorbing nutrients so well. You become nutritionally depleted then your low nutritional status worsens your mood issues.

Receiving easily absorbed nutrients at this point is vitally important for reversing the pattern. Once the tipping point has been passed, you should start on an upward cycle of improved mood, better digestion, and boosted nutritional status. If you have a mood disorder of any description, it's highly likely that you're deficient in one or more essential nutrients.

8.2.4 Nutrient Depletion Contributes to Sleeplessness

Your body uses hormones and chemicals to control when you're asleep and when you're awake. For this to work well, the right hormones need to be made in the right quantities and they need to be released at the right times.

It's a complex system that only functions properly when all the necessary nutrients[233] are readily available.

The master hormone for sleep is melatonin[234]. It's released from the brain in the evening to signal your body to fall asleep. If your body can't

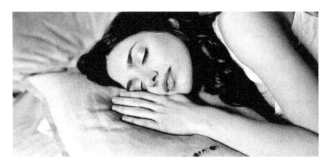

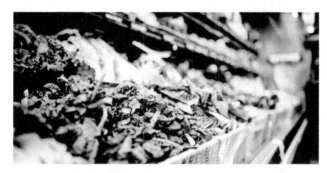

make enough melatonin, you simply won't be able to get to sleep.

When you do sleep, it'll be light and unrefreshing. Some of the nutrients involved in getting good sleep include magnesium, calcium, B vitamins, and zinc. If you have trouble getting to sleep or staying asleep, it's likely you have at least one nutrient deficiency.

8.2.5 Your Skin Will Often Show Nutrient Deficiencies

Your skin is a highly visible organ and it's one of the first to be neglected if your body is short on nutrients. This is because your body needs to prioritize its use of vitamins and minerals, and vital functions such as breathing and pumping blood are more essential for survival than having perfect skin.

Nutrient depletion contributes to acne, eczema, psoriasis, and sensitive skin. Zinc, essential fatty acids, vitamins C, D, A, and E are all important for skin health[235].

Your body uses these to make healthy skin cells that are able to resist infection and can hold the correct amount of oil and moisture to keep skin soft and supple.

Nutrient deficiency can make inflammation worse

Inflammation has been called the root of all disease because it's associated with almost every illness you can get. It's a fundamental driver of heart disease, cancer, chronic digestive diseases[236], and immune conditions. Nutrient

deficiency makes inflammation worse by restricting your body's ability to overcome infections and recover from injuries.

Inflammation can also lead to nutrient deficiencies as your body burns through vitamins and minerals in its attempt to heal itself and quiet down the inflammation. Many plant foods are powerfully anti-inflammatory because of their ability to prevent the inflammatory response.

They do this by interfering with the processes that result in inflammation. They also influence the environment that chemical reactions are occurring in, inside your body. This is where the concept of alkalizing foods[237] comes from. Your body is much less prone towards inflammation when it's more alkaline.

8.2.6 Chronic Illnesses Can Result from Long-Term Nutrient Deficiency

Your body's organs need nutrients to work properly. The building of healthy cells and tissues requires vitamins and minerals. If your body is deficient for a long time[238], it will struggle to function normally and eventually it will show symptoms.

Sometimes living cells get replaced by scar tissue when cells are too badly damaged or dysfunctional. This is what happens in liver cirrhosis, heart disease, and arterial disease. By the time you have scar tissue instead of healthy cells, it's difficult to reverse the process. Taking action early is really important.

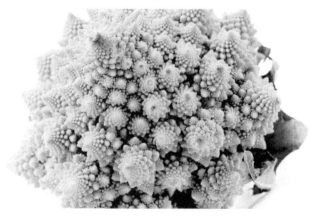

Certain nutrients act as antioxidants which protect your body from oxidative stress. Oxidative stress can be caused by infections, injuries, chemical exposure, the sun's rays, mental stress, and emotional tension.

Without anti-oxidants to cancel their actions, these stresses can turn into serious dysfunctions. The nervous, muscular, digestive and immune systems can all be compromised by oxidative stress, leaving you vulnerable to disease.

8.3 Why You Should Take Supplements Daily

8.3.1 Everyday Life Depletes Your Nutrient Stores

Modern life is filled with circumstances that threaten your nutritional wellbeing. Even though each occurrence is small when viewed alone, they all add up to impact your health. When you combine nutritionally deficient food with constant exposure to chemicals and stress, your lifestyle puts you at risk of becoming depleted[239] over time.[240]

8.3.2 Consistent Small Dosing Leads to More Effective Replenishment

Your body needs to process nutrients in small doses. If you try to correct a deficiency in one hit, most of the nutrient will be expelled because your body can't digest large doses. Anyone that's had side effects from taking supplements probably got them because the dose was too big and their system was overwhelmed.

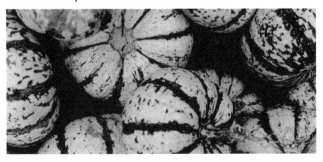

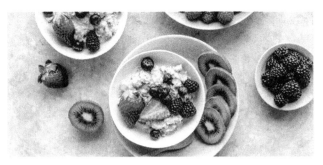

Supplements used for detoxification are often started at a low dose and increased over a few days. This is to minimize the side effects that can come from detoxifying too quickly.

Your body needs time to process things, especially if you're unwell or severely depleted. As you gradually get healthier and rebuild your nutrient stores, your body will be able to process more.

8.4 Do's and Don'ts When Choosing Supplements

8.4.1 Organic Vegan Whole Food Supplements are the Best

The ultimate supplements are made from vegan whole foods. This means they are whole plant extracts, with the entire edible plant part processed. Processing can be as simple as drying and powdering.

Maca powder is an example of a supplement that's processed in this way. Such a minimal amount of processing ensures that you get the benefit of the whole extract.

8.4.2 Whole Food Extracts Contain Many Nutrients that Work Together

A whole food extract contains every compound found in the plant. Plant chemistry is complex and most plants used for medicine contain hundreds of different chemicals in their leaves, roots, stems and flowers.

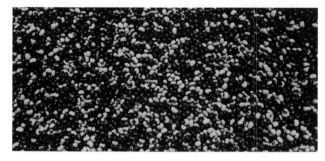

Using it as nature has provided it allows synergy to take effect. Synergy[241] is the combined action of all the chemicals found in the plant. They all work together to provide nutrition, reduce your symptoms, and minimize side effects.

When manufacturers take out one chemical and use only that in their supplements, they lose the synergistic effect. The single chemical that has shown itself to have the desired effect is called the active constituent.

Often the active constituent produces the outcome hoped for regarding the specific symptom or disease being treated. But just as often it creates side effects. And it doesn't work as effectively as the whole food extract.

8.4.3 Organic Supplements Provide the Purest Nutrition

Certified organic supplements are superior quality because their purity level is higher than conventionally farmed foods. Certified organic foods don't contain highly toxic residues because they haven't been sprayed with chemical pesticides and herbicides.

Organic farming standards stop farmers from using a vast range of chemical sprays. Instead, they use crop management practices. And when they do use sprays, they choose products with a very low toxicity rating.

Organic farms use organic fertilizers that contain more trace elements and a broader range of nutrients than the chemical fertilizers used by regular farmers. The food that's grown in this soil naturally contains a better nutritional diversity[242].

This transfers on to the supplements made from this food, which are more biologically active in your body. This nutritional density and diversity gives you better results.

8.4.4 Supplements Without Fillers are Better Quality

Fillers are used in supplements to bulk out the product. This is necessary if the active ingredients are required in very small doses. Trace minerals and some vitamins have an active dose measured in micrograms, which is so tiny that it would be lost in a capsule.

Sometimes the filler is used to make it easier for the manufacturer to measure out the correct dose. This is known as a bulking agent. There are other additives used in the making of supplement products, for reasons like stopping the product from sticking to manufacturing equipment (flow agent) and holding tablets together (binding agent).

A supplement made from whole food shouldn't need fillers because the active constituent is only one small part of the product. It's present in perfectly balanced, naturally occurring levels.

The remainder of the bulk is made up of supporting nutrients and inactive plant parts like fiber. This natural balance is what makes whole food supplements superior because they can act synergistically in your body.

Some manufacturers use fillers unnecessarily[243], as a way of reducing their costs and increasing their profits. Fillers are a cheap substitute for health-giving nutrients. The highest quality

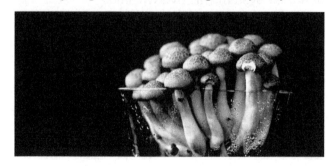

supplements only contain whole foods and active ingredients.

Not only do fillers take away from the healing potential of a supplement, some of them can also have a negative impact on your health.

Although you should try altogether to avoid supplements that contain fillers, some are considered worse than others and it's worth noting which ones are most likely to cause side effects. Many fillers are controversial, with the science still unproven and people on both sides of the argument holding strong opinions.

Here's a list of common fillers to watch out for:

1. **Carrageenan** – Carrageenan[244] is extracted from seaweed and used as a thickening agent. It's often used a vegan alternative to gelatin. It's been suspected of causing digestive inflammation, exacerbating digestive allergies and contributing to serious digestive issues.

   It's also believed by some to encourage the formation of cancerous tumors. Because it's sourced from the sea, it has the potential to be contaminated by ocean pollution, including radioactive material, such as that leached by the Fukushima disaster.

2. **Magnesium Stearate** – Magnesium stearate[245] is a flow agent and binder. It keeps materials from sticking to manufacturing equipment and helps to hold ingredients together.

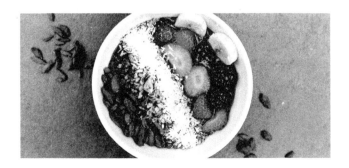

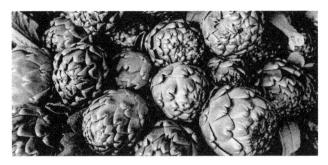

The debate is ongoing about whether this filler is safe. Some believe that it reduces nutrient absorption and irritates the digestive system. When it's sourced from genetically modified or hydrogenated oil, it may be toxic.

Some magnesium stearate is guaranteed to not be genetically modified and sourced from non-hydrogenated oil.

3. **Magnesium Silicate** – Magnesium silicate[246] is also known as talc, or talcum powder. This filler is used as bulking agent and flow agent. It's similar in composition to asbestos, which is a known carcinogen, and it's often mined from the same locations as asbestos.

   It's been found to be contaminated with asbestos and isn't a food grade product according to the FDA.

4. **Hydrogenated Oils** – Hydrogenated oils[247] are used as bulking agents for fat soluble ingredients. They've been chemically altered in a way that makes them toxic. They're also commonly derived from soybean oil, which makes it likely they're genetically modified, unless they come from certified organic soybeans. Genetically modified food has been linked to cancer and other serious illnesses.

When you supplement with plant-sourced vitamins and minerals you are feeding your body with a form of nutrition that is most bioavailable and most similar to its original form.

Taking capsules ensures that you have the correct dose every day, regardless of any

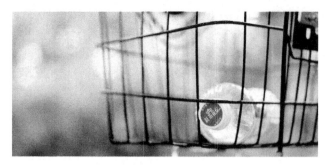

variations in your diet. By using only super clean supplements with no fillers, dairy, soy, or gluten, you're guaranteed purity and effectiveness.

8.5 Everyday Supplements for Optimum Living

Now that you know what to look for when choosing supplements, and what to avoid, here's a selection of premium products you can add to your daily routine for optimum health.

These are our personal choices for our own use. We don't make money from selling any of these products. We're sharing them with you because we genuinely believe they're the best on the market.

Using the following whole food supplements will optimize your digestion, leading to better nutrient absorption and improved nutritional status. This leads to stable blood sugar levels, a healthy weight, more energy, a clearer mind, and better focus.[248]

With each item we want to talk about benefits and also mention any contraindications. The Synergy powder at the bottom of the list contains two dozen different things. Almost all of the supplements are just literally food - not any processed stuff.

8.5.1 Korean Ginseng (*Panax ginseng*)

Korean ginseng[249] is a traditional Chinese remedy for fatigue, weakness, lethargy, and a compromised immune system. The name itself (Panax) comes from the Greek word "panacea",

meaning cure-all. The range of illnesses it has been used to treat is vast and fascinating. It strengthens your immune system and promotes longevity.[250]

Ginseng has a unique action in the body, unlike any other herb or pharmacy drug. It works on the whole body rather than any one particular organ or system. In traditional terms it's a tonic, meaning that it improves overall vitality and your body's ability to withstand stress.

Ginseng improves physical and mental performance - increasing stamina, resistance to stress, and focused thought. It's not recommended during pregnancy, lactation, or times of severe depletion, because it can be too stimulating.

8.5.2 Glutathione

Glutathione[251] is a powerful antioxidant that's used by many different organ systems and biological processes in your body. It helps to regulate your immune system, encouraging powerful immune responses when necessary but also ensuring that your immune system shuts off once it's done its duty. This helps to prevent the development of autoimmune diseases.[252]

One of glutathione's important antioxidant functions is in protecting red blood cells from degradation and early death. Red blood cells have the important purpose of carrying oxygen to cells, which all cells need to function optimally.

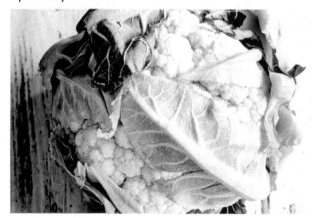

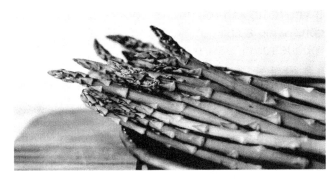

Red blood cells circulate in your bloodstream for around 4 months[253] when you're healthy. If you have anemia or an infection, your red blood cells can die as soon as 2 weeks after being manufactured. Glutathione can help to preserve their integrity, keeping them alive for longer.

Glutathione is a great aid to detoxification. It's active in your liver and helps to preserve vitamin C for reuse. It has been shown to help with the removal of many different toxins from your body, including DDT, chemicals in glues and resins, xenobiotics, and carcinogens.

Glutathione protects your body against damage from environmental stress, chemical stress, mental, and emotional stress. It benefits your skin and immune function and is an ideal supplement if you're concerned about aging. It's not recommended during pregnancy.

8.5.3 Choline

Choline[254] is usually classified as a vitamin. It's essential for healthy cell function, and it's very active in the nervous system. Choline is especially important for nerve signaling because it helps to maintain the protective coating on the nerve fibers (the myelin sheath).[255]

Nerve signaling is necessary for every basic function of your body, including muscle contraction and digestion.

Levels of fat and cholesterol in your blood are regulated by choline[256] as it works to break fat particles apart. Choline suspends fat and cholesterol in your blood as tiny separated particles, instead of large clumps.

These smaller particles are much less likely to attach to your artery walls or cause blockages in your blood vessels. This means a lowered risk of diseases that are associated with high cholesterol, such as atherosclerosis and coronary thrombosis.

Choline is a brain food that helps with mood balance. It's suitable for use during pregnancy and breastfeeding to ensure baby's brain and nervous system develop correctly. It's also useful for the aging brain as it can support memory and mental focus.

8.5.4 Turmeric (Curcuma longa)

Turmeric[257] has become something of a superstar recently. This powerful antioxidant spice is being recommended for virtually every health condition imaginable. And it deserves its reputation as a cure-all. In its native India, turmeric is regarded as a blood purifier and tonic.[258]

Traditional Indian medicine recommends turmeric for poor digestion and liver conditions. By improving the function of your digestion and liver, turmeric helps your body to extract all available nutrients from your food and keep your blood pure.

This leads to increased energy and better general health as your body receives everything it needs for optimal functioning.

Turmeric's ability to reduce inflammation has been celebrated in India for thousands of years and it's now been validated by rigorous scientific studies. It's especially useful for pain and chronic diseases but is also being used by athletes and everyday people to improve overall health.

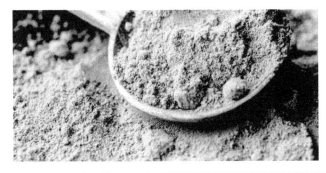

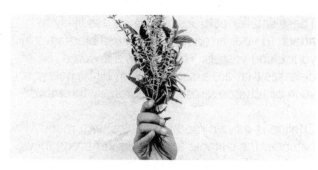

As an antioxidant, turmeric protects fats in your brain from damage. This means improved brain function and a lower risk of developing illnesses associated with oxidative stress, including Alzheimer's disease and multiple sclerosis.

Studies have also shown that turmeric is capable of protecting DNA from breakdown caused by free radicals.

8.5.5 Maca (Lepidium meyenii)

The root of the maca[259] herb is a traditional Peruvian remedy that has proven itself a worthy addition to modern natural medicine. It's usually sold as a dry powder that's easy to add to food or smoothies.

People that don't like the earthy, slightly bitter taste, can take it in capsules. Less commonly it can be processed into a liquid extract.

Maca is a nutritional tonic, containing the minerals iron, potassium, and manganese in good quantities. It has a lot of other unique plant nutrients, like glucosinolates and polyphenols.[260]

Glucosinolates are being studied for their ability to shrink cancerous tumors and have shown promising results.

The rich nutrients found in maca are a perfectly blended combination for increasing energy and stamina. Maca is especially useful for strengthening your libido, balancing your reproductive hormones and improving fertility. You need to take maca every day for at least 6 weeks to see a lift in your libido.

If you're hoping to improve your chances of conceiving a child, make maca part of your daily routine for at least 6 months.

Maca also has a reputation as a reliable aid to natural beauty routines. It improves the condition of the skin, restoring moisture and a youthful glow. This is likely to be due to its effect on hormone balance along with its nutritional qualities.

As a bonus, this useful herb also positively influences the menstrual experience by supporting estrogen levels and reducing symptoms such as hot flashes and insomnia.

8.5.6 Luna Natural Sleep Aid

This sleep aid contains a synergistic blend of herbs, minerals and amino acids to give your body everything it needs for a deep, relaxing sleep. It comes with 2 different variations on the formula, one with melatonin[261], and one without melatonin[262]. This is because some people are intolerant to melatonin supplementation.

Luna Natural Sleep Aid is non-addictive and non-drowsy, making it a safe option if you're concerned about the side effects of pharmacy sleep medicines.

Luna Sleep Aid is a carefully crafted blend of magnesium, L-theanine, valerian, chamomile, passion flower, lemon balm, hops, and the neurotransmitter GABA. GABA is a key part of keeping your nerves and mind quiet.

Most GABA is made inside your nerves and there's contention over whether it can be

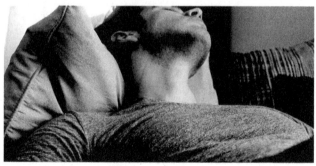

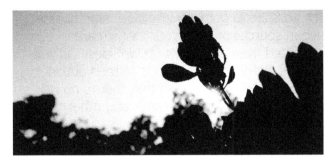

effective as an oral supplement because it needs to be inside your brain to have a relaxing effect. Studies suggest that when you take GABA orally[263], only a very small amount makes it to your brain.

However, it's certainly not going to do any harm at the safe dosage found in Luna Sleep Aid.

The mineral magnesium is well known for its relaxing properties in muscles and nerves and L-theanine is an amino acid that reduces stress. On its own, L-theanine is relaxing[264] without being sedating. But when used in combination with other herbs and nutrients, it's a useful part of a sleep aid formula.

It helps with hormone and neurotransmitter balance.

The herbal extracts in Luna Sleep Aid all have similar properties. They're sedating, calming, and soothing. Valerian and hops in particular are popular and well researched for their ability to induce sleep without causing addiction or drowsiness the next day.

While valerian[265] is extremely effective for most people, it's worth noting that around 10% of the population respond differently to it and are actually stimulated by this herb. If you think this could be you, try valerian alone to see whether it sedates or stimulates.

8.5.7 Nopal

Nopal cactus[266] is native to Mexico where it has a long history of use for reducing inflammation[267]. This makes it useful for almost every condition imaginable because most illnesses have inflammation as a major driving force. As such, it has a reputation as a cure-all. It's likely that nopal's anti-inflammatory action is largely due to its complex antioxidant components[268, 269].

Nopal also helps to balance blood sugar levels and manage cholesterol. So if you're working towards losing weight, it can be a great aid to reaching your goals sooner. And if you have diabetes or high cholesterol, it can become one part of your daily protocol.

Nopal cactus hasn't been tested for use during during pregnancy or breastfeeding so it's best avoided under these conditions.

8.5.8 ZMA

ZMA[270] contains a balanced and highly bioavailable blend of zinc and magnesium. The combination is useful for muscle building and recovery following sports and workouts. It also helps with testosterone production and sleep quality.[271]

The formula is designed for males, however female athletes and bodybuilders can also benefit from it. It's not recommended for use during pregnancy and breastfeeding.

8.5.9 Essential Fatty Acids (Omega-3 / DHA / EPA)

Omega-3 oils are essential for brain, heart, joint, and reproductive function, protecting against diseases in all of these body systems. They're commonly deficient because they're found in

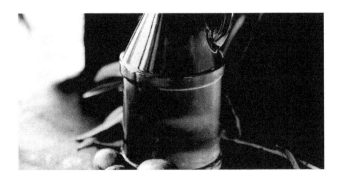

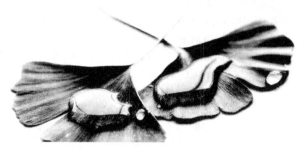

high concentrations only in oily fish and not many people have diets that include a lot of fish.[272]

People who live near the ocean and eat fish often are less likely to be deficient. Japanese and Alaskan populations are examples of people who have plenty of omega-3 oils in their diets.

It's possible to get omega-3 from vegetable sources but it's in a form called ALA. Your body has to convert ALA into DHA and EPA, which is a complex process involving a lot of supporting nutrients such as zinc, B vitamins and vitamin C.

If you're lacking in other nutrients, your body will struggle to convert enough ALA to DHA and EPA. This will leave you deficient in DHA and EPA even if you're eating plenty of vegetarian omega-3 foods.

The problem with fish oils is that they are often extracted from fish that's contaminated with ocean pollutants, including plastics, heavy metals and even radioactivity.

Fish oils are also very delicate and can easily be damaged by light, heat and oxygen. So, manufacturing, transport and storage are important factors in whether you have a quality product.

Good quality fish oils are extracted, transported, and stored without exposure to light, heat or oxygen. They are also sourced sustainably and tested for purity. Nordic Naturals[273] are known for producing high quality fish oil. They harvest only for oil, not as a byproduct of fillets. And they keep the product protected through the entire process.

It's possible to get very effective, high quality vegan sources of Omega-3[274] which are extracted from algae. It's grown specifically for its oil content and the crop is farmed outside the ocean environment so that there's no risk of contamination from plastics and other ocean pollutants.

8.5.10 Vitamin B Complex

B vitamins are often recommended and sold as individual remedies. Vitamin B6 is especially common as an aid to hormone balance and sleep. While it is useful for these conditions, there are others from the B vitamin group that are also effective and can be used along with B6. Vitamins B1, B2, and B3 are essential for good sleep[275], while B9 and B12 are indicated for menopause, PMS and other hormone imbalances[276],[277]

So the most effective way to take B vitamins is to use them all in combination. They all work together and they need to be in balance for optimum functioning. If you only take vitamin B6, you'll still be impacting your health positively because it helps with cellular division.

It's used by every body system and organ to keep making new cells. So skin, digestive and reproductive membranes, and the immune system all benefit from vitamin B6 supplementation.

But you won't experience the same broad range of benefits that you get from a B complex supplement. If you add vitamin B9 to your B6 supplementation, you also benefit from

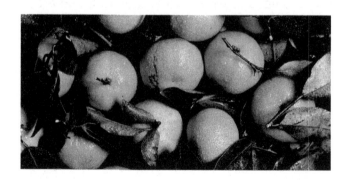

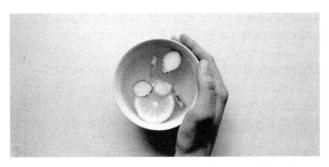

increased DNA synthesis. And if you add B12, you then benefit from better energy production.

So you can see how these work together – manufacturing cells, making DNA, and producing the energy to fuel these processes. These are basic biological functions and the B vitamins are essential for them to occur. B vitamins work on the foundations of your health.

Pure, vegan, raw B vitamins[278] provide the ideal balance of these essential nutrients for improved mood, sleep, energy, and mental focus. B vitamins are processed quickly in your body, making them non-toxic and safe to take at all times. Dosage should be reduced if pregnant or breastfeeding.

8.5.11 Ginger (Zingiber officinale)

The root of the ginger herb contains a unique complex of medicinal oils. With a spicy, sometimes sharp and intense burst of flavor, Gingerc[279] is an excellent herb to take daily as a warming, energizing tonic. It increases circulation to your extremities, so it's good for people who have cold hands and feet.

The increased blood flow also benefits congested colds, influenza and other respiratory issues including asthma, pleurisy and pneumonia.[280]

Painful, achy conditions[281] like arthritis, cramps and period pain can be helped by ginger's gentle heat. It's also anti-inflammatory so can act in more than one way to give you relief from symptoms as well as reversing some of the underlying damage.

Ginger improves digestion[282] and it's often used for seasickness and nausea during pregnancy. Other digestive problems such as colic, cramping, bloating, and flatulence can also be helped by decent doses of ginger. It's available as a liquid extract in glycerin or alcohol, and you can get it dried in powder form.

Although it's safe to take for morning sickness[283], the stimulating properties of ginger mean that some authorities are cautious with its use during pregnancy. For this reason, a maximum dose during pregnancy is set at 2 grams daily of dried ginger. If you have any doubts or concerns, speak to a health professional before use.

8.5.12 Probiotics

Probiotics[284] are one or more strain of beneficial bacteria that you take by the billion. They're so tiny that even 15 billion of them can fit into a small capsule. Beneficial bacteria are being studied more and more as scientists begin to realize how profoundly the bacteria in the gut can impact human health.[285]

Gut bacteria are heavily involved in maintaining your nutritional status, a fact that has been understood since the mid-20th century. More recent discoveries show that they also have intimate connections with your immune heath and your nervous system.

The full implications of this are still being unraveled, but what is becoming obvious is that your gut bacteria is a major player in your health.

Probiotics can replace beneficial bacteria that have

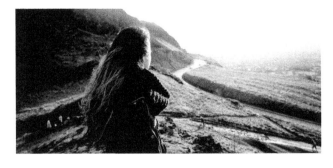

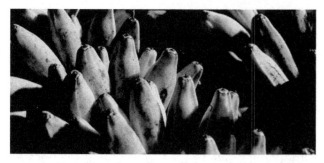

died off following infection or antibiotic use. This keeps your gut bacteria in balance and prevents disease causing bacteria from taking hold.

This means your gut health is better, you can absorb more nutrients, and your immune health will be stronger.

Certain nutrients such as vitamins B9 and B12 are manufactured in the gut[286] with the help of your gut bacteria. Having adequate beneficial bacteria lowers your risk of developing cancer and assists you in aging well.

Most diseases can be helped by probiotics because they have such a positive impact on digestion, and digestion is an absolutely fundamental process for staying healthy.

Probiotics are especially useful for digestive conditions, inflammation, and allergic illnesses. Any time your immune system is overworked or under-performing, probiotics can help. They also have a place in maintaining your mood, sleep, and energy, because of the connection between your gut and your brain.

If you're taking probiotics at the same time as antibiotics, be sure to take them at least 4 hours apart.

8.5.13 Digestive Enzymes

Digestive enzymes[287] help you to digest difficult foods and foods that could potentially cause allergy, such as dairy and gluten.

Sometimes your body simply doesn't produce enough enzymes to effectively digest your food.

This can be a genetic difference, as digestive enzyme balance is different for everyone.

But it can also be a nutrient deficiency that's causing inadequate enzyme production. If this is the case, then taking digestive enzymes will help your body to better absorb the nutrients it needs to make more enzymes.

This becomes a positive cycle of improved digestion and improved nutritional status, which leads to more energy and better health.

The boost you get from taking digestive enzymes also triggers your body's own healing and rebuilding processes so that your stomach and gut wall become stronger. They're an essential supplement for anyone suffering digestive issues, allergies, immune conditions, or diseases with an autoimmune cause.

Digestive enzymes are safe to take every day.

8.5.14 Multivitamins

A daily multivitamin[288] supplement is your ultimate insurance policy. They contain small amounts of all essential vitamins, and often they will have minerals, herbs and co-factors as part of their formula too. This broad approach to nutrition ensures that you will get a boost regardless of your specific health concerns.

Without having to conduct complicated or expensive tests to find out which nutrients you're lacking, you can cover all bases in one formula. Many multivitamins are manufactured from synthesized vitamins, often including hidden animal products, and all sorts of surprise ingredients.

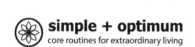

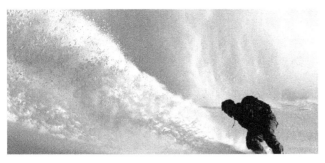

This is one supplement where you need to read ingredient labels carefully and talk to a professional if you're uncertain.

Working on your whole body, multivitamins are active on your digestion, immunity, brain, nerves, muscles, and skin. A good quality multivitamin can improve all parts of your wellbeing.

They're especially useful for improving mood, increasing energy, and helping to keep you feeling youthful and fit well into your older years. Gentle, whole food multi vitamins are safe to take during pregnancy and breastfeeding.

8.5.15 Super Smoothie Powder

A daily smoothie is a great way to really boost your nutrient and antioxidant levels without taking handfuls of capsules. A good super smoothie powder[289] should be made from natural extracts only and will usually be based on super foods, sometimes with medicinal herbs, proteins, and co-factors.

It will give you a huge hit of antioxidants in a great tasting formula.

Increased antioxidants help to keep you fit, healthy, youthful, and energetic. They protect skin, nerves, brain, and internal organs from conditions associated with stress and aging.

There's no better way to reduce your chances of becoming ill than to get a daily boost of all-natural, high potency antioxidants.

8.5.16 Vitamin C

Vitamin C[290] offers many different health benefits. Its principle function is in producing collagen, which is the main protein used for holding your body structures together. Collagen is found in your skin, joints, muscles, and around your internal organs. It's absolutely essential for health.[291]

Vitamin C is useful for building healthy skin, strong immunity and an appropriate stress response. It gets depleted easily and it's entirely non-toxic so replacing it daily is a great idea. It's safe to take at all times, and big doses are recommended when there's infection.

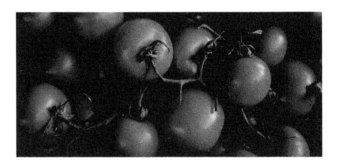

9.0 Principles of Detoxification

Every second 310 Kg (21 billion pounds annually) of toxic chemicals are released into or air, water, and soil by industrial facilities around the world.[292]

Your body has its own built-in methods of detoxification, but with the onslaught of chemicals we're exposed to today, it might need a little help.

9.1 Everything You Need to Know for Ultimate Cleansing

9.1.1 What is Detoxification?

Detoxification is a natural process that happens within your body all the time[293]. Your internal organs are in a continuous cycle of absorbing nutrients and utilizing them to make energy, then expelling the waste products that are left behind.

Your detoxification organs are also busy ridding your body of things that aren't nutrition and shouldn't be there to begin with. This includes alcohol, tobacco, and other drugs - pharmacy or recreational.

Chemicals can be picked up as environmental residue or contamination[294]. For example, if you work with paint, cleaning products, or building

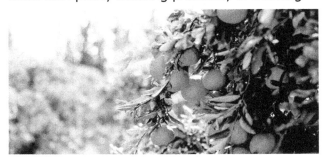

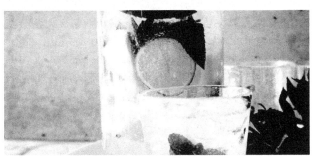

materials, you'll absorb a small amount of those substances from your workplace.

Your health is determined to a great extent by how well your body is able to remove its own metabolic waste products as well as the chemicals it comes into contact with. Your toxic burden describes how much waste is built up in your body because it hasn't been able to process all of it.

When your body can't remove waste and chemicals fast enough, it stores them in your body tissues.

Fat cells are especially prone to being used as storage for your body's toxins[295]. This is why you often get side effects and symptoms when you lose weight. The fat that's released from your fat cells carries toxins with it that go back into your blood circulation.

The balance between levels of toxin exposure and effectiveness of detoxification processes is what creates your toxic burden.

If you live a clean lifestyle and your health is basically good, your toxic burden is likely to be light. But if you eat unhealthy food, drink alcohol often, work with chemicals and have an underlying health condition, it's likely that your toxic burden is heavy enough to reduce your wellbeing.

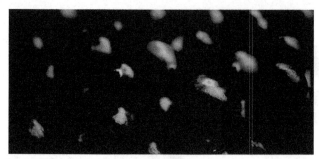

Your liver, bowel, kidneys, bladder, lungs, and skin are all involved in detoxification. The vast majority of chemical processing in your body is done by your liver. Your liver carries out more than 500 vital functions[296] and you certainly wouldn't be healthy if your liver isn't working well.

It takes nutrients from your food and alters them so that they're the right form for your body's cells to use. It takes poisons out of your blood and neutralizes them so that they can't harm your body. It then dumps them into your bowel for removal through feces.

Your kidneys are another major detoxifying organ.[297] They filter your blood as it passes through them, removing waste and turning it into urine. This is then removed through your bladder and urinary tract. Your lungs remove waste through your breath and your skin removes waste through the oils it makes.

Skin conditions quite often appear in people with a toxic overload.[298] This is because your liver and kidneys are overwhelmed and can't process any more. Your skin is a sort of backup detox organ, where damaging chemicals are stored or pushed through as a way of protecting the rest of your body.

9.1.2 Why Would I Need to Detox?

When your body can't keep up with the toxic burden it's under, you can change the balance by altering your diet and lifestyle. Although there are many different plans and protocols for detoxification, they all work on the same principle.

The principle is that when you feed your organs better quality nutrients, they're better able to perform their natural detoxification processes.[299] And when you reduce or remove the environmental toxins you're exposed to, your organs are able to work on stored toxins and have the opportunity to cleanse your body at a much deeper level.

Detoxification as a health protocol involves eating a very specific diet for a prescribed number of days. Often it also incorporates supplements and there may be lifestyle practices such as yoga or meditation, depending on which protocol you follow.

The increased nutrition and lowered stress triggers your body's detoxification organs to work harder and get more cleansing done.

A build-up of toxins can lead to a broad range of symptoms and conditions, depending on how your body responds to the toxic burden. In general, toxins are inflammatory[300] and damaging to your body's cells and organs. So if you have a condition associated with inflammation, you will most likely benefit from committing to a detox protocol.[301]

Inflammatory conditions and symptoms associated with toxicity and inflammation include the following:

- Parkinson's disease
- Multiple sclerosis
- Alzheimer's disease
- Mental illness
- Learning difficulties
- Regular headaches or migraines

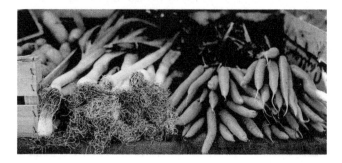

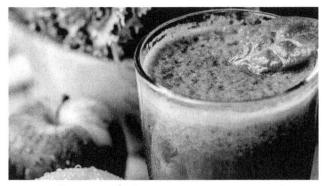

- Constant fatigue
- Infertility and other reproductive issues
- Heart and artery disease
- Acne, eczema, and psoriasis
- Asthma and allergies
- Cancer
- Obesity and diabetes
- Diverticulitis, gastritis, and constipation

If you have a family history of any of these diseases, or if you have increased risk factors, for example high blood pressure, you can make detoxification part of your regular self-care routine. It's important to maintain a generally healthy diet and lifestyle all the time.

If you eat terribly most of the year, and then try to detox once or twice yearly, you'll probably have a strong reaction when you detoxify. This is because inflammatory chemicals that have been stored away in your cells will be released into your bloodstream and flood your body in overwhelming quantities.

As your blood is pumped around your body, it carries these inflammatory chemicals with it, to your tissues and organs. As this impure blood passes by, it can damage parts of your body on its way, causing symptoms. These are called detox symptoms, detox side effects, or sometimes referred to as a healing crisis[302].

Usually these symptoms last for one or two days at the beginning of your detox program. People commonly feel nauseous and may have temporary changes in bowel motion, quite often diarrhea but constipation can happen too. You may experience headaches or a worsening of any symptoms you had before the detox, for example, eczema can flare up.

The experience of feeling worse instead of better during a detox is very common, but once the symptoms have passed, you'll likely feel better than ever. If you haven't done a detox before and you're worried about the side effects, you can choose to make your first detox quite gentle. This is especially useful if you know you tend to overindulge.

If your detox program is very strictly prescribed, you may need help adjusting it. You can talk to a health professional about it and they'll be able to advise you. Otherwise, you can take half doses of the recommended supplements, or half the duration of the detox program.

This will give you the opportunity to experience any side effects at a level where you're still comfortable. This is great for keeping you enthusiastic about your detox because it can really put you off if you feel absolutely rotten for the duration of your program.

By starting slow and gentle, you get to gauge as you go whether you need to repeat your next detox at the same level or whether you could make it more powerful. Your symptoms are a good indicator of how much you needed the detox. But unfortunately, the more you need it, the worse you'll feel.

If you eat well all year-round and then do a detox as well, your detox side effects are likely to be much less severe. Because you haven't had a heavy toxic burden to begin with, you haven't had a huge crisis when it comes to doing

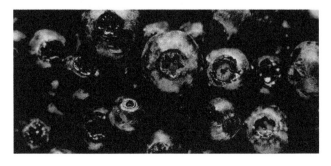

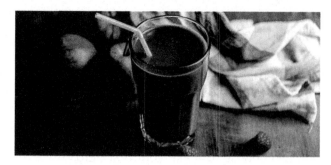

some deeper cleansing. So aiming to eat well and live right every day is essential.

9.1.3 How Can I Tell if I Need to Detox?

Detoxification programs are often recommended by health professionals as part of an overall treatment plan. But it's easy enough to decide for yourself that it's something you need and do it without professional guidance. Make sure you take the time to research it before you do it though, so that you know what to do and what to expect.

Many people choose to do their detox program when they're not at work and can take time out. This makes it much easier to cope with the side effects because you can lie down when you need to, go for a walk to get fresh air when you need to, and generally use it as "you time", where your only commitment is to your own health.

It also takes away the temptation to cheat because you can control what food is in your environment. When you're out and about, temptation's everywhere. All the stores, restaurants, and even your friends' houses will be filled with delicious sweets and treats.

You'll be going home to eat another meal of lightly steamed veggies. It's much easier to stick to your plan if you don't have this psychological barrier to overcome.

Even the healthiest person can benefit from a regular detox. It gives your body a chance to catch up on important background cleansing processes. The fact that you're always eating

dense foods is enough to keep your liver and kidneys quite busy. The liver works tirelessly in digestion, pulling food fragments apart to extract the nutrients from it and make them available to the rest of your body.

When you give your liver these nutrients in a partially digested state, or in a highly available form, it doesn't have to work so hard to provide your body nutrition. It can then occupy itself with other tasks that aren't usually a priority, but are essential for long-term health[303], such as the removal of hormones, cholesterol, bacteria, viruses, and other toxins.

If your liver didn't perform these functions, you could develop hormone imbalance, your cholesterol levels might spike, or you could become unwell with a chronic infection and toxic overload. So much of your health depends on the proper functioning of your liver.

To give your body the opportunity it needs to thrive, detox protocols should be followed at least twice yearly for at least 7 days each time. You'll see detox programs designed from between 3 days and 21 days. And you'll see recommendations for detox frequency from once yearly to once weekly.

The most important part of choosing how to incorporate detox into your life is to make sure that it fits with your lifestyle so that you can commit to doing it regularly. If one week's holiday from work twice yearly is what works for you, then do that.

If you like the idea of a juice fast every Sunday, then do that. Just be sure to commit and follow

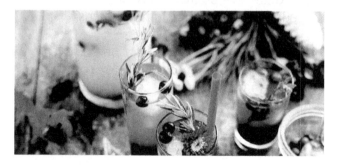

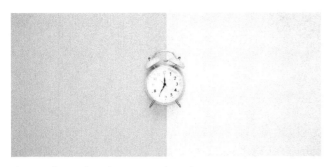

through with what you decide.

Of course, if you're unwell, you'll need more. You'll need to detoxify more often and it's essential you look at long-term changes to your diet and routine. If you're already healthy and you just want to maintain it, you'll need a less intensive program of detoxification.

The traditional time for detoxification is in the springtime. After a long winter of eating comfort food and cold weather crops, fresh spring greens are just what your body needs[304] to regain its vitality. Full of enzymes and chlorophyll, green foods stimulate your digestion and your detoxification processes.

9.1.4 When is the Best Time to Detox?

It's possible to get greens all year-round, and the idea of eating seasonally is now a choice rather than a necessity. But there is no substitute for freshly picked green vegetables that have been grown in natural sunlight.

The alternative is to transport these delicate foods from somewhere far enough away that they're genuinely grown in season. Or to eat greens that have been grown under artificial lighting. Even the most careful grower with a greenhouse full of technology will struggle to recreate real spring growth in their controlled environment.

Some people recommend that you should only stimulate detox processes when you're reasonably strong. This is because it can temporarily weaken your system when you're going through a healing crisis. The extra stress of your body's cells being exposed to toxins and inflammatory chemicals can be overwhelming for someone who's already depleted.

The idea in this situation is to build your body up before you undertake to detoxify it. This means eating lots of nourishing food and using wholefood, vegan supplements. How long you spend building up your strength is going to be different for everyone, but as a guide, at least 4 weeks, and it could be up to 3-6 months.

Detoxification is also better suited to some health concerns than others. It's not necessary or appropriate to use detoxification protocols for someone who has an eating disorder or is malnourished.

The only exception to this is when someone has lost their appetite or their digestive function because of heavy metal poisoning. In this circumstance, it can be very difficult to rebuild the body without addressing the underlying toxicity. You simply can't rebuild without digestion.

Pregnant and breastfeeding women should also avoid detox because the healing crisis can be a risk to the baby. Exposing a developing child to all your stored up toxins is a risk you don't want to take.

Having said that, detoxification can be an effective strategy for improving fertility, and a program of 6 months' duration has given many infertile couples the child they've been wanting.

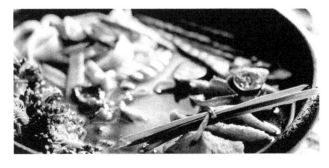

This needs to happen before conception.

9.2 Guidelines for Successful Detoxification

Detoxification programs focus mainly on your liver because it's the most important organ for removing waste products from your body. The special foods and supplements you eat while you're doing a detox are mostly aimed at improving the functioning of your liver and bowel.

Three distinct processes are involved in detoxification, and each needs to be addressed for optimum results:

9.2.1 Cellular Detoxification

The first part of detoxification is about releasing waste from your body cells into your bloodstream. This is absolutely necessary for your liver to be able to neutralize toxins because the only access your liver has to the rest of your body is through your bloodstream. Blood is flowing through your liver all the time and that's how detoxification begins.

If you've been living an unhealthy lifestyle, eating the wrong foods or living with stress for a long time, then your body will have toxins stored away. It does this because it can't keep up with processing all the chemicals, hormones and other waste that circulate in your blood.

Leaving you with bad quality blood would lead to inflammation and damage to your organs. Your body stores waste in cells as a way of protecting itself.

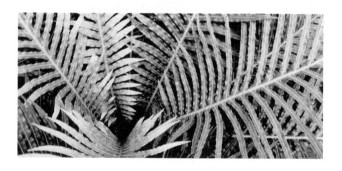

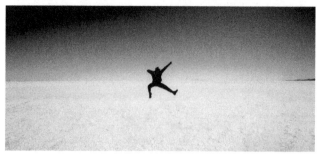

Your cells are incredibly sensitive and active. They respond to every hormone and chemical that flows past in your blood, and they're constantly exchanging oxygen, nutrients, and waste.

They are kept healthy by having access to abundant oxygen and nutrients. The idea of cellular detox is that you give your cells more oxygen and nutrients and then they're better able to expel waste products.

Chlorophyll is the only cellular detoxifying agent you need. It's what makes plants green and it's a powerful cleanser. You can take it as a powder, liquid, or tablets. Or you can get it directly from fresh food by eating leafy greens.

The green algae chlorella contains very high amounts of chlorophyll and it's also the main ingredient in many heavy metal detox formulas.

Chlorophyll works in many different ways at once[305]. It increases the oxygen carrying capacity of your blood, which gives your cells what they need to function optimally. It also protects the DNA inside your cells from oxidative damage, by reducing the activity of enzymes that break down DNA.[306]

And chlorophyll is a chelating agent. Chelation is an incredible natural process that is used specifically for heavy metal detoxification. If you have mercury, lead, or any other hazardous metal inside your body cells, you need to use chelation to remove them.

Chelating agents such as chlorophyll are able to physically attach to heavy metals and other

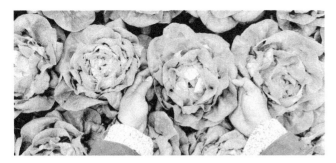

toxins, neutralizing them and carrying them out of your body. To really cement its place as the absolute best cellular detox agent, chlorophyll also helps your liver out with its chemical detoxification processes.

This encourages optimum cleansing not just at the level of your body cells, but also at the next stage of the detox process, which is liver detoxification.

9.2.2 Liver Detoxification

Your liver is like a big filter. All your blood passes through the liver, coming into contact with your liver cells. These cells remove toxins as the blood flows by[307], ensuring that blood leaving the liver is cleaner and safer than blood entering the liver.

Once the toxins are captured in the liver, it has to process them. This is the essence of liver detoxification. It's a series of complex chemical reactions that alter and neutralize toxins.

Because your liver is directly connected to your gut through the portal vein, all food particles pass through your liver before entering your blood circulation[308]. This is a vital level of protection between the outside environment and your bloodstream.

Blood that has been through your liver re-enters your general circulation and will eventually pass through your kidneys. At this point, it includes the metabolic waste that your liver has neutralized and prepared for removal.

Your kidneys are able to extract much of this and expel it harmlessly through your urine.

Unless you understand biochemistry quite well, the mechanics of liver detoxification won't mean much to you. What's more important to understand is that there are nutrients, foods, and herbs that encourage detox processes to happen much more effectively.

All antioxidants support good liver function. This is because your liver uses antioxidants as a major detoxifying agent[309]. Antioxidants can chemically alter toxins captured in your liver cells, so that they're no longer able to cause damage at a cellular level.

Antioxidants that support liver detox include:

- Saint Mary's thistle herb (*Silybum marianum*)
- Schisandra herb (*Schisandra chinensis*)
- Turmeric root (*Curcuma longa*)
- Dandelion root (*Taraxacum officinale*)
- Vitamin C
- Vitamin E
- Selenium
- Carotenoids

Foods and supplements that contain sulfur also encourage optimum detoxification[310]. Again, this is because your liver uses sulfur for its chemical detox processes. Your liver cells can actually attach sulfur onto a toxic molecule, changing the function of that chemical and preventing it from causing damage to your body as it continues to circulate in your blood.

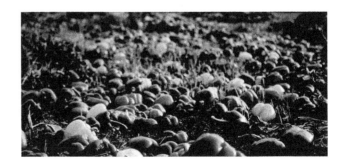

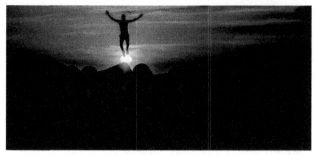

Sulfur can be found in:

- Cruciferous vegetables (broccoli, cauliflower, cabbage, kale, etc.)
- Garlic and onion
- Sulfur-containing amino acids – taurine, glutamine, glycine, cysteine, glutathione and methionine (often incorporated into liver-supporting supplements)

B vitamins are the final key to ensuring effective liver detoxification. They're essential for proper functioning of your liver, and they're often deficient because your body can't store them very well, but will use them up quickly when under stress.

Vitamin B6[311] and B9 are particularly important for liver detox, but it's always best to take B vitamins as a complex because they all work together. Take B vitamins in supplement form as a tablet, capsule or liquid.

Or increase your dietary intake of the following B vitamin-rich foods:

- Nuts
- Seeds
- Whole grains
- Leafy greens

9.2.3 Bowel Detoxification

The final stage of detoxification that you need to understand is bowel detox. Your intestines are your barrier between the outside world and the environment of your body. They're there to absorb nutrients and expel waste, but they're also there to protect you from bacteria, viruses and parasites that could be in your food or water.

If your intestines aren't working well, they can let foreign particles have access to your bloodstream and internal organs, and that's when you can become really unwell. It's a delicate balance, because your gut wall needs to allow nutrients to into your body. But it also has to stop everything else.

One of the things that can go wrong is that your bowels can move food through too slowly. You would notice this as constipation, which occurs when the bowel fills with too much fecal matter, causing pain and discomfort. The other thing that happens is your gut contents become too dry and hard, which adds to the feeling of unease.

What's happening at the cellular level is your body is absorbing more and more water from your gut contents. This is a normal process that's necessary for mineral and vitamin balance. But when it continues without bowel movement, toxic particles can be pulled into your bloodstream along with the essential vitamins and minerals you needed.

This contributes to your toxic burden and can hinder your attempts to detoxify.[312] The way to avoid this is to increase soluble fiber in your diet, which will add bulk to your gut contents and keep them well formed. When your gut contents press against the smooth muscles in your gut wall, it stimulates movement through your bowel. Soluble fiber also feeds your good gut bacteria, helping to keep your digestive system functioning optimally.

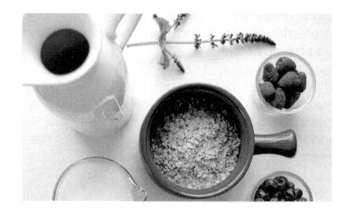

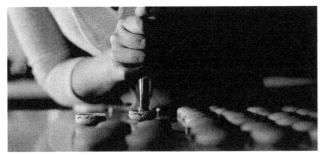

The role of your gut in your health is much bigger than how much fiber you eat. Your bacterial population plays an essential part in giving the right instructions to your body for manufacturing hormones, immune cells, and neurochemicals. It's important to address your gut health in any thorough self-improvement plan.

9.3 A Simple 7-Day Detox Program

A detoxification program doesn't have to be complicated. It could be simple as committing to one day each week of juice fasting. Juice fasting is much easier to do if you're at home and own your own juicer. If you prefer, you can buy fresh vegetable juices that will be almost as good.

Choose organic vegetables if you can, and include greens such as kale or spinach. Vegetables such as carrot and beetroot contain minerals in dense amounts and are low in sugar, so they make the best bases for juice fasting.

Fruit juices have high sugar content and can cause havoc with your blood sugar levels, causing spikes and crashes of energy through the day.

For a full week cleanse, start the first day with the juice fast described above. That means no other food apart from fresh juices. It gives your digestive system a rest because it doesn't have to work hard to extract nutrients from juice.

Your liver is a hard-working organ and as soon as you stop feeding it huge amounts of food

to process, it will start on deeper cleansing processes.

For the rest of the week, restrict your diet to the following foods only:

- Fresh raw or lightly steamed vegetables, especially leafy greens and cruciferous vegetables
- Fresh juices
- Superfood smoothies
- Small amounts of high quality, lean protein foods such as fish, nuts, seeds, and eggs
- Plenty of fresh water

Include each day the following supplements:

- Chlorella, chlorophyll or spirulina, 500-1000 mg daily
- Vitamin C, 1000 mg daily
- Multivitamin/mineral supplement, 1 capsule daily, with a meal
- Antioxidant or liver support formula, 1 dose daily, in the morning, as directed
- Bowel support formula, 1 dose daily, in the evening, as directed

Make yourself a meal plan and supplement plan, so that you know what to do and when. Make sure you drink at least 4 cups of water daily to keep your kidneys actively moving toxins out.

If you find you have detox symptoms following this protocol, add a small amount of carbohydrate food to your daily meal plan. Choose something nutritious and low sugar such as brown rice or quinoa.

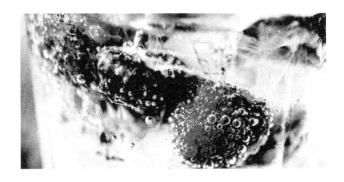

If you still don't feel great (i.e. have a Herxheimer reaction caused by harmful pathogen die-off and the elimination of toxins faster than your body can get rid of them), stop all supplements except the chlorophyll.[313]

Be ready to adjust your plan as you go, because it can be difficult to predict how your body will react to the changes. If this is close to your regular diet, you might not feel very different. But if it's a total overhaul, you could have some quite powerful reactions.

If you have any doubt at all about the protocol, contact a health professional for some personal guidance. You can repeat this protocol, or a variation of it, once every 3 months or as often as you think you need it.

You'll likely never feel better than after a great detox!

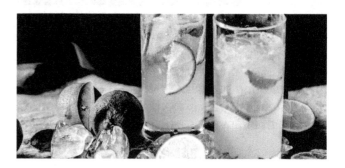

10.0 How Exercise Heals

If it doesn't challenge you, it doesn't change you." – Anonymous

If you just looked out of your window and saw people jogging, skateboarding, or biking, and it inspired your to just close the blinds, then you're missing out on one of the most compelling reasons to exercise.

Movement heals.

10.1 You Know Exercise is Good for Your Health, But Why?

Your body is made to be used. The ultimate purpose of digestion and all your internal organs is to nourish your skeleton and muscles so that you can move. That saying – use it or lose it is not a lie when it comes to both your physical and mental health.

When you exercise[314], your body directs nutrients, oxygen, and energy towards your heart, lungs, and muscles. This keeps these essential body parts healthy by nourishing and strengthening them. If you don't exercise, your body won't spend the energy it takes to maintain them in peak condition.

Of course, we all need to move at least a small amount just to live. Every day you get out of

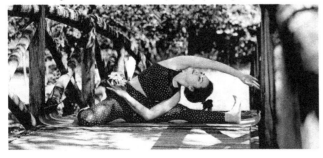

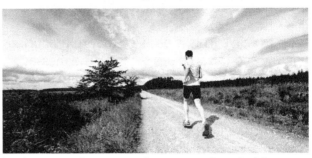

bed, move about your house, and probably maintain a moderate level of activity as you go about your daily routine. However, one of the biggest problems people face in the modern world is that so much time is spent sitting down[315].

If you work in an office or another job where you're sitting a lot, you might be spending 8 hours or more every day in a sedentary state. In other words, your brain is working but your body isn't. It's difficult to get enough exercise if you live like this.

But there are some small changes you can make to your routine that mean you're exercising without even realizing it. Try walking or biking to work. Or take the stairs instead of the elevator when you have the choice. Make sure you get up out of your seat at least once every hour. Walk the long way to the bathroom or go around the block quickly in your lunch break.

If you feel short of breath after any of these activities, it means you've pushed your body to the point where it's starting to respond positively. Assuming you don't have an illness that could cause shortness of breath, the need to take deeper breaths is a good sign.

It means your muscles have had to work and they're demanding more oxygen so that they

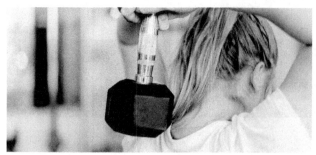

keep working. This is because they're producing energy, and this requires oxygen. The message goes from your muscles to your brain to your lungs, and you start to take deeper, fuller breaths. Your lungs are able to pull in more oxygen-rich air by expanding fully and exhaling sooner.

10.1.1 Exercise Supports Heart Health

Your heart also starts to work harder to pump oxygen-rich blood to your muscles quickly[316]. The extra oxygen is meant for your muscles but it doesn't just go straight to your legs. It flows through your entire body, which means that your brain and all your internal organs also get the benefit of additional oxygen.

Oxygen enables cells and organs to function effectively. It feeds into the energy-generating systems of your body, speeding up cellular reactions and improving the efficiency of your metabolic processes. This supports your health on all levels.

10.1.2 Exercise Supports Metabolic Detoxification

At the same time as oxygen is increased throughout your body, the extra movement of blood through your system also improves your body's ability to remove waste products from cells and organs. Your body's waste products are substances that it no longer needs or that are toxic to it. Collectively, they're called metabolic waste[317,318].

Metabolic waste is the breakdown products of your body's normal functioning. It's made up

of a range of different substances, including carbon dioxide, nitrates and sulfates. Removing metabolic waste is vital to keeping your cells healthy and functioning well.

Carbon dioxide is removed directly through your lungs every time you breathe out[319]. Most other waste is removed through your kidneys in the form of urine. One of the reasons you get thirsty when you exercise is because your waste removal processes have been stimulated, and your kidneys are asking for extra fluid to flush your body out.

10.1.3 Exercise Aids in Weight Loss

Exercise is well known to assist with weight loss[320]. The main reason for this is because it uses energy to exercise. You get energy from your food, and if you don't have a use for it, your body stores it as fat. When you exercise, your body releases energy from your fat cells so that it can power your muscles.

There are other reasons that exercise helps with weight control. Exercise affects your hormone balance, and hormones play an important part in whether your body stores fat or not. Hormones also dictate where in your body fat will be stored[321]. Most people would agree that having fat around your belly is not desirable but having a bit extra on your butt wouldn't be so bad.

When you exercise, your muscles are asked to work harder than usual and they respond by requesting more oxygen and nutrients. This is so that they can continue to do their job because they need oxygen and nutrients to make energy.

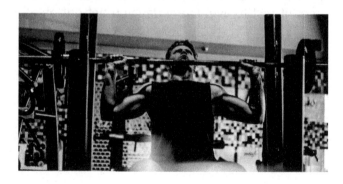

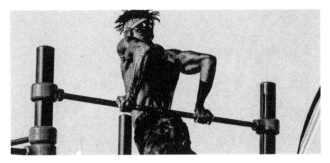

The energy they make is used to power your muscle cells, allowing you to keep moving with the speed and strength you want to.

10.1.4 Exercise Builds Strength

If your muscles are struggling to keep up with the demand you're placing on them, they'll also respond by creating more muscle cells[322]. That means that next time you exercise, they'll be able to function better because there will be more of them. This is how muscle building works. Muscle building is the goal if you want to become more toned and shapely.

10.1.5 Exercise Boosts Your Mood, Aids Sleep, Reduces Stress

But physique isn't the only reason you might want to exercise. It's also been proven that exercise helps with mood, sleep, stress and hormone balance. It's likely that it does so through its combined effects on multiple body systems. As we've already discussed, exercise brings highly oxygenated blood to your entire body, including your brain.

Your brain is like the rest of your body in the way it's able to function much more effectively when it's well oxygenated. That's one way that exercise instantly improves your brain function. But it's the discovery of endorphin release that has really fascinated exercise scientists. Endorphins are also called "feel-good hormones".[323]

The feel-good hormones are responsible for maintaining your mood and making sure that when stressful events do occur, you feel like you can cope with them. Endorphins released during exercise include dopamine and serotonin, which are both important for mood balance[324].

Exercise stresses your body, which is the main reason you feel fatigue and stiffness the next day. But the stress also seems to be an important part of why exercise makes you feel good emotionally.

It's like a practice run for responding to a stressful situation, creating the opportunity for your body's coordinated stress systems to work together. When you're stressed, your brain and adrenals have to work together. The more they do this, the more streamlined their activity becomes, and the more resistance to stress you develop.

Combine this with the waste removal benefit of exercise, and you have a powerful tool for balancing stress hormones. Stress hormones such as cortisol and epinephrine circulate in your blood and are eventually broken down by your liver.

When you exercise your liver gets a boost of oxygenated and nutrient-rich blood so it can process stress hormones faster, getting them ready for removal from your body by your kidneys. The net result is your stress levels go down and your happiness levels go up[325].

10.2 What Happens When You Exercise?

Your muscles are made up of long cells shaped

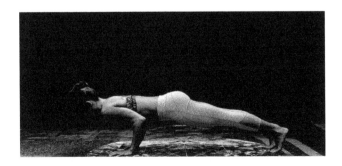

like a cable with fibers inside them. The cables are organized into bunches which band together to form the large shapes we think of when we imagine muscle.

Your muscles are moving all the time. Every movement you make is caused by your muscle cells' contraction. Even when you aren't thinking about it, your heart muscle is pumping blood throughout your body.

When you exercise, your heart pumps faster and harder to supply more oxygen to your body. At this point you'll usually notice it because you can feel it and hear it. Your lungs also get busy during exercise, drawing in extra air to oxygenate your blood.

Both your heart and your lungs are powered by muscle. Your heart is basically one big muscle and your lungs rely on your diaphragm, which is a wide muscle that sits across your abdomen under your lungs. When your diaphragm contracts, it pulls your lungs down, forcing air to rush into the space. Your blood vessels also contain muscles that are helping by pushing the blood through.

The muscles in your arms and legs, your heart, blood vessels and diaphragm all use ATP (adenosine triphosphate) to make energy[326]. Muscle cells can store a little ATP for immediate use. They also store glycogen, which can be quickly made into ATP. These are used for sudden bursts of activity such as sprints or lifting weights.

But once they run out, a few minutes into exercising, your muscles have to find another

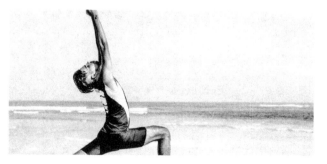

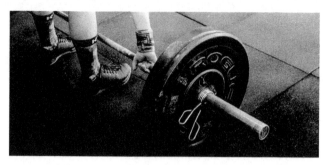

source of energy. They can make ATP from sugar (glucose) directly from food in your gut, or they can extract it from your liver where it's stored as glycogen. Your muscles can also convert fat to ATP, through a process called ketogenesis. Ketogenesis is the basis of the ketogenic diet, which forces your body to use fat for energy instead of carbohydrate.

Producing energy from glucose or ketones is the essential muscle activity that occurs when you exercise. The more you ask your muscles to do this, the more they will create the means to respond. When you're really fit, you can create huge amounts of energy on demand. As your energy levels increase, your overall health improves and it can have a profound impact on your attitude and motivation.

10.3 How Often Should You Exercise?

When you're reasonably healthy, you can exercise vigorously every day or every second day[327]. If you're serious about getting fit, you can follow a schedule that will give you the right mix of workouts and rest days. When you first start, it's a good idea to have two days of exercise then one day of rest.

As your fitness increases, you can increase this to three days of exercise with one day of rest -- until you have only a single day of rest each week. Resting in between workout days is important because it gives your body a chance to recover.

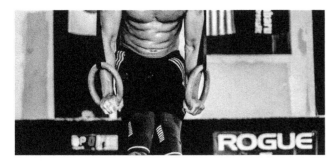

Recovery after exercise is a key part of building your fitness successfully. When you work your muscles hard, you create microscopic tears in your muscle fibers. The reason your muscles are sore the next day is because of these tiny injuries.

Your body creates inflammation in the injured tissue as its way of healing the area, by bringing increased blood flow and nutrients to the damaged muscle. It can then reconstruct the muscles' fibers, making them stronger and tougher so that next time you work them, they're more resilient and less prone to injury.

Of course, it doesn't exactly work that way in practice because you'll just work even harder the next time and then have sore muscles all over again. But you will get bigger muscles over time as you keep doing this. This is how you tone your body. The tiny injuries to your muscle fibers are a normal part of exercising and getting stronger.

When you're recovering from an illness, whether it's a serious condition or just a simple head cold, it's important to pay extra attention to getting the rest you need. There's no golden rule for how often you should exercise and how often you should rest, but aim to find a healthy balance between the two.

If you don't exercise enough, your body won't be getting all the benefits of increased oxygen and circulation, which can be a great aid to healing and recovery when you've been ill. Especially if you've been spending extra time in bed and haven't been active. Your circulation will be stagnating, with metabolic waste building up.

If you exercise too much while you're recovering from an illness, the inflammation can be too much. While it's natural and normal to experience inflammation following exercise, it can also cause further damage if too extreme.

And if you've been unwell, it's likely that you already have inflammation in your body. When you combine the inflammation from your illness with the inflammation from your workout, it can reach damaging levels. Excessive inflammation can increase your healing by days or even weeks.

This is especially true if you've been suffering from an inflammatory condition. And because most illnesses have inflammation at their root, it's highly likely that you need to consider inflammation levels when deciding how and when to exercise.

If you're currently ill and haven't reached the recovery stage of your illness yet, it's even more important to watch your activity levels and don't engage in over-exercising[328]. You will benefit from movement even if you're seriously unwell, but the amount and frequency need to vary based on your health.

Remember that the amount of exercise you need is unique to you. Don't try to compare yourself to anyone else or try to keep up with the routine you would follow if you were completely healthy. If you have a chronic illness, you need to pay even more attention to how much inflammation your exercise is causing.

Chronic illnesses are those that have been ongoing for three months or longer.

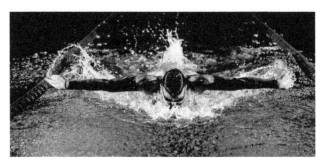

Degenerative conditions such as arthritis and multiple sclerosis are chronic. They're not going to get better, but their progression can certainly be slowed down. And you can manage them in a way that enables you to live the best life possible.

Other chronic illnesses that are debilitating, but not necessarily permanent, include chronic fatigue syndrome, digestive issues, and mood disorders, to name a few.

If you have a chronic illness, you need to closely monitor your exercise. In the same way that you might need to try different dosages and times for a medication, you need to try different exercise routines.

It's normal to feel a bit tired, sore, and stiff after exercising, but if you wake up the next day feeling like you've been in an accident, you've pushed your body too far. Over-exercising can cause a flare-up of your symptoms, as your inflammation levels spike.

You may also experience extreme fatigue, insomnia, loss of appetite, and a weakened immune system. A weakened immune system can manifest as a cold, cough, flu, cold sore, asthma, allergic reaction, or eczema. If you notice any of these symptoms after exercising, you need to take a rest day and re-evaluate the intensity of your activity. You could try an exercise that's more gentle, or you could shorten your workout duration.

When you're acutely ill, with a cold or a flu for example, it's a good idea to take extra rest days. Especially at the start of an illness, when

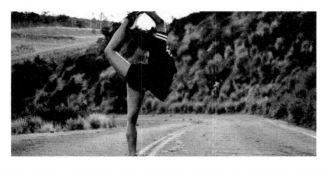

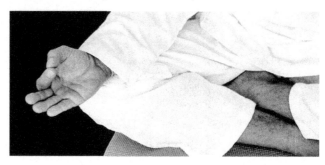

you have symptoms of inflammation such as achy muscles and a headache, it's a good idea to restrict your exercise to a short walk or something equally gentle. Getting fresh air and raising your heart rate slightly is enough to give you a circulation boost but won't overwhelm you with inflammation symptoms.

10.4 What Type of Exercise Should You Do?

It depends on your goals. For healthy people, an appropriate goal is to stay healthy, to age well, to tone up, or to get fitter and stronger. Getting clear on your goals is the first step in any good exercise plan, because you need to have something to aim for.

Once you know what you're trying to achieve, you can work backwards to make a plan that's going to get you there. Write your goals down. Then break them down into small components. Use specific and realistic goals. And make a plan that contains all the support you're going to need.

For example, if you want to lose weight around your belly, your goal might be to "lose four inches from my belly in the next six months". This is achievable. And when you break it down, it means losing just under an inch each month, just a fraction of an inch each week.

Your plan might start with contacting your local gym to inquire about regular classes, or signing up with a personal trainer who can keep you on track. If you want to tackle it by yourself, your plan could go straight to organizing a weekly schedule.

Your initial weekly exercise plan for losing belly fat could look something like this:

- Monday – gym class
- Tuesday – Pilates at home
- Wednesday – rest day
- Thursday – walk to work
- Friday – swim
- Saturday & Sunday – rest days

Whatever it is that you decide to do, make sure that it works for you in your current lifestyle. If you need to turn your entire life upside down to fit in an exercise regime, it's unlikely you'll be able to follow it for very long.

You might start with great enthusiasm, but it'll fade quickly if your scheduled exercise times are always encroaching on your normal life. The more you can integrate exercise into your regular routine, the more likely it'll become a permanent addition to your lifestyle.

Exercise is broadly divided into strength building and cardiovascular training. Most exercise programs balance resistance training with cardiovascular training. But if you have a specific illness or a definite goal, then one or the other can become the focus. Strength building uses weights and resistance to build muscle tissue on your frame. This is what you need to focus on if you want to tone up and get in shape.

Cardiovascular means heart and lungs, and it's about training these parts of your body to function optimally so that you have stamina

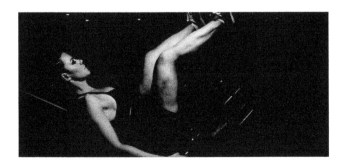

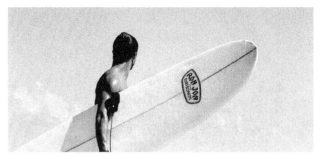

and good health. Cardiovascular fitness is really important for staying well as you age and reducing your risk of developing chronic diseases. Along with eating a balanced diet, cardiovascular exercise is the best thing you can do to make sure you don't get heart or arterial diseases late in life[329].

For people who are chronically unwell or over the age of 70, gentle, low-resistance exercise is better than an intense workout. This is because resistance training puts a lot of strain on your joints and can encourage inflammation. Walking, swimming, kayaking (or the use of a rowing machine), as well as yoga and Pilates are all suitable for people who need to avoid intense exercise.

Strength building exercises are good for people who want to shape up[330]. This requires resistance, which could mean walking up a steep hill, carrying weights while you walk or run, and working with weights at the gym. Squats, lunges, push-ups, planks, and jumping jacks are all strength building exercises that don't require any special equipment. You can do these exercises anywhere you have space.

Cardiovascular exercise is really important for people who are at risk of developing heart or arterial disease. If you have a family history, if you've been a smoker, or if you're overweight, then you need to focus your efforts on this type of exercise.

Running, cycling, dancing, swimming and kayaking (or rowing) are the most common ways to specifically exercise your heart and lungs. Any activity that gets your heart rate

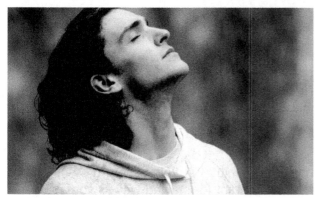

up and your breathing faster is working your cardiovascular system. Taking the stairs instead of the elevator counts.

If you're fairly robust and in reasonable health, you can afford to push yourself when you exercise. This means finding your limit of comfort and endurance and then working past it. If you stay within your comfort zone when you exercise, you'll maintain your current level of fitness but you won't improve.

Remember your muscles grow and strengthen in response to being challenged. You have to ask them to do more than they can currently cope with so that they will direct energy towards being able to cope with more.

If you have good health, you have the luxury of trying virtually any type of exercise and using different combinations. This means you can find something you really enjoy and it will seem like less of a chore and more like fun. This will help to keep you motivated to keep up your efforts over the long term. Be sure to mix resistance training with cardiovascular exercise for optimum results.

10.5 How Do You Reduce Muscle Stiffness and Aches?

Having stiff, achy muscles after you exercise is normal. But it doesn't feel very good. And it can make you want to take a day off even when it's not your scheduled rest day. Luckily, there

are natural ways you can counter the ache that will help to keep you enthusiastic about your exercise regime.

Some people suggest cold water and some suggest hot water on your aching muscles. Both can help but they should be used at different times. Cold water is best used immediately following your workout[331]. Take a cool shower or have a tepid bath straight after you finish exercising. This will reduce the inflammation in your exercised muscles by reducing circulation to the area.

Then soak in a hot bath or hot tub the day after. Hot water increases circulation so it's good when you want to speed up your body's natural healing processes. The trigger for inflammation is gone by this time and all that remains is to rebuild your muscles bigger and stronger. Improving circulation at this point can help your body rebuild muscle faster.

Anti-inflammatory, anti-oxidant and muscle-building supplements can help a lot with exercise recovery[332]. There are many good quality supplements to choose from, and as long as you buy from a trustworthy company they should be effective. Turmeric extract (curcumin), astaxanthin, glutamine and BCAAs (branch chain amino acids) are among the best choices for reducing muscle stiffness after exercise.

10.6 Summing it Up

Exercise is an essential tool for health and healing. Whether you're in good shape and want to stay that way, or recovering from an

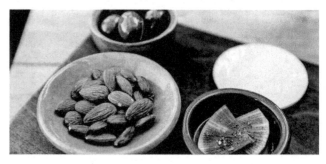

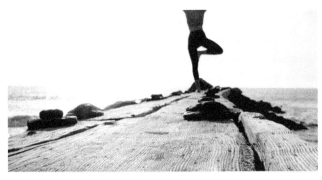

illness, exercise can help in every situation. You just need to vary the type and amount of exercise you're doing so that it suits your unique situation.

Over-exercising can be harmful because it encourages inflammation and can make your existing symptoms worse. It can also give you different symptoms associated with inflammation, such as extreme fatigue and loss of appetite.

Some inflammation is to be expected after you've exercised. This is what gives you sore muscles the next day and it's an indication that your muscles will rebuild stronger and bigger. Stronger, bigger muscles mean improved shape and tone.

Exercise benefits your health by increasing your energy levels and your body's capacity to deliver oxygen and nutrients to your vital organs. During exercise, your entire body receives an oxygen boost through increased circulation.

Increased circulation also helps to remove metabolic waste and stress hormones from your body, leaving you feeling clearer and more relaxed.

Additionally, your brain releases endorphins and other feel-good hormones when you exercise, helping to lift your mood and improve your sleep. It also benefits your concentration and mental function.

Every time you get your heart rate up you're working the muscles in your heart, lungs and

blood vessels. These organs are essential for good health, especially as you age. Keeping them in good condition means you'll be much less likely to develop heart and artery diseases as you age. If you're at risk of these conditions, you need to follow a diet and lifestyle plan that incorporates cardiovascular training.

Cardiovascular training keeps your heart and lungs healthy and resistance training builds muscle. Both are important for health and both occur when you exercise. But you might want to focus on one or the other depending on your personal situation and exercise goals.

It's important to have goals when you start exercising, so that you stay motivated and keep on track. Once you know what you want to achieve, you can create a plan for yourself, or get someone to help you plan, so that you get to where you want to be with your health.

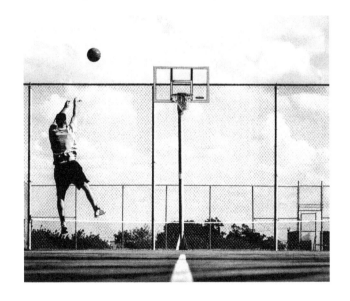

11.0 The Kick-Ass Morning Routine That Makes Your Whole Day Amazing

If you are like most people your morning starts in chaos, likely an extension of the night before.

You simply wake up, slam the alarm a few times and dash out the door.

You have no set routine or ritual that will prepare you for a day of success.

Here's the difference between you and a successful person: you set yourself up to fail with your current morning routine, while successful people have a routine in place that practically guarantees that they will thrive throughout the day.

Why is a morning success routine so important?

According to research conducted by Kelly McConigal, PhD, the author of "The Willpower Instinct", and one of Forbes' most inspiring women, our "will" to succeed each day is finite, but most of us don't even use the willpower that we *do have* at our disposal.[333]

If we *start* our day with a routine, we don't have to use up our willpower. Our routine is simply a set of habits that ensure we succeed in every way, including:

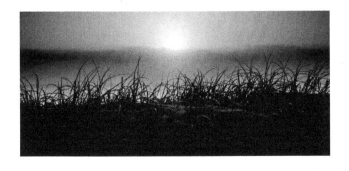

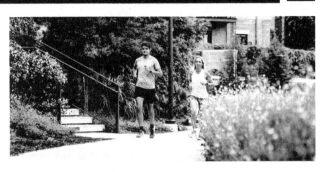

- Keeping us in forward-momentum no matter how we feel.
- Nourishing our mind and spirit so we feel motivated to tackle anything that comes our way.
- Giving our body the energy it needs to get through a 12-hour plus day, and still thrive.
- Building resilience.
- Anchoring us in a set of positive actions that frees up mental and emotional real-estate for other things.
- Motivating toward pre-determined goals.

A kick-ass morning routine will sustain you on the mornings you wake up feeling uninspired, tired, or listless.

And we all know that these mornings will happen.

Some of the most successful people have morning routines, because they simply work.

11.1 Morning Rituals of Famously Successful People

Famous artists, musicians, and scientists throughout history have had their own morning rituals, too.

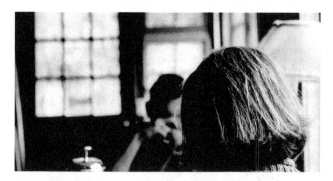

Good habits, ignited in the morning hours, helped to fuel the genius of Beethoven, Sartre and Marx.

The famous writer, Toni Morrison, considers waking with the morning light a mystical experience that helps fuel her creativity.

Novelist Nicholson Baker gets the benefit of two mornings. He rises to write at 4:00 AM, accomplishes as much as he can, and then goes back to sleep for a spell. He rises again at 8:30 AM to start the rest of his day.

Wolfgang Mozart still rose early every day, even after working on his compositions until sometimes 1:00 AM at night, as this was the only time he had with his other responsibilities and performances to compose new material.

Ludwig Van Beethoven was so precious about his morning routine, it is rumored that he would instruct his coffee to be made with exactly 60 beans, to fuel his daily ritual.[334]

Benjamin Franklin was a bit unorthodox in his morning ritual. He would sit in his room completely naked for an hour or so every morning so he could take an "air bath."

Jeff Bezos, Founder and CEO of Amazon, hates morning meetings. He prefers to stay home and have a healthy breakfast with his family before heading out to face the day's demands.

The globally-acclaimed Japanese writer, Haruki Murakami, chose to move to a more rural area to indulge in his morning ritual. He routinely rises at 4:00 AM, works for several hours, then spends the afternoon running and swimming. He allows his mind to calm down listening to music and spending time in nature before he goes to sleep at 9:00PM.

Howard Schultz, the CEO of Starbucks, does start his morning with a cup of French-pressed coffee, but he also gets up early and walks his dogs every day.

Steve Jobs, co-founder of Apple, would look at a written-down axiom: "If today was the last day of my life, would I be happy with what I am about to do today?"[335]

There are a variety of morning routines that work for different people, but we have observed some commonalities that can help you to succeed as others do.

Are you ready to create your own morning routine?

11.2 The Elements of a Successful Morning Ritual

They key components of a morning ritual will vary, but most of them contain:

- Quality sleep the night before, often with a schedule that allows an early – to—sleep, early – to—rise habit.
- A healthy, plant-based breakfast to give you energy for a full day.
- A moment or several to reflect, meditate, express gratitude or consciously design the rest of the day.

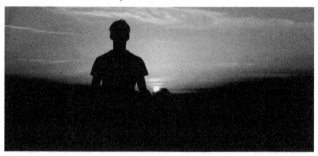

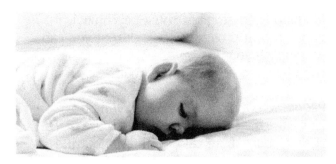

- Exercise. Walking or multi-tasking by reading on a treadmill are common.
- Coffee is used by many, but we will show you non-caffeine options that are better for creating sustainable energy.
- Time with loved ones.
- Spending time in nature.

Each of these habits has a specific way of nourishing our minds and bodies so that we can accomplish all that we desire on a daily basis. This leads to the creation of positive habits that act synergistically to fuel our creativity and passion for living a full and fulfilled life.

11.2.1 The 24-Hour Qi Cycle

For example, great sleep is tied directly to the human circadian cycle which is connected to the rise and fall of the sun behind the horizon. When we wake with the sun, it is easier to go to sleep as night falls. Our bodies make the appropriate levels of melatonin, serotonin to help us fall asleep easier when we see daylight during the day, and have complete darkness at night.

Though some highly successful people like to burn the midnight oil, it is generally considered better to rise early. This ties us to the natural light-dark cycle. From both a Chinese Medicine perspective and the ancient science of Ayurveda, rising early and retiring early also allows us to tap into the purest energy of nature – when all is quiet and still. The meridians can absorb "qi" from nature more easily when we are still and the morning is fresh. This is part of the 24-hour qi cycle which is likely connected to our own biorhythms.[336]

11.2.2 A Healthy Plant-Based Breakfast

Though many people skip breakfast, or simply grab some coffee and a donut on the road, this is one the worst mistakes you are making when it comes to your morning routine.

What you put into your body first thing in the morning is breaking your fast – the time from dinner until you wake that your body has used to rest, repair, and detox. While your has been diligently metabolizing toxins, repairing cells and damaged tissues, and replenishing your energy stores as you sleep, it has been busier than it is even during waking hours. Yet, after all this hard work, we expect to down some caffeine and sugar and expect our bodies to perform like a Ferrari all day – racing to meetings, make calls, drop off the kids at childcare providers, and fight morning traffic.

It's a recipe for disaster.

It's also no wonder that our blood-sugar levels start to crash at around 10:00 or 11:00 AM, and by the time we get to lunch we make yet *another* bad choice about what to eat because we are ravenous and grouchy.

Having a high-quality, plant protein-based smoothie is one of the easiest ways to jump-start your energy and replenish your body after it has been hard at work overnight. You can go straight to the end of this book to find dozens of recipes for a morning breakfast that will fuel you well into the afternoon, without putting you on a blood sugar rollercoaster, and sabotaging your ability to think straight,

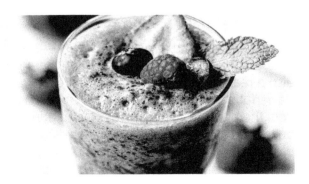

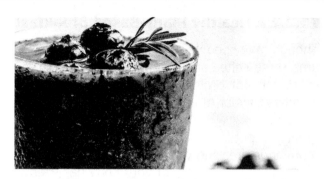

accomplish your goals, and do everything that is required of you in a busy day.

11.2.3 Quiet or Solitude to Consciously Plan Your Day

Whether you actually take twenty minutes to meditate every morning, write in a gratitude journal, look at your ultimate goal, like Steve Jobs did, or simply sit quietly and consciously plan out the steps of your day, you are participating in a conscious design for your day.

This differs drastically from someone who wakes up, stuffs some food in their mouths, and runs around all day putting out fires and *reacting* to life. If you do this you are likely to become the guinea pig for someone else's life goals, and stray from the actions that will bring your closer to your own goals.

You can meditate, write in a journal, re-familiarize yourself with next steps, look at your big goals, or write down the actions you want to take to make the day productive. As long as you take a few moments to realize your day begins with *you*, then you will act and respond to life in a completely different way than if you did not do this.

11.2.4 Exercise

There is a reason that great writers like Emmerson or Keats took long walks. There is also a reason why heads of state, CEOs, and powerful people start their days with exercise. It gets the blood pumping, gives you an adrenalin boost and sustained energy for the rest of the day, and even ensures that your fitness goals don't get pushed aside by other demands.

Morning exercise gives you a psychological boost, too. It proves to yourself that you can accomplish your fitness goals, which fuels your confidence to achieve other goals.[337]

People who exercise in the morning also kick-start their metabolism so they are more likely to burn more calories throughout the rest of the day. Morning exercise also inspires healthier choices at breakfast time.[338]

If you save your exercise routine until the evening, it can also interrupt your sleep cycle, since we tend to get a boost of energy caused by an endorphin rush right after doing cardio or intense training.

11.2.5 Alternatives to Coffee

We know the drill.

Some of you will say, "Don't even talk to me before I've had at least one cup of coffee it he morning."

We understand.

It isn't as if coffee is *completely* bad for you.

Small amount of caffeine, and the rich antioxidants available in a single cup of your favorite organic brew (without added sugar, milk, soy, artificial flavors, etc.) can boost your health, however, most people abuse caffeine.[339]

Too much caffeine can fry your adrenals, and cause you to crave more caffeine (and sugar) in order to function, which eventually leads to a health death-spiral. You know you've

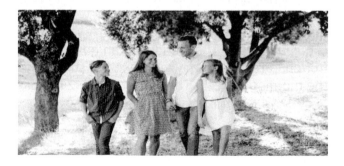

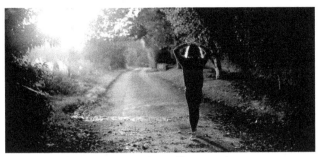

been drinking too much caffeine when you get withdrawal symptoms like headaches or irritability. Clean energy doesn't do this to you.

Instead of coffee, try these alternatives to jump-start your day:

- Matcha green tea (less caffeine and 10 times the antioxidants).
- Teecino is a great substitute if you are coming off a heavy caffeine addiction. It is full of prebiotics called inulin which comes from the chicory root.
- Ginger tea supports digestive health and can give you a swift kick in the morning when you need one. It also reduces inflammation, and has no calories.
- Green smoothies (these are full of phytonutrients that naturally fuel a balanced and sustainable energy cycle)
- Yerba Mate is helpful for people who have insulin issues (which may appear as low blood sugar in the morning). It contains a vasodilator called theobromine which can help with blood flow, too. It offers some of the buzz of coffee but with a few added nutrients.
- Kombucha drinks. These can help to balance your gut flora with healthy microbiota, which always leads to greater, sustainable energy.
- Coconut water has loads of potassium and less sugar than most fruit juices. It has a few extra calories, but the health benefits off-set them.
- Turmeric tea is great if you need mental clarity first thing in the morning. It is anti-inflammatory and with its active ingredient, curcumin, it offers some cerebral get-up-and-go.

11.2.6 Time with Loved Ones

Ever since human beings cohabitated across the plains of Africa, we've proven that we are highly social creatures. We came together as Homo Sapiens to hunt, cook, and share wisdom. In order to feel happy, we need to bond with others. It is hard-wired into our DNA so that we can survive.

Dr. Lisa Berkman of the Harvard School of Health Sciences conducted a study that observed 7000 people for nine years. People who lacked strong social support were more likely to die earlier than those who had strong family or social ties.[340]

Spending time with our loved ones at the start of our day can remind us why we are willing to work long hours, deal with challenging situations, and strive to be a better person.

11.2.7 Time in Nature

Time in nature is paramount in importance to your well-being. Forests, mountains, oceans, streams, and wild nature connects us with natural biorhythms and adds to our mental clarity. Spending time in nature also:

- - Improves your short-term memory
- Boosts your concentration skills
- Increases your creativity
- Restores mental fatigue
- Reduces anxiety, depression, and other mental health issues
- - Relieves stress
- - Boosts your immune system
- - Reduces inflammation

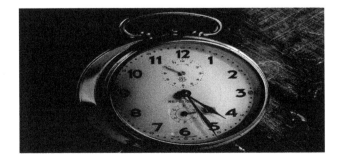

- - Reduces cancer risk
- - Reduces the risk of developing myopia (sight problem), especially in adolescents
- - Minimizes the risk of early death[341]

11.3 Sample Successful Morning Ritual

Your morning ritual might look this, but feel free to adjust it to meet your personal goals:

- Rise at 6:00 AM
- Practice Vipassana meditation for 15 minutes
- Write down ideas from meditation in journal for 10 minutes
- Look at daily targets for larger goals to refresh mind
- Have green protein smoothie for breakfast and sit with family
- Walk or hike for 30 minutes in nature Mon, Wed, Fri; gym on Tues, Thurs, Sat.
- Shower, get dressed for rest of day
- Take turmeric tea with you on the road
- Drive kids to school, and head to work

11.4 Summing it Up

Your morning ritual should contain elements that enhance your spiritual, physical, emotional, and social well-being. Each of these aspects fuels the others to create a synergistic set of habits that will ensure every day is a successful day. The faster you can put one into place, the sooner you will start seeing positive results.

When you first start a morning ritual, be willing to stick to it for a week or so before you tweak it, as any new habit can take time to solidify.

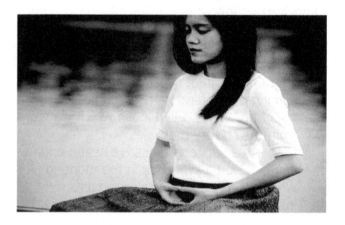

12.0 Hacking Sleep

I love sleep. My life has the tendency to fall apart when I'm awake, you know?" – Ernest Hemingway

Your life is much less likely to fall apart when you get sufficient sleep, yet we live in a world where most people are sleep-deprived. Even in hospitals – where people ostensibly go to get better – 100,000 deaths occur simply due to sleep deprivation.

More than 40 million adults are trying to get by with less than six hours of sleep a night. Though some people are biologically wired to need less sleep than others, good rest is key for numerous physiological responses in the body to occur.[342]

Sleep lets us heal, clean-house, and rejuvenate ourselves. We simply can't live without it.

12.1 How to Get Better Sleep: Causes, Cures, and the 6 Best Hacks for Insomnia

How terrible does it feel to get up early after a sleepless night?

You see the world through a haze of exhaustion. You mindlessly go about starting your day, fighting with lethargy and the heaviness of your

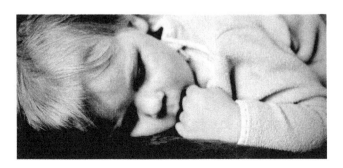

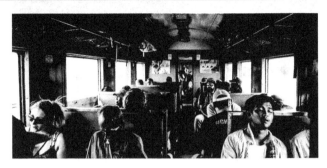

body while simply going through the motions. You have achy muscles and joints because your body simply hasn't had the rest and repair that sleep provides, and is that a cold coming on? Surely your allergies can't be acting up again!

12.1.1 Your Body is Actively Repairing and Rebuilding While You Sleep

You need to switch off for eight hours every night. It might seem as though you're doing nothing during that time, lying perfectly still and serene, but studies show that your body is very busy with repair and rejuvenation while you're asleep[343,344].

It's when most of your new cells are manufactured, and your body has a chance to catch up on housekeeping duties. Rather than spending energy on thinking, talking and moving, your body spends it on reducing inflammation[345,346] rebuilding injured tissues, and strengthening your immune system[347]. It is also busy getting rid of pathogens like bacteria and viruses that can make you sick. It's no wonder you always feel run down, and on the verge of another sickness if you aren't consistently getting ample sleep at night.

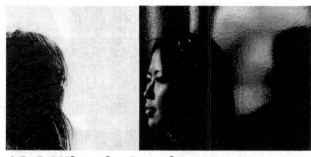

12.2 What is Causing Your Sleeplessness?

12.2.1 Symptoms of Sleeplessness are Usually Caused by Inflammation

When you don't get enough sleep, your body falls behind on these important repair and rebuild processes, and you feel the result of the stress and inflammation it causes. Inflammation is what causes the broad range of symptoms that can come with sleeplessness. Brain fog, drowsiness, aches and pains are just the start of it. If insomnia continues for a long time[348], it can also lead to stress, anxiety, depression, allergies and chronic illnesses.[349]

12.2.2 Identifying Causes of Your Sleeplessness

Understanding the cause of your sleeplessness is the key to changing your disturbed sleep pattern and creating a new routine that puts you on the path to optimum health. Sleeplessness has many causes, and they each need a different approach to be resolved.

As an example, if you're waking in the night because of low blood sugar, then it's vital you take steps to re-balance your blood sugar levels through the day as well as at night.

There are times when you might not be able to pinpoint the source of your sleeplessness. You can use a combination of techniques at these times, to gently push your body towards a better sleep routine. Complementary therapies always work better when you use multiple strategies at once.

12.2.3 Stacked Complementary Therapies Provide the Best Sleep Results

The simple act of using blackout curtains might not be enough to make you fall asleep quickly. However, if you stack the use of black-out curtains with turning off all digital devices an hour before you go to bed along with taking a high quality nutritional supplement, you'll sleep better.

If you then eat the right food at the right times, as well as reduce your caffeine and alcohol intake, then you're very likely to see an even better improvement in your sleep.

Stacking each of these remedies will give you the best results, and reduce insomnia for good.

12.3 If You Can't Get to Sleep: Causes and Cures

12.3.1 Sleep Onset Insomnia

When you can't get to sleep after you've gone to bed, you likely have sleep onset insomnia.

If it takes you longer than an hour to fall asleep after you've shut your eyes, you also qualify for having sleep onset insomnia[350]. If you fall asleep in a reasonable time but then wake very soon after, or just don't fall into a deep sleep but stay somewhat awake, that can also be considered sleep onset insomnia as well.

Your bedtime routine and sleep environment are very important factors if you have this type of

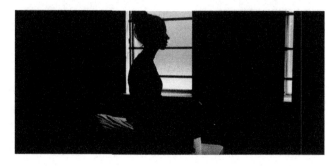

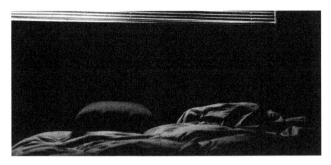

sleeplessness. If your routine around going to bed is disturbed, or if it's different every night, your body can fail to recognize that it's time to shut down.

Your body needs routine and regularity at bedtime.

There is a hormone in your brain called melatonin[351] that is also called the sleep hormone. It's released at night to make you tired and encourage you to fall asleep. Being in a low light environment encourages melatonin release[352]; this is why dimming or switching off lights can help you to sleep.

Melatonin is usually low in people who have sleep onset insomnia.

It's a good idea to learn more about the sleep hormone melatonin and how to encourage its production. Throughout this article, you'll read about the nutrients, foods and environmental factors that your body needs to make melatonin.

Tension and stress contribute to sleep onset issues.

Tension, stress, and emotional disturbance[353] are very common in people who have sleep onset insomnia. If you think these could be a factor in your sleeplessness, then you really need to address them as their own separate issue. It's no coincidence that many strategies for sleeplessness are also useful for stress because the two conditions go together so often.

Proper nutrition and cutting out stimulants can help you to fall asleep more easily.

Nutrients such as magnesium and B vitamins[354] are prescribed for stress as well as insomnia. Foods that encourage production of your happy hormones (serotonin) and your sleep hormones (melatonin) are also useful for both conditions.

Caffeine[355], alcohol, nicotine, and other stimulants can disrupt your sleep pattern because of the way they influence your hormones. It's best to eliminate or at least reduce these substances from your diet and your lifestyle as much as possible.

Certain pharmaceutical drugs can also upset your sleep hormone balance, including appetite suppressants, anti-depressants, anti-seizure medication (phenytoin) and thyroid hormone replacement drugs. Obviously if you're taking these particular drugs then there's a real need for them, and you shouldn't try to give them up. But knowing that they're contributing to your sleeplessness can give you some clues about which measures you could take to counter their effect.

12.3.2 Chronic Pain May Be Causing Your Insomnia

If pain is keeping you awake you need to address it separately

Chronic pain can also make it difficult to get to sleep[356], and the only way to make this better is to address the pain itself. Sometimes pain relief is needed before going to bed as part of your overall pain management strategy. And

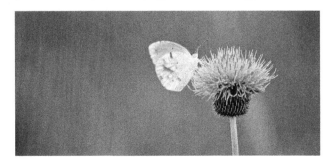

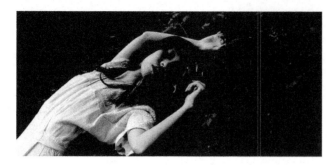

sometimes it's worth looking at other options like using mechanical aids such as braces or pillows to make yourself more comfortable. If you can work towards better health and less pain by treating the cause of your pain, then your sleep will likely improve without much further effort.

Increasing melatonin helps you fall asleep.

Sleep onset insomnia has a specific pattern of hormone disturbance. As you would expect, the vital sleep hormone melatonin is often lower than normal. Melatonin can be gradually increased, over a period of around 6 weeks, by taking tart cherry extract[357] daily. Tart cherry contains a compound called phytomelatonin, which basically means plant melatonin.[358]

Phytomelatonin adds to your flagging melatonin levels, bringing you back to balance. It also contains potent antioxidants that can help to protect you against the inflammation caused by sleeplessness.

Reduce stress and support your liver.

Stress hormones, including cortisol and epinephrine, are often higher than usual in people dealing with sleeplessness. Making an effort to remove yourself from stressful circumstances is ideal, but it's not always possible so sometimes you have to work around the situation. Do what you must to support your body in its efforts to get you through.

Cortisol and epinephrine need to be broken down in your liver, so caring for your liver health[359] is really important during stressful

times. This could mean taking a liver-supporting supplement such as Saint Mary's thistle seed extract -- or cutting out alcohol or drugs as you can. There are many commercially available nutrient formulas for liver support. Again, make sure you buy from a trustworthy manufacturer.

When someone is suffering sleep onset insomnia, feel-good hormones serotonin and dopamine are often depleted. Magnesium, zinc, vitamins C and B help to restore these important hormones back to their normal levels. Your body simply can't make happy hormones without all the necessary building blocks.

Passionflower to the rescue.

Passionflower[360] is specific for sleep onset insomnia. It's calming and mildly sedating with a pain relieving action. It's especially good for restless, irritable sleepers. It can be taken as an herbal tea, a tincture, or in capsules. You will find it in many herbal formulas, including Luna sleep aid.

12.3.3 Sleep Maintenance Insomnia

Sleep maintenance insomnia is when you have trouble sleeping through the night.

You may fall asleep exhausted, often earlier than you intended, only to wake between the hours of 3 a.m.-5 a.m., unable to get back to sleep. When you wake in the morning, you feel exhausted.

Adrenal fatigue often causes sleep maintenance insomnia.

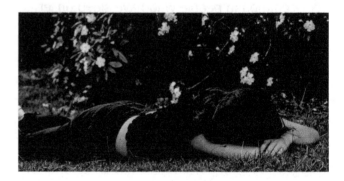

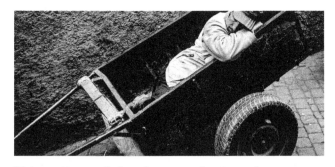

This pattern of sleeplessness is strongly associated with long-term stress, anxiety and adrenal fatigue. If you have this type of insomnia, it's important to learn more about adrenal fatigue and how to recover from it.[361]

With adrenal fatigue[362], your adrenal glands are overworked, and you're likely to feel edgy, anxious, and exhausted.[363]

Blood sugar balance is important for staying asleep.

Low blood sugar levels[364] is another common cause of sleep maintenance issues. Usually your body is alright when you go to bed because it hasn't been too long since you last ate. But if you're suffering from blood sugar fluctuations, it's very likely to get worse through the night as your body struggles to maintain its normal balance point.[365]

By the time you've woken up due to your low blood sugar level, it's likely you really do need to get up and eat something. A small portion of carbohydrate-rich food is usually enough to allow you to go back to sleep. You might need only one cracker or a single piece of fruit and you'll fall asleep as soon as you lie back down.

12.3.4 Menopause

Menopause can cause sleeplessness.[366]

Hormone imbalance associated with menopause[367] is another common cause of sleep maintenance insomnia. If you're menopausal or perimenopausal, your hormones are fluctuating so suddenly and to such extremes, that your body hardly has time to adjust before the next wave hits it.

This means blood sugar levels can soar and crash and your body temperature can go from sweats to shivers. Your energy level can swing between excited and lethargic and your appetite can go from ravenous to anorexic. None of this contributes to a long, refreshing sleep.

If you have menopause-related sleeplessness, you need to treat it as menopause rather than insomnia, by aiming to balance your hormones.

12.3.5 Is Alcohol Causing Your Insomnia?

Drugs and alcohol can wreak havoc on your ability to stay asleep.[368]

These substances can really mess with your body's normal rhythms. Whether it's pharmacy or recreational, drugs and alcohol can influence your hormone balance[369], nervous system function, and digestion. That means mood, energy levels, hunger, and sleepfulness are all at risk of getting out of balance.

Of course, sometimes you need pharmaceutical drugs, and you should never stop your prescribed medication without talking to your physician. But you might find that talking to them can help you get clear about which you need, which you can reduce, and whether you can eliminate any of them.

If alcohol or recreational drug use is affecting your sleep, you really need to look at that separately.

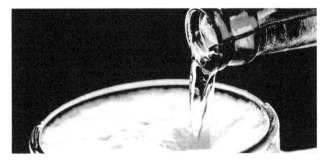

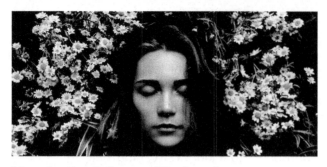

Licorice herb is specific for sleep maintenance insomnia.

When you get to sleep fine, possibly even falling into bed exhausted, but you can't stay asleep all night, licorice[370] is your go-to natural medicine. It's nourishing to the adrenal glands, so if you've been under stress for a long time, licorice is the perfect herbal extract. It tastes very much like the candy.

It can be used as part of a blend to mask the taste of other, more bitter herbs. If you want to use the dried root, you need to boil it for 10-15 minutes before drinking it to really bring the good compounds out.

Calcium and magnesium are useful nutrients for supporting sleep maintenance as well. You can get them from your diet or you can take them as part of a supplement formula. Magnesium is a major ingredient in Primaforce ZMA[371], designed for optimum absorption.

12.4 Six Healthy Habits for Great Sleep

Not all sleep hacks are specific to sleep onset or sleep maintenance.

Many will work regardless of the cause or pattern of your insomnia. Developing healthy habits around your sleep times will help you get the foundation right so that when you face a bout of insomnia, you've already done most of the hard work.

Making sure your environment and lighting are conducive to good sleep can go a long way to hacking your way to better sleep. Eating the right food, taking nutritional supplements, and using medicinal herbs complete the picture of setting yourself up with the best possible chance of getting quality sleep.

12.4.1 The Importance of Timing for Sleep

Have you heard of a circadian rhythm[372]? It's basically your daily rhythm - the patterns of waking, sleeping, and eating that shape your life. Your circadian rhythm is your body clock, and it's controlled by a complex interplay of nervous and hormonal signals.[373]

Different hormones are released at different times of the day, stimulating you to wake up in the mornings, feel hungry and thirsty, get tired in the evenings, fall asleep when it gets dark, and repair and rebuild your body during the night.

As much as you might like spontaneity in your life, your body prefers to follow the same routine every day. The more you can work with that and support it, the better your body will perform. This means going to bed at the same time every night, so your body can adjust to it and make a habit of it.

It also means making sure you get enough sleep every night, which should be around 8-9 hours[374]. So if you know you have to get up at 6 a.m. in the morning, your bedtime should be no later than 10 p.m. Set your phone alarm to tell

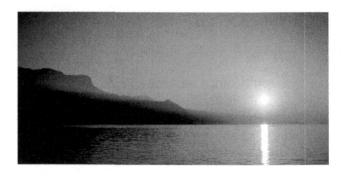

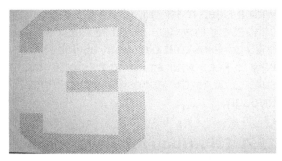

you it's time to go to bed. Better yet, set your alarm to tell you when you're half an hour away from bedtime, so you have time to get ready before sleep time.

The timing of your eating can also influence your sleep. Your body takes around 3 hours to digest a meal, and it digests much more effectively if you're upright during this time. Especially if you suffer heartburn or indigestion, lying down with a full belly can really make it worse. Eating your main meal just before sleep can also contribute to weight gain and problems with blood sugar balance.

Try to have your evening meal at least 3 hours before bed time[375]. And if you get hungry again before sleep, have a light, healthy snack that will help to balance your blood sugar. Eat a handful of nuts, seeds, or dried fruit. Or have a small portion of a carbohydrate food such as a piece of toast or a couple of crackers.

12.4.2 Electromagnetic Frequencies and Sleep Disturbance

Computers, phones, televisions and other electronic devices emit electromagnetic frequencies (EMFs). You're exposed to more EMFs now than anytime in history. While there is still no certainty about their effects on human health, a couple of studies[376] have pointed towards EMFs disturbing sleep.[377]

Until there is further evidence one way or the other, the effect of EMFs on sleep remains an unproven theory. However, many people report that they sleep better after taking steps to reduce EMFs in their sleeping environment.

Other health concerns possibly linked to EMF exposure include cancer, reproductive issues, and mental health conditions.

So for the small effort involved in minimizing EMFs in your home, you don't have much to lose. It's as simple as switching off all electronic devices before sleep. They need to be powered off, not just on standby or hibernate. Wireless internet routers also emit EMFs and these can be put on a timer so that they automatically switch off for the night and come back on in the morning.

It's also important to try to avoid them as you get nearer to bedtime. This means turning off your computer or TV an hour before bed. You could spend your evening wind-down time with a book to read or a board game to play.

12.4.3 Light Sources Can Keep You Awake

The sleep hormone melatonin is released in low light[378]. Your eyes send the message to your brain that it's night time, and your brain sends melatonin through your body to cause sleepiness. During the day when you're in bright sunlight or indoor lighting, there's no message to release melatonin so you don't get sleepy.

Indoor lights can have an effect similar to sunlight in preventing you from feeling tired. Warm white (soft white) light bulbs give out a frequency of 2700K. This is similar to an evening light, and it has a warm, yellow tone with a cozy feel. This bulb is the least likely to disturb your melatonin production[379], so it's really good for your bedroom, lounge area, and other

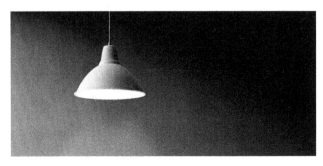

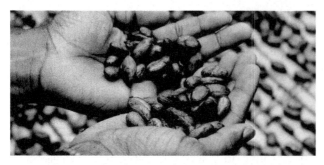

places you spend your evenings. If you haven't got warm white bulbs in these places already, consider swapping them.

Cool white (bright white) bulbs at 4100K are good for kitchens and areas where you need to see well and stay awake. Daylight bulbs at 5000K are best for bathrooms and places where you need really good visibility such as home offices and studios. They're good for reading, applying makeup, and working on intricate projects, but when you're trying to wind down towards sleep in the evening, these color bulbs need to be switched off so they don't disrupt your melatonin release.

Blue light[380] eliminating glasses can also help with preserving your circadian rhythm and melatonin release. These glasses selectively block the blue light frequencies that disrupt your body clock. So you can still see your computer and other screens, but you're not risking the loss of a good night's sleep. These glasses have other benefits associated with them such as improving mood and protecting your eyesight.

LED lights and fluorescent lights emit a lot of blue light, which is the most disruptive light frequency to proper melatonin balance. If you need to leave them on at night, consider dimming them or covering them with a blackout filter. If at all possible, switch off these light sources at least half an hour before bedtime.

Blackout curtains[381] are an essential part of any sleep hack. As we've already discussed, your eyes need darkness to send the right messages to your brain for the sleep hormone melatonin to be released. Even if you sleep in a light room with a sleep mask on, you'll still be exposed to light every time you take the mask off. Having solid curtains that block out all light is the best way to keep your sleep hormones in balance. Be sure to cover the edges too where light filters through.

12.4.4 Nutrition for Sleep – Which Food to Eat

Don't neglect the importance of proper nutrition – include key nutrients and their food sources including magnesium, calcium, and B vitamins. Also, increase tryptophan and decrease tyramine.

Of course you can't make the right hormones without the right nutrients. The best place to get nutrients will always be by eating a wholefood diet. When necessary, supplements can be used to boost and support your healthy diet. Your body needs the right type of protein to make melatonin and its precursor serotonin. It then also needs the right combination of nutrients to make serotonin into melatonin.

Tryptophan[382] is the key protein used as the building block for making sleep and mood hormones. If you don't have enough tryptophan in your body, you simply won't be able to make the right hormones for getting good sleep.

Tryptophan abides in abundance in:

- Garbanzo beans (chickpeas)
- Cocoa
- Sunflower seeds

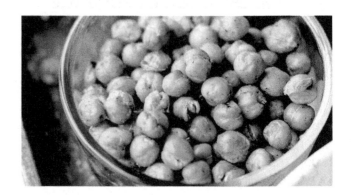

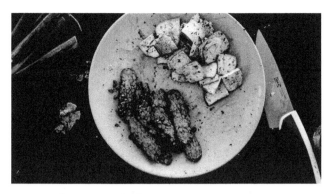

- Sesame seeds
- Spirulina
- Pumpkin seeds
- Watermelon seeds
- Almonds
- Peanuts

Other important nutrients for good sleep include magnesium, calcium, and B vitamins. Magnesium[383] is well known as a muscle relaxant and sleep aid. It helps with stress, tension, anxiety, and other mood disorders. And it works for both sleep onset and sleep maintenance insomnia.

The best magnesium food sources are:

- Spinach and other leafy greens
- Pumpkin seeds
- Almonds
- Black beans
- Avocado
- Banana
- Dark chocolate

Calcium[384] is important for sleep because your nervous system needs it to send messages. These nervous messages include muscle relaxation and slowing down thoughts. Calcium is also needed to convert tryptophan into melatonin. If you don't have enough calcium, you won't have enough melatonin.

To get calcium from your diet, choose these foods:

- Spinach and other leafy greens

- Tahini (sesame butter)
- White beans
- Broccoli
- Figs
- Oranges

B vitamins[385] are essential for good sleep. They're very active in the nervous system and work in many different ways. But one of their most important functions is to assist your body in producing mood and sleep hormones, including serotonin and melatonin. Even though people talk about vitamin B3 and vitamin B6 the most when it comes to sleep, it's actually best to consume all the different B vitamins in combination. This is because they work together and need to be in balance in your body.

Get B vitamins in your diet from:

- Whole grains
- Nuts
- Seeds
- Mushrooms
- Leafy greens

Melatonin is found in many plants because they use it to regulate their circadian rhythms just as humans do. Foods that contain decent amounts of natural melatonin include:

- Goji berries
- Tart cherries
- Walnuts
- Almonds
- Pineapple
- Tomatoes
- Bananas
- Oranges

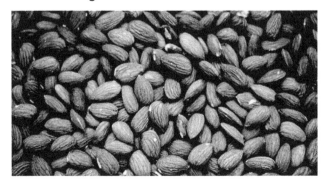

12.4.5 Supplementation for Sleep – Best Supplements to Take

Supplementing for better sleep is just as effective as supplementing for better overall health.

Primaforce ZMA[386] is a combination of zinc, magnesium, and vitamin B6, designed to provide the ideal ratio of these important nutrients. It can help with hormone balance, including sleep and mood hormones. It also acts as a nerve and muscle relaxant. The formula is pure and potent with no fillers, for maximum absorption and effectiveness.

Nested Naturals Luna[387] is a combination of medicinal herbs and L-theanine. The herbs work together to induce a state of relaxation and encourage a long, deep, refreshing sleep. L-theanine is a protein with proven calming effects.

12.4.6 Herbs for Sleeplessness

Medicinal herbs contain a vast array of active plant compounds. A a single herb can contain hundreds of different chemical compounds and often a few that don't even have names yet. Scientists are still discovering medicinal plants, and have yet to glean how every constituent within each plant supports our health, but they do.

It's not surprising that herbs can affect your body in potent and effective ways with all those amazing ingredients. The different chemicals work together synergistically to alter the way

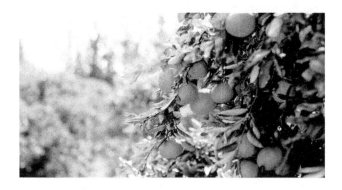

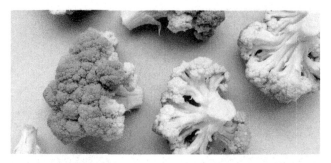

your nerve signals are being sent, and the way your hormones are being produced.

Passionflower is specific for sleep onset insomnia, and licorice is specific for sleep maintenance insomnia. These herbs can be taken alone or mixed with other herbs to make a formula unique to your needs.

If you see an herbalist, they'll most likely prescribe you a mix of herbs extracted into alcohol that will include sedating herbs with others that match your symptoms. An herbal tonic blended skillfully can be a powerful sleep hack.

Valerian Root[388] (*Valeriana officinalis*) is very popular as a sleep aid. It's non-addictive and effective as a sedative. Valerian has been the subject of many scientific studies which have shown that it relieves tension, stress, and anxiety as well as encouraging longer, deeper sleeping. Valerian is very bitter to taste and it's the root that's used for medicine so it needs to be boiled if you're going to use fresh or dried herb. It's most often given in a capsule to avoid the bitter taste and the effort of boiling.

Chamomile Flowers[389] (*Matricaria recutita*) are a gentle sleep aid, useful for relieving sleeplessness that's associated with digestive upset. Certain people with anxiety often feel it in their gut as a twisting or knotting sensation or changes to their appetite. This is a result of the brain-nerve-gut connection, also called the gut-brain axis. If this sounds like you, then chamomile is your new best friend because it works on the gut as well as the nerves.

Lemon Balm[390] (*Melissa officinalis*) is clarifying and soothing. If your mind's just too busy and full to fall asleep, then lemon balm is perfect for you. It's a member of the mint family and has an uplifting, refreshing taste when made into an herbal tea. It's best used fresh because much of the delicate oil that gives it such a sweet flavor evaporates when the herb is dried. If you want to use lemon balm for sleeplessness, it's best to grow it at home. It's easy to grow in the garden or in a pot and once you've planted it, it will establish itself almost like a weed, bringing you many years of soothing herbal infusions.

12.5 Summing it Up

Your sleep hygiene is just as important as brushing your teeth every day. You need sufficient sleep so that your body can complete important tasks, like getting rid of waste, ridding itself of toxins and pathogens, and repairing cells and DNA.

Be sure to:

- Turn out the lights (make it as dark as possible) so that your natural sleep-wake cycles are triggered.
- Eat the right food. A plant-based diet will help support better sleep.
- Eliminate stimulants, alcohol, and drugs.
- Take good supplements like Valerian root, Chamomile, or Passionflower.
- Address hormonal changes like menopause.
- Minimize the use of cell phones, computers, and other electronic devise which emit blue light. This interrupts your circadian rhythms.

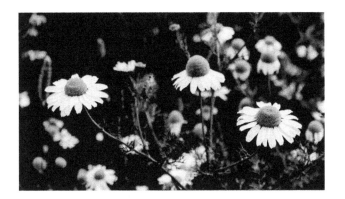

13.0 Hacking Stress and Anxiety

"Have you been busy?"

It's a simple question. It shows you're interested in someone's life, curious about what they've been doing with their time. But it also contains a message, because the expected answer is yes.

Yes, I've been really busy. This contains a message too. The message is that being busy is normal and expected. If you're busy, you must also be happy, productive and successful. And if you aren't busy, you must be lazy, depressed - a useless sponge on society.

But busy can also mean stressed, anxious, worn out. A victim of impossible social and personal expectations – work hard, strive for greatness, don't stop until you've achieved your ultimate dream. Truthfully, I find it exhausting to think about the greatness I haven't achieved. Because there's a lot of it!

You only have one life, and there are only 24 hours in each day. If you want to spend it working yourself to the ground, in pursuit of your goals, you can take that option. Hopefully you enjoy it. Hopefully it's what gets you out of bed every morning, excited and looking forward to your day.

But if not, if you just feel stressed and worn down by the daily grind of your life, then read on. Ultimately, success is different for every person. And if yours looks like living a long,

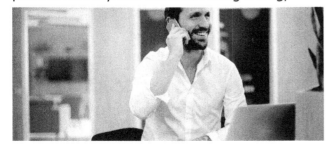

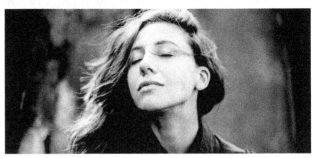

stress-free, healthy life, then you need to let go of your own expectations of superhuman accomplishment. And the next time someone asks you if you've been busy, you might be in the enviable position of being able to say a genuine, comfortable "No, actually I've been taking my time with life and it's been great."

All that energy that's been going into stressing, feeling anxious, being constantly busy, feeling guilty every time you let yourself rest... You could free it up to spend on the things that really matter to you. Whether it's your family, friends, hobbies, or even being more effective and more efficient at work, once you dampen down your stress response, you will have energy to burn.

To start with, you need to understand the mental, emotional and physical responses that you go through when you're stressed or anxious. And then we can look at how to hack those responses into a healthier, calmer sequence.

13.1 Understanding Your Stress Response – Brain, Nerves & Hormones

13.1.1 How Your Brain Creates Stress

Have you ever wondered how stress works? It's actually the result of many complex interactions

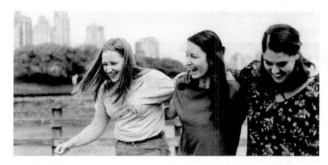

between your brain and your body. But it all starts with your thoughts. I'm sure if you tried it now, you could think about something stressful or unpleasant in your life and you would notice that you are actually creating a stressed feeling in your body.

I can do this by thinking about the last job I had. There was one lady in particular who I had a really strained relationship with, and I used to get anxious about going to work because I didn't know how to improve things with her. Eventually I left that job, in part because of her, but two years later I can still feel the stress and anxiety when I think about it.

Your thoughts create your feelings[391]. Did you know it's that way around? Some people think that feelings come first. It's not! Your thoughts generate electrical and chemical impulses in your brain that then become emotions. So if you're having negative thoughts, it will lead to stress and other bad feelings. If you're having positive thoughts, it will lead to happiness and other good feelings.

What tends to happen is that people get into habitual thought patterns[392]. So as an example, if you're used to thinking that work is a generally negative experience, you'll probably keep on thinking that. Even if you have a few good days and you enjoy yourself, by the time the weekend is over you'll be back to your default thought pattern: that work is a negative thing in your life.

There are many techniques and strategies for "reprogramming" your brain - changing or updating your thought patterns to more positive

thoughts. Or at least thoughts you actually want to have, that leave you feeling comfortable with the situation you're in. Some examples of strategies for improving your habitual thought patterns include neuro-linguistic programming (NLP)[393], mindfulness practice[394] and cognitive behavioral therapy (CBT)[395]. If you want to learn more about reprogramming your mind to be more positive, look into each of these in more detail.

For the purposes of this article, all you really need to understand is that thoughts create emotions. And emotions drive behavior. What I mean by behavior is actions. This includes the words you choose to say and how you use your body – whether you want to be closer to someone or feel the need to distance yourself, whether you want to be affectionate or feel the need to protect yourself. Your internal body responses are also noticeable – whether you feel relaxed or tense, comfortable or awkward.

13.1.2 Getting the Message To Your Body

To get back to understanding the stress response: your thoughts create electrical and chemical responses in your brain. You experience these as emotions but you also feel them as a physical reaction in your body. Stress and anxiety create tension and unrest in your body[396].

If you think of a time you've been really stressed, you can imagine what was going on with your body. You might have been agitated and unable to sit still, pacing around. Or if you were sitting you may have been trembling,

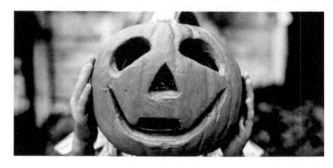

shaking or wringing your hands. You were holding tension in your body, maybe with your jaw clenched, fists balled, or your shoulders held up tight around your neck. Your breathing was likely shallow and fast as all the muscles in your chest and around your lungs were clenched.

This is all a result of instructions from your brain. Your brain sends electrical messages along your nerves to your muscles, telling them to tense up. It puts your nerves themselves into a state of agitation, so that it's difficult to calm down even if you want to. Your brain also hijacks your bloodstream, using it to send chemical messages through your body. This brings us to how your body reacts to these chemicals on a physical level – the fight or flight response[397].

13.2 Ready for Stress - Fight or Flight

You may have already heard of fight or flight? A lot of people are talking about it because it's a key impulse in the stress response. And it can cause a lot of health problems associated with stress. Fight or flight is essentially what happens when your body listens to your stressed brain. Your adrenal glands secrete stress hormones such as cortisol and it creates a whole range of physical changes in your body.

If you really were in danger, you'd be glad you had a fight or flight response because it can actually keep you alive in an emergency. It redirects and increases blood flow to your brain and your muscles, so that you can think yourself out of a dangerous situation, or use

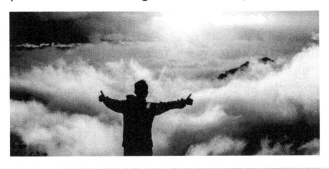

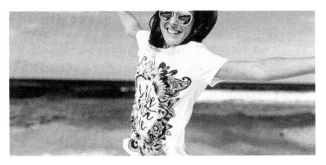

physical force to get to safety. If you've read or heard stories about people who have shown superhuman strength in an emergency, that's the fight or flight response in action. Reaction time is faster than normal and your heart and lungs are pumping lots of highly oxygenated blood through your muscles.

Sounds great, right? Except that there's a cost to your body. It doesn't matter too much if you just get a sudden fright one time and then go back to your usual state of calm. But if you live with constant stress or anxiety over a long time, the effects can accumulate, and it really can impact your health[398].

For one thing, the hormones and chemicals saturating your blood are pro-inflammatory. Every organ they come into contact with is going to become slightly inflamed. This includes your blood vessels, heart muscle, lung tissue, digestive system and even your brain.

This is why high-flying corporate executives so often develop high blood pressure: their blood vessels are inflamed from all the stress hormones they've been exposed to for months or years. Your body will try to protect itself in this situation, by placing plaque into damaged areas of blood vessel walls. It's the beginning of heart and arterial disease for many people as arteries become hardened by all the plaque and the blood vessels can't expand and contract like they need to.

Constant stress and an overactive fight or flight response also affects your digestion[399]. All that extra blood flow has to come from somewhere. It makes sense if you think about, digestion doesn't matter much when your life is in danger and you really need to just keep yourself alive, say, when you're outrunning an avalanche - just one of the times you would be very grateful for fight or flight. Your body redirects blood flow away from your digestion when you're stressed, so that you can think more clearly, or utilize every bit of physical strength you have.

But what about day to day living, when digestion is an essential part of living a long, healthful and vibrant life? You may have already guessed, your digestion suffers if you're under constant stress. You may be eating all the best food possible, filled with vitamins and minerals, but if your digestion isn't working optimally, you won't be absorbing all available nutrients from your food.

This can become a perpetual cycle of stress and malnutrition because your body can't function properly without all the vital nutrients it gets from your food. It simply can't manage your stress level and your fight or flight response, if it doesn't have all the key components it needs to build healthy nerves, organs and hormones.

And it's not just about digestion. All of your body's important repair and rejuvenation processes occur when you're relaxed[400], when your brain recognizes that it's safe to switch off fight or flight, and direct energy towards health maintenance. This is when your body has a chance to repair cellular injuries, generate new cells, check and correct immune function, and clear away inflammation. If you don't get on top of your stress, your body just doesn't get to take care of itself.

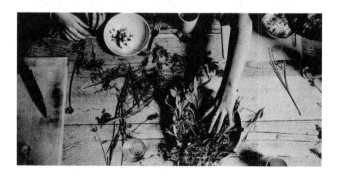

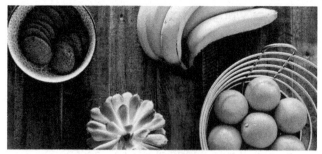

If you start to become malnourished from under-functioning digestion and your cellular repair processes are impaired, your stress gets even more out of control, and your digestion and repair get even more dampened down. You can see how this cycle can easily get away on people, especially if they're not aware of it or don't know what to do to stop it. Luckily, there are lots of points in the cycle you can intervene, and lots of different strategies you can use to tip the balance back the other way and start to reverse the cycle. We'll look at some of these techniques now.

Remember with natural remedies, you're much more likely to get a good result if you combine more than one strategy at a time[401]. Some of these you can even combine with pharmacy medicine. Just watch out for highly bio-active herbs or nutrients as some of these can interact with drugs. If you're at all uncertain, check with your physician.

13.3 Best Hacks For A Stressed Mind And Body

Harness The Power of Your Mind

We've already touched on the idea that stress starts with your thoughts. Now we're going to take a deeper look at how you can use this knowledge to your advantage. It makes sense that we should address stress from its root cause and then build up other layers of support around that. If you miss out the part about changing your thoughts, the other strategies that you try to use for reducing stress are much less likely to be effective.

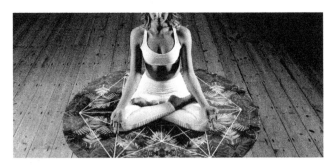

1. Get Curious About How Your Mind Works

The idea of using your mind to improve your health is definitely not new. Traditional cultures around the world have been talking about it, writing about it and teaching it for thousands of years. If this piques your curiosity, start by looking further into Eastern traditions such as Hinduism and Buddhism[402]. You'll find their ancient texts refer often to the concepts of mindfulness and self awareness.

Self awareness and mindfulness are also taught by modern psychologists and therapists. The basic idea[403] is simply that you become aware of your thoughts, feelings and responses. This is in contrast to letting them run on autopilot, unchecked and unconscious. It sounds like a fairly simple practice, and it is. But it's very easy to switch off without even realizing it, slipping back into old habits. The challenge is not in being mindful, the challenge is in remaining mindful at all times.

2. Learn This Basic Self Awareness Exercise

One easy exercise you can do to get a feel for how mindfulness works is to take 2 minutes just to tune into your self. Stand, sit or lie somewhere where you won't be disturbed, and just observe your self. You'll probably notice you're holding tension in your body somewhere, you might become aware of your posture or some pain that you've been ignoring. Noticing these things about yourself is all you have to do. You don't have to try to correct them. And you definitely shouldn't berate yourself for being less than perfect.

The idea is only that you observe yourself. If you can't stop the chattering mind, and it's determined to have a say about the things you're noticing, don't let it go to a place of judgment. Say to yourself something like, "Hmm, my jaw is clenched, that's interesting." You're consciously choosing to keep your opinion neutral, rather than letting your thoughts spin away.

You only need to practice this exercise once or twice daily. At first, practice it when you're feeling neutral, not when you're stressed. Just by increasing your awareness, you'll begin to make adjustments with no effort at all. Of course when you notice your back is slouched and you have pain in the area, your instinct is to straighten up.

3. Use This Advanced Self Awareness Exercise

As you get more comfortable using this basic technique, you can start to apply it to other situations. When you're under stress, you can use it to become aware of how you're responding. As soon as you bring your attention to your own responses, you create the opportunity to choose whether to continue as you are or whether to change something. It starts with self awareness.

4. Take Up Regular Practice

There are many other practices, strategies and techniques you can use to harness the power of your mind to reduce stress. Some popular practices combine mindfulness with physical exercise, including yoga[404], tai chi[405] and other martial arts.

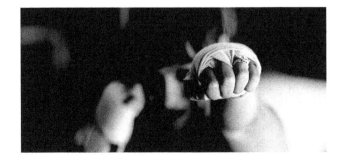

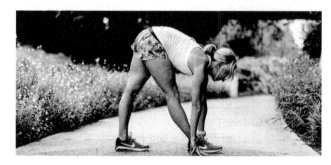

Hack Your Fight or Flight Reflex

As we talked about earlier, stress and your body's response to it can get locked into a cycle of perpetuating more and more stress. As well as intervening at the level of your mind, where stress originates from, you can also interrupt the cycle at the physical level. There are 3 ways of doing this: through exercise, chemical intervention (pharmacy and/or supplements), and diet. We'll look at each in turn.

5. Use Exercise To Calm Your Body

Physical exercise has been shown many times over to greatly improve health. Just by moving your body, enough to get your heart rate up, you instantly improve circulation, delivering vital oxygen and other nutrients to all your body cells. At the same time, the increased blood flow takes metabolic waste products away from those same cells, leaving them powered up and functioning optimally.

This increases your body's ability to process stress hormones and reduce the fight or flight response[406]. So you're breaking the stress cycle at the point of physical stress hormone metabolism. A body that is exercised regularly has higher levels of feel-good hormones and lower levels of stress hormones.

Other benefits of exercise contribute to the reduction of stress too. It makes sense when you think about it, that your body is preparing to run away from danger during flight or fight. So if you give it what it's prepared for, a good burst of physical exertion, it can use up all that energy that it's been directing to your muscles,

in a positive way. It can then go back to a state of "rest and relax", confident that danger has passed.

As a bonus, regular exercise keeps you fit, strong and shapely. Research shows that people who stay active are likely to live longer[407], happier, healthier lives. The "green prescription" as it's now being called, is being recommended by physicians of all modalities. Exercise is particularly effective for mental health issues such as stress, anxiety, and depression, because of the positive influence it has on the hormones that control your mood and energy levels.

6. Take Pharmacy Medication With Care

Pharmacy drugs can be useful for people who are under intense, ongoing stress. In acute or extreme circumstances they can be a great relief and can help to break the stress cycle at the physical level. But some of them have side effects[408] and can even be addictive[409], especially when used long term. For these reasons, it's a good idea to keep working on mindfulness, diet and lifestyle improvements even if you have your stress controlled by pharmacy medication. If you get to a point where you can stop the pharmacy prescription and carry on managing your stress using other strategies, that can be a very positive step to take, provided you have the right support and supervision when making the transition.

7. Supplement Your Stressed Body

Using whole food, vegan nutritional supplements is an effective strategy if you're stuck in a stress

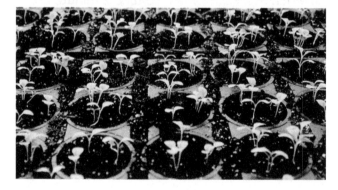

cycle. I say whole food, vegan because this is the purest, most effective supplement form available. Supplements need to be used as a boost to a healthy diet, if you want really good results.

There are a small handful of nutritional supplements that can genuinely replace diet entirely, but these are usually reserved for very ill patients whose digestion is so impaired that they can't actually eat properly. If you have a functioning digestive system, you should use it to its limit, by eating all the health-giving food you can get your hands on.

Of course, it's not always practical to eat the perfect diet every day. If you have a lifestyle that's causing you stress, you probably have very little spare time, and don't want to spend it in the kitchen making home cooked meals. But as long as you do your best with diet, then using nutritional supplements to fill in the gaps can benefit you greatly.

8. Relax With Magnesium And Calcium

Specific nutrients are known to be essential in keeping stress under control. These are used in maintaining nerve health, so that your overworked nerves can carry on sending messages clearly between your brain and your body. Magnesium[410] and calcium[411] are in this category. These 2 nutrients also work in your muscles, making sure that they can contract and relax as instructed. The relaxation part of muscle function is especially important when you're stressed, and magnesium is a key nutrient for

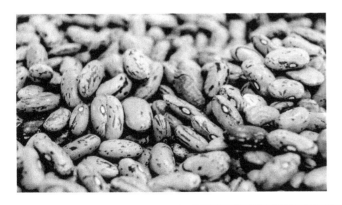

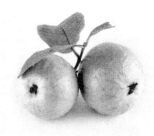

muscle relaxation. Magnesium is often found to be deficient in stressed people. It also helps with sleep, an important aspect of keeping stress levels down.

9. Feed Your Adrenals With Vitamin C

Other nutrients are used by your adrenal glands, those poor neglected organs of yours that are constantly working to produce and release stress hormones, responding to every little stressful thought you have with a rush of hormones into your bloodstream. Vitamin C is the key nutrient for keeping your adrenals healthy[412]. This one gets easily used up, being water soluble and relatively delicate. So taking it daily is quite important. Unlike magnesium and calcium, which can be stored in reasonably large amount by your body, vitamin C doesn't store very well, so your reserves can be easily depleted. Take between 1,000mg-5,000mg daily, depending on your stress level.

10. Feed Your Nerves With B Vitamins

B vitamins[413] are also well known for their use in treating stress, anxiety and mood disorders. There are different B vitamins and they're all active in your nervous system. They work together so you should always take them in a complex, rather than single B vitamins. Even if there's one particular B vitamin you think you need more than the others. The balance between the different B vitamins is really important. Like vitamin C, they're water soluble and not well stored by your body, so taking a small dose daily is preferable to taking big doses at irregular intervals.

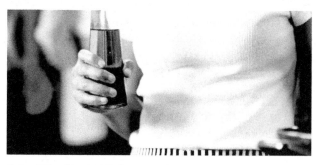

11. Alkalize With Powdered Greens

To really get the benefit of whole food vegan supplementation, you can use spirulina[414], chlorella[415] and other powdered greens as a multivitamin, multi-mineral boost. Greens in particular are potent anti-inflammatories and anti-oxidants as well as nutritional powerhouses.

Whole Food Nutrition Is The Best Medicine

This brings us to our final strategy for hacking your stress using complementary strategies. Last, but definitely not the least, diet is the foundation of your natural stress management, along with harnessing the power of your mind. If you do nothing else after reading this article, commit to improving your diet and try the mindfulness exercise. These 2 actions alone can be extremely effective in managing stress and anxiety.

12. Power Your Health With Fresh Greens

As hinted at above, greens are the key to using your diet to manage your stress and anxiety responses. Recall we were talking about the damage that long term stress can cause in your body, with stress hormones generating inflammation in every cell they come into contact with. Well, fresh green vegetables are the perfect antidote to all this inflammation[416]. They're naturally anti-inflammatory, powerfully anti-oxidant, and they alkalize your body fluids. All of this adds up to greater health and a resilient body that can perform its repair and relaxation duties even during stressful times.

Greens and other fresh food is relatively easy for your body to digest too. So it bypasses the influence of your stagnant digestion by providing nutrients in an easily absorbed form. Even when your stress level is high, you can rely on delicate green vegetables such as broccoli, spinach, silver-beet, kale, green beans, peas and salad greens to provide you with instant, concentrated nutrition. They're particularly rich in the minerals magnesium and calcium.

13. Vary Your Diet For Optimum Health

Once you've determined that nutritionally-dense vegetables are going to make up the foundation of your diet, then you can add in some variety. Fresh fruit[417] is a great source of vitamins (including vitamin C), enzymes, co-factors and phyto-nutrients. Nuts, seeds, beans and legumes can provide you with B vitamins in a natural, highly bio-available form. They're also a great source of vegetarian protein, which your body needs to build new tissue. With all the inflammation and cellular injury that comes form being chronically stressed, protein is an essential part of getting back to health. Your body needs these building blocks for its repair and rejuvenation.

14. Eat Good Oils Daily

Making sure you have enough good oils in your diet is also important for keeping your response well-tuned. This means eating a variety of cold-pressed vegetable oils, such as olive oil, avocado, sunflower oil, flax-seed oil, and hemp-seed oil. These oils are best eaten raw so that they're biologically active in your body. If they've been exposed to heat, light or oxygen then they're probably rancid and won't give you much health benefit. Look for a vegan source of

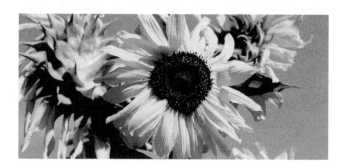

omega-3 oil[418], because this is one of the most active oils in your brain. Along with the other good oils, omega-3 helps with nerve signaling, hormone production for good mood and good sleep.

15. Avoid Toxic Food Groups

Avoiding foods that contribute to your toxic burden[419] or increase inflammation is equally as important as making sure that you're eating lots of the good foods. Try to avoid or minimize your intake of deep fried foods, carbohydrate-dense meals, baked goods, confectionery, and high sugar foods. This includes fizzy drinks and foods that have hidden sugar, for example many salad dressings contain a lot of sugar, somewhere you probably wouldn't think to look. Stick to whole food, plant based meals for the most part, and you'll have gone a long way to hacking your stress and anxiety the natural way.

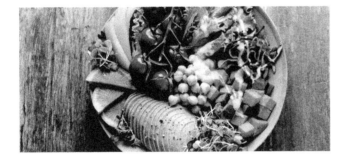

14.0 The Science of How Gratitude Changes Everything

One looks back with appreciation to the brilliant teachers, but with gratitude to those who touched our human feelings. The curriculum is so much necessary raw material, but warmth is the vital element for the growing plant and for the soul of the child." (Carl Jung)

"Gratitude makes sense of our past, brings peace for today, and creates a vision for tomorrow." (Melody Beattie)

"There are only two ways to live your life. One is as though nothing is a miracle. The other is as if everything is a miracle." (Albert Einstein)

Gratitude is like water for a growing plant, as the famous psychologist, Carl Jung so eloquently understood. It is among qualities like compassion, warmth, and empathy that make life more meaningful. However, gratitude has a special ability to help us feel content, even in the face of some of life's most enduring trials and heart-breaking failures.

Dr. Robert A. Emmons, now considered the world's leading researcher on the subject of gratitude, has looked extensively at what this mental state can do for us. He found that it has profound effects on our self-esteem, our psychological well-being, and even our *physical health*, but the benefits of gratitude don't stop there.

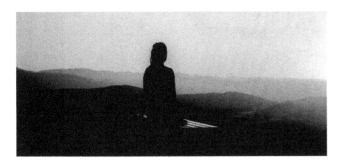

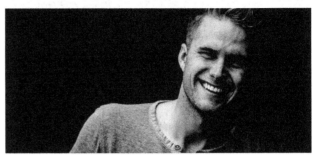

In fact, gratitude may be *most* helpful when we are in the midst of adversity or emotional suffering. When everything is going our way in life, it isn't hard to count our blessings. We naturally feel grateful for all the good that comes our way.

When we're facing tough times though, being grateful isn't only possible, it is vital! Consciously practicing gratitude can help us see the big picture and not get bogged down with temporary setbacks. Cultivating an attitude of gratitude can also shift us into the appropriate mindset to feel motivated to tackle challenges head-on.

A study led by Philip Watkin, published in the Journal of *Positive Psychology* proves how gratitude can help us be more resilient during moments of stress or emotional duress.

Participants in the study were asked to recall an unpleasant, unresolved memory. They were asked to pick a time when they were betrayed or deeply hurt. The group was then randomly divided into three sub-groups. Each sub-group was assigned a writing task.

One involved focusing on the positive aspects of the upsetting experience, and how they might feel grateful for it.

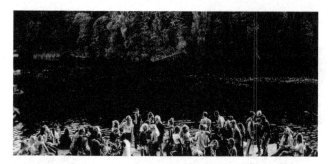

Another sub-group of writers were told to deny the negative aspects of their memory, and one group was instructed to write on a neutral topic.

The group that faired the best was the one that wrote about their negative experience with a tinge of gratitude for its positive aspects. They felt more closure, fewer unpleasant emotions, and were more resilient in the face of their negative experience.[420]

14.1 Gratitude Isn't Just Positive Thinking

Before you assume that gratitude is just a Pollyanna form of positive thinking, and a way to ignore negativity, pain or suffering, the evidence proves this just isn't true. It isn't a vacant, banal attempt at glossing over life's challenges.

Being grateful requires us to give credit to others for the kind things they do or say. It requires us to recognize our *inter*-dependence (notice we didn't say dependence) on others. To be grateful we must accept the responsibility of living in a web of social relationships which are all affected by our actions and thoughts. This requires us to be humble, which is a positive quality, but it may also inspire feelings of indebtedness and obligation, which only emotionally mature people can tolerate.

This feeling then inspires reciprocity, a cornerstone of any highly functioning society. It is also a key component of emotional development – not a Pollyanna philosophy – that causes us to accept our part in creating a reciprocal relationship. This quality requires our awareness, time, and personal, inner work to develop.[421]

Another clue that gratitude is not *just* positive thinking or a form of denial is that while it creates mostly positive feelings it can also challenge us to face real-life, extremely challenging issues with greater clarity. Pollyanna thinking dismisses that there are challenges at all. Gratitude clearly addresses the challenge, but re-frames it in a way that serves us so that we can get through it with greater acumen.

Luckily, the field of positive psychology has introduced much more scientifically-backed research to support what we've known in our guts for centuries or perhaps observed in our better moments – through a quiet thankfulness of the leaves of an Oak tree blowing in the wind, or a warm feeling that arises when a friend helps us out in a time of need.

Specifically, gratitude offers these astounding benefits:

14.2 Psychological Benefits of Gratitude

14.2.1 Gratitude Creates Stronger and More Consistent Positive Emotions Like Joy, Contentment, Pleasure, and Happiness.

Harvard Health researchers, including Emmons researched gratitude and found out that it makes people feel happier. In one study a group

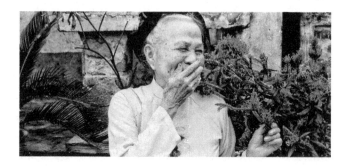

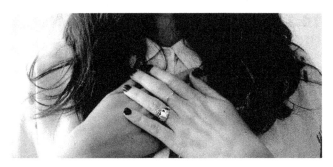

was asked to write about daily irritations or things that displeased them (without emphasis on positive or negative feelings) and another group was asked to write about things they were grateful for during the week. Both groups conducted this exercise for 10 weeks. Those who had written about things they were grateful for reported feeling more optimistic about life, exercised more, and had fewer visits to physicians than the people who wrote about things that irritated them.

Dr. Martin P. Seligman from the University of Pennsylvania conducted another gratitude study involving 114 people which was compared to a control assignment involving writing about early memories. The 114 people were directed to write and personally deliver a letter of gratitude to someone who had never been properly thanked for his or her kindness. The results were phenomenal. The people who did this had a huge increase in their happiness score, and the results lasted for over a month, outweighing the positive results from any other intervention.[422]

14.2.2 Gratitude Inspires Productivity

In the workplace, managers often struggle to inspire their team to put in extra effort, but research has shown that gratitude may be their biggest ally.

According to Medium Corporation, "Expressing gratitude creates a positive cycle – where the person showing thankfulness feels good and the person being appreciated does, too – is an important one for managers, leaders, and culture builders. It's too easy to focus on what

needs to be accomplished (by definition, what's lacking) rather than acknowledging what we already *have*. But failing to acknowledge workers has a clear impact on productivity and job satisfaction."

14.2.3 Gratitude Helps Us Feel More Optimistic About Life

Feeling optimistic about life has reverberating effects, and when we are grateful we tend to be more optimistic. Multiple studies have indicated that when we are grateful for other's actions, we tend to feel more optimistic about our own life. It may simply be because we acknowledge that other people contribute to our goals or desires, and thus we don't feel so alone in trying to achieve a challenging endeavor.[423]

14.2.4 Gratitude Gives Us a Greater Feeling of Control

Research suggests that gratitude helps us feel more in control of our lives. In one study, researchers administered a difficult test and told the study participants that they could win money for doing well on the test. Then the participants received a helpful hint that would help them get a high score.[424]

All the participants regarded the hint as helpful, however, only those who felt personally responsible for their own score felt grateful for the hint. Gratitude was actually associated with a greater sense of personal control over one's success.

Grateful people give credit to others, but not at the expense of acknowledging their own

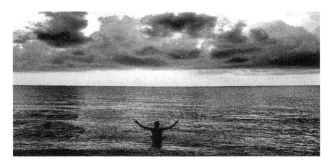

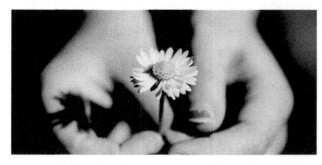

responsibility for their success. They take credit, too. It's not either/or—either I did this all myself or somebody else did it for me. Instead, they recognize their own feats and abilities while also feeling gratitude toward the people—parents, teachers—who helped them along the way.

14.3 Social Benefits of Gratitude

14.3.1 Gratitude Allows Us to be More Generous, Helpful and Compassionate

Recent studies have shown that generosity[425] and gratitude go hand in hand both at a psychological and neurobiological level. Generosity and gratitude are symbiotic in nature. We can kick-start a neurobiological feedback loop—an upward spiral of well-being—that is triggered by small acts of generosity and gratitude each and every day of our lives.[426]

14.3.2 Gratitude Encourages Patience

Research conducted at Northeastern University reveals that people who are grateful for everyday little things tend to be more patient and can make sensible decisions.

When 105 undergrads were asked to choose between receiving a small amount of money immediately or a larger sum at some point in the future, the students who had shown more gratitude in earlier experiments were able to hold out for the larger sum of cash.[427]

14.3.3 Gratitude Allows Us to Be More Outgoing

Another benefit of gratitude is that it tends to help us reach out to others be more gregarious, and connect with others socially so that we tend to be less isolated and lonely.

Gratitude also fosters trust, makes forgiveness easier, and generally supports healthy interpersonal relationships.[428]

14.4 Physical Benefits of Gratitude

The physical benefits of gratitude are all well documented. Among the benefits gratitude offers are:

- A stronger immune system
- Less physical pain[429]
- Reduced blood pressure
- Better, more restful sleep
- A tendency to take better care of our bodies and stick to a work-out regime

This single positive emotion can help reduce stress and depression, combat heart disease, reduce inflammatory markers in the body, foster better relationships, and help us achieve our goals – so how do we develop more of it?[430]

14.5 How to Cultivate Gratitude

One of the first ways to get a baseline for your level of happiness, against which you can measure the effects of a gratitude-cultivation

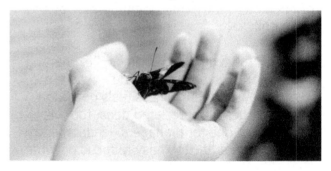

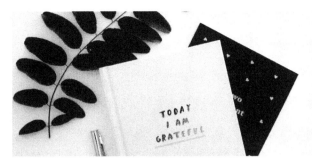

practice over time, is by taking the Oxford Happiness Test available at http://happiness-survey.com. This will tell you how happy you are today.

After practicing the following gratitude suggestions for three weeks, take the Oxford Happiness Test again and see how much your score improves. You'll likely be pleasantly surprised.

Try these gratitude tricks to boost your mental, physical, and social health and well-being:

1. Write in a gratitude journal for ten minutes every morning when you rise or before you fall asleep. Write down at least twenty things you are grateful for. This can start with the fact that you are breathing, and extend out to what others do for you.
2. Hand-write thank you notes to 3 people who have done something above-and-beyond for you this week. One of them might be to your spouse for taking care of the kids or supporting you, day after day, year after year.
3. Mentally count your blessings three times during the day. When you are driving is a great time to practice this gratitude practice.
4. Start a random act of kindness chain as a way to express gratitude externally. Buy someone's drink anonymously, or pay someone's toll on the highway.
5. Write a letter to someone who you can't talk to for whatever reason (death, geographic distance, etc.) and thank them for all the ways that they helped you in your life.
6. Take a picture of something you are grateful for and place it where you can see it every day.
7. Practice not complaining about *anything* for the next 24 hours. (It isn't as easy as it may sound.)
8. Take notice of three small, seemingly inconsequential things that you are grateful for right now which you normally overlook.

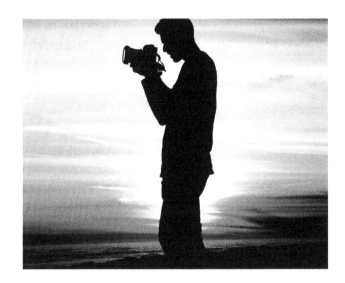

15.0 Take Charge of Your Health: Detox Your Home

The first three industrial revolutions created a toxic world. The World Economic Forum suggests that while technologies have made our planet faster and more efficient, the industries responsible for these technologies left an environmental Armageddon[431] in their wake – and our health suffers all the more for it.[432]

The Environmental Protection Agency has categorized over **4 million chemical compounds**, and at least three new chemicals are introduced by industry every day.

In a 1992 study the EPA[433] published the results of 7000 randomly sampled Americans who were tested for chemical residues, and the results were shocking. **Some** chemical residues[434] **were found in blood samples that haven't been used for more than 100 years**.[435,436]

Additional research has discovered that there are more than 700 chemical contaminants in human adipose tissue and blood that have never even been identified – likely byproducts of chemical synergies[437] when multiple chemical compounds interact with one another in our bodies and the environment.[438,439]

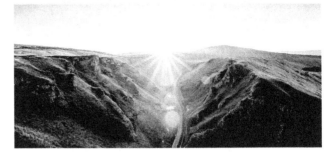

Another study found 40 additional carcinogenic substances in human blood and adipose tissue[440].

Human stem cell[441] toxicology tests have discovered that cellular, molecular, and tissue changes happen due to toxic overload.[442]

Additional research suggests that we have grossly underestimated[443] the toxicity of several known toxins, too.[444]

Forbes[445] recently published an article stating that chemical toxicity from BPAs, weed killers like Atrazine, and other industrial chemicals are causing early onset puberty, cancer, and neurological and reproductive defects.[446]

But that's only the beginning of the health challenges we face with an abundance of toxicity in our air, water, soil, and even in our homes.

And while we've been subjected to chemical warfare outdoors, many of us unwittingly participate in poisoning ourselves while living inside our own homes.

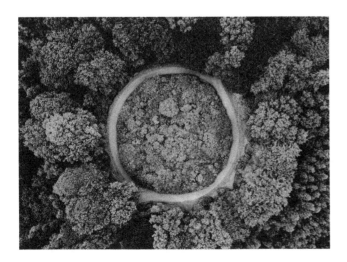

15.1 Symptoms of Toxic Overload

Following are just a handful of symptoms and disorders associated with toxic overload:

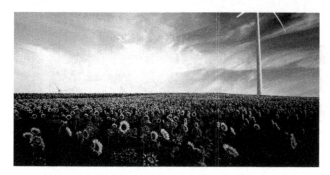

- **Reduced immunity**. Chemical toxicants alter our immunity[447] from a young age, making disease later in life more probable, but in real-time, our immune system becomes compromised and unable to defend against pathogens and bad bacteria. Autoimmune diseases are on the rise, largely due to toxin exposure. One study[448] found that genetics add to autoimmune disease, but that environmental toxins, gut alterations and dietary components cause 70% of all cases![449,450]

- **Chronic Fatigue**. Many doctors struggle to pinpoint a single cause of chronic fatigue in their patients, but it is likely that toxins are the white elephant in the room that everyone is ignoring. Diseases like CFS and fibromyalgia have a basis in chronic inflammation, which is caused by toxic overload.

- **Physical reactions**. Our bodies tend to speak up when we expose them to toxins, and sometimes they completely revolt. Symptoms such as skin rashes, headaches, or increased respiratory difficulty like allergies or asthma can be due to perfumes, exhaust, shampoos, cleaning products, and other environmental toxins.

- **Childhood cancers and birth defects**. Childhood cancers[451] are on the rise – a disease which used to be considered very rare – is now becoming commonplace even in toddlers. As an article published by Business Insider[452] details, birth defects are on the rise – and multiple studies[453] point to toxicity as a prevailing reason.[454,455,456]

- **Infertility and miscarriage**. Infertility[457] rates in both men[458] and women[459] are on the rise due to toxic overload. Sperm counts[460] in Western men are lower than ever, and women are finding it more difficult to carry pregnancies to term, or even become pregnant[461,462,463,464,465].

- **Adult cancers**. Cancer is now one of the leading causes of death globally. Every type of cancer from gastrointestinal to breast cancer to testicular cancer is linked to toxic exposure. The U.S. Department of Health and Human Services along with the National Cancer Institute state that more than two-thirds[466] **of all cancer cases can be linked to environmental toxins**.[467]

- **Cognitive issues and neurological disorders**. Many people are unaware that their inability to focus or that their poor memory is a result of exposure to chemical toxins. Even "sub-critical[468]" toxic exposure can lead to diseases like Alzheimer's, Parkinson's, and depression[469] as well as brain-fog and lesser evils.[470,471]

- **Chronic digestion problems**. If you have irritable bowel syndrome, leaky gut, or one of myriad other digestive ailments, it is likely that your gut flora[472] has been altered by toxic chemicals.[473]

- **Candida infections**. Candida is a fungal overgrowth which thrives in a toxic body. This single-celled organism feeds off dead tissue and sugar which you are more likely to crave when your detoxifying organs[474] (liver, stomach, pancreas, skin, digestive tract, etc.) become overburdened.[475]

- **Thyroid and endocrine conditions**. One of the sneakiest ways for toxic overload to harm your health is through an interruption of your hormonal balance. The negative feedback of an endocrine system swamped

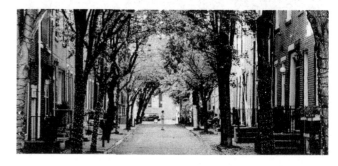

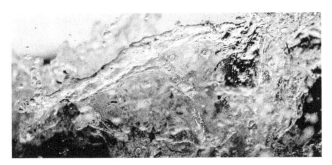

with toxins can cause your body to make more stress hormones, and even send signals to trigger the immune system's inflammatory response to ignite chronic inflammation. When a hypothalamic-release[476] is not in concert with the other endocrine glands, including the thyroid, adverse conditions develop.[477]

15.2 10 Steps to Reduce the Toxic Load in Your Home

With so many adverse health effects linked to chemical toxins, it becomes imperative to do whatever is possible to reduce exposure.

While there is only so much you can do about the chemical toxins in the external world, you can remove a huge burden from your body by removing chemicals from your home.

Here are some actionable steps you can take immediately to make your home less toxic:

1. **Swap out all toxic cleaning products**. This includes oven cleaners, furniture and floor polish, rug and upholstery cleaners, window and bathroom cleaners, air fresheners, chlorine bleach, dry cleaning chemicals, and anything else used to clean your home. Almost every cleaning product can be replaced with non-toxic essential oils like rosemary, sage, or citrus, a little vinegar and water, olive oil, and aluminum-free baking soda. You'll remove a host of indoor pollutants just by getting rid of toxic house-cleaning products.
2. **Use a high-quality water filter**. Some newer homes are being built with high-quality water filters in them, but since all environmental toxins eventually end up in our waterways, and municipal water supplies are doing a horrible job at removing pollutants, you need to do it at home. Aquagear, PureWaterFreeodm and other brands offer water filters[478] that can remove pharmaceuticals, fluoride, heavy metals, and biological pathogens.[479]
3. **Get a HEPA air filter**. Some studies suggest that indoor air[480] can be even more polluted than outdoor air. People who live in cities also spend around 90 percent of their time indoors, which means they are breathing in toxic air all day every day. They will help to capture dust, mold, and some chemicals, but not VOCs (chemical off-gasing caused by the use of other products or even by your carpets or paint on your walls). HEPA filters are best at removing biological pollutants[481] from the air, but you may need to remove chemical toxins by using greener products to begin with or an industrial air purifier.
4. **Find better personal care products**. Does your toothpaste contain fluoride[482], a harmful neurotoxin that has been linked to a lowered IQ? Does your shampoo[483] contain one of more than 15 harmful toxic chemicals like parabens, sodium laureth sulfate, polyethelyene glycols, formaldehyde, dimethicone, synthetic fragrance, cocamidopropyl betaine, etc.? Does your favorite moisturizer, mascara[484], or blush contain toxic chemicals[485]? Even your baby's soap[486] can contain harmful ingredients. The best way to weed through all your personal

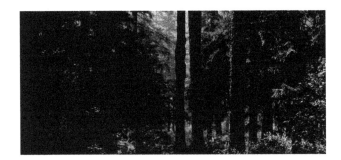

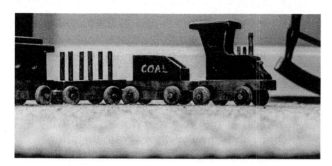

care products is to look at the label, and if you can't pronounce something, or it contains more than 5 ingredients (that you can't pronounce) then throw it out and find a better substitute. The Environmental Working Group has a great list[487] of personal care items[488] that are non-toxic, too.

5. **Don't purchase products (rugs, paint, vinyl flooring, treated wood, etc.) that will off-gas VOCs**. Volatile chemical compounds that are harmful to your health are used in tons of household items, from a simple throw-pillow that you put on your sofa to the paint that is used to coat your walls. Look for environmentally-safe, non-toxic alternatives whenever you can. Also look for organic bedding (sheets pillows, even mattresses) and steer clear of chemically treated rugs, fabrics, or furniture. Many "stain-resistant" or synthetic fabrics are notoriously toxic, so ask when in doubt, or seek out products that have the Global Organic Textile Standard Seal[489]. Additionally, rugs made from organic cotton or wool will also last much longer, as well as not spew VOCs into your home. These can be much more expensive, but consider them an investment in your health, and something that will last long enough to pass down to your grandchildren.[490]

6. **Replace plastics**. Plastics are a big endocrine disruptor, and even the "BPA" versions used in children's toys can cause health problems. Moreover, there are millions of consumer products containing phthalates[491] that are not even labeled as such. Even school supplies for children contain phthalates and other harmful toxins! When possible, opt for natural versions. Wooden toys are preferred (they also last longer), and non-toxic substitutes for plastic bath toys, blocks, etc. can be found online[492]. Also, start removing plastic bins and storage from everywhere in your home, especially in the kitchen where it can leach into your food, and replace them with glass or wood alternatives[493].

7. **Switch out toxic cookware**. There are still lawsuits pending for Dow chemical, and the makers of Teflon, the brand name for a chemical concoction used to coat pots and pans to make them non-stick. Most non-stick cookware is coated with from perfluorochemicals (PFCs). Enameled cast iron is expensive, but if you invest in a few quality pieces you can remove this toxin completely from your kitchenware, and the cancer[494] risk that comes with PFC exposure.

8. **Use naturally cleaning plants**. In addition to using essential oils from plants to clean your home, you can also put some indoor plants around your home to naturally freshen and detox the air. Even NASA scientists[495] have discovered that a home filled with plants can help to reduce airborne pathogens, and reduce sickness. Some plants even remove chemical contaminants like benzene, formaldehyde, and trichloroethylene. Try Spider plants, Dracaena, Ficus or Weeping Fig trees, Peace Lily, Snake Plant, Boston Ferns and more.

9. **Replace toxic chemicals in your garage.** Most people's garages are a smorgasbord of toxic chemicals[496]. Paint, paint thinner, herbicides, pest-control, caulking, adhesives, batteries, fertilizers,

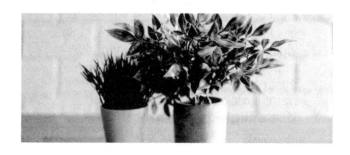

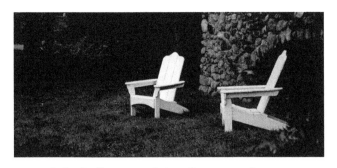

light bulbs containing freon, and more are a veritable cornucopia of health hazards. Contact your local chemical disposal agency to properly dispose of these toxins so that they aren't off-gasing in your garage. Replace them with non-toxic paints, and organic fertilizers wherever possible.

10. **Grow a healthier lawn**. Moving to the outer boundaries of our homes – the lawn, we can do so much better to remove carcinogenic chemical exposure. As Gardeners.com[497] elucidates, "Our love affair with lawns comes with a cost. Each year U.S. homeowners apply more than 3 million tons of synthetic fertilizers and 70 million pounds of lawn pesticides and herbicides. To make matters worse, it's estimated that 65 percent of these chemicals find their way into our lakes, rivers, and underground aquifers." If you want a greener, non-toxic lawn, add organic compost to the soil, stop fretting over weeds (dandelion leaves are actually an incredible detoxifier and cancer-fighter), or look at them as an indication of what needs to be added to your soil:

- Moss may mean that you have too much shade, or overly acidic soil
- Nutsedge indicates your soil isn't draining properly
- Crabgrass may mean that the turf is too dense and you are mowing too often

15.3 Summing it Up

By detoxing your home, you can greatly reduce the toxic burden on your body, and reclaim your health. Though we are exposed to toxins when we are outside via air, water, and soil

contamination, just greening our homes and removing or replacing toxic products can greatly enhance our quality of life and overall health. The laundry list of diseases and symptoms caused by in-home toxicity can start to be eliminated with actions that you take.

Don't get overwhelmed – because there is truly a toxic product everywhere you look in your home when you first start this process – but do be diligent about replacing one source of chemical toxins at a time. You'll be rewarded with your efforts, and your family will be safer, too.

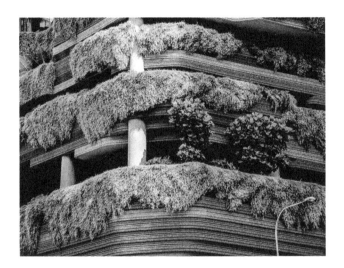

16.0 Suggested Reading List

"*A reader* lives a thousand lives before he dies. The man who never reads lives only one." – George R.R. Martin

Do you want the experience of a thousand lives lived before this one has even started? If you do, then you need to read. There are so many people who have lived through bucket loads of adversity and ecstasy, and they've got tons to share from those experiences.

What's more – every high-performance person has learned from the mistakes and success of others. While you can't duplicate hands-on experience just by reading a book, you can learn what other successful people do to make their lives work at peak performance levels.

The following is a list of books we highly recommend reading or listening to with an app like Audible in your down time, while driving, while waiting in line at the airport, or while doing your grocery shopping or morning workout.

If you think you don't have time to read every single book on this list, you're mistaken. Just listening a few minutes to the insights and habits in these books every day – instead of wasting time on social media or sitting in front of the television – will transform your life.

By reading through the titles and summaries, some will jump out at, practically call your name. Those are the ones to start with. Don't think you need to start at the top and work your way through, one-by-one. You're Greater Intelligence knows which book or books contain the information you need RIGHT NOW.

These authors provide scientifically-backed research and impeccable life experience on how to live better, happier, and more efficiently, while motivating you to live better *as* you achieve your goals.

If you want another way to shed a mediocre level of living, this is the way to do it. Use your mind, to save yourself a lot of time and energy – like that old advertisement for the Yellow Pages – but let your ears and eyes do the work instead of your fingers.

Without further ado, here is our preferred reading list with a summary of each title. Have fun and dig in.

Suggested Reading List (Numerical-Alphabetical by Title):

The 5 Second Rule by Mel Robbins

Get rid of all your excuses. Robbins tells you how your brain can be harnessed to take massive action in 5 seconds, since that is how long it usually takes us to talk ourselves *out* of doing something good or different. By using her 5-second rule, you can bypass the inner critic so that you can accomplish more than you ever thought you could before.

The 10x Rule by Grant Cardone

Most people operate with only three degrees of action: no action, retreat, or normal action. This won't cut it for achieving bigger goals. Success isn't luck, and *extreme* success requires a lot of effort. Cardone tells you how to keep extending this effort throughout your life so that you don't just succeed in baby steps, but by quantum leaps. If you've experienced some moderate success, but you're all too familiar with burnout, this book is a great read.

Abundance: The Future is Better than You Think by Peter Diamandis

The basic needs of every person on earth will be met in our near future. An exhaustively researched, bold peek into the future shows us that we will have much more than we ever imagined. The statistics in this book alone will make even the most stalwart pessimist change their tune. And when you're having an "eh" day, it will make you feel more positive about just about anything.

Bold by Peter Diamandis

This book is radical. Diamandis has described how Fotune 500 companies make massive waves in their respective industries. He tells you how single human beings change the trajectory of a company or project in unthinkable ways. If you've ever wanted to take that moonshot – go for the impossible – but didn't know how to go about it, then Diamandis is your guy. The impossible *isn't*. It's that simple. His words have impacted the lives of billions of people – you should be one of them.

Code of the Extraordinary Mind: 10 Unconventional Laws to Redefine Your Life and Succeed On Your Own Terms by Vishen Lakiani

Lakiana challenges you to reframe your views on everything – culture, family values, religion, politics, self-limiting beliefs, and more because most of those paradigms are worn out B.S. Lakiana offers a blueprint of laws to break us free from the shackles of an ordinary life. Get rid of limiting rules that are ruining your chances for success.

Daring Greatly: How the Courage to Be Vulnerable Transforms the Way We Live, Love, Parent, and Lead by Brene Brown

Dr. Brown has been on the New York Times best seller list multiple times because everyone can use great advice about how to stay vulnerable and yet be impenetrable when it comes to achieving goals. This book tells you how to master the razor's edge between the two.

Enlightenment Now by Steven Pinker

We may face incredible problems every day, but human beings are smarter, healthier, happier and living longer than ever before. Arguably, we're becoming enlightened. Pinker takes your attention away from the latest dismal news headlines and re-focuses it on seventy-five, in-your-face scientific graphs proving that human beings are flourishing on every level: prosperity, peace, safety, knowledge, and happiness notwithstanding.

Extreme Ownership: How US Navy Seals Lead and Win by Jocko Willink and Leif Babin

Willink and Babin, two of the most decorated officers in the special operations unit of the Iraq War, share jaw-dropping tales from their time in combat and Navy Seal training that apply to every aspect of life, from business, to personal relationships. When your mission is to help U.S. forces secure a violent city deemed, "all but lost," you learn a thing or two about how to cope with adversity.

Fat for Fuel by Dr. Mercola

There isn't a foodie or health nut that hasn't heard of Dr. Mercola by now. This book tells you how healthy fats can fuel the fire to achieve endless energy and astounding health without ever having to succumb to the sugar-carb, yo-yo, roller-coaster again. This book contains advice that should not be overlooked. How else are you going to power through 12-hour days without sound nutrition?

The Four Agreements by Don Miguel Ruiz and Peter Coyote

This book explores Toltec wisdom to teach you about the source of your self-limiting beliefs which prevent you from achieving your life's goals and heart's desires. In a nutshell, the four agreements are: Be impeccable and do what you'll say you will do, **don**'t take anything personally, **never** make assumptions, and always do your very best work.

Grit by Angela Duckworth

A pioneering psychologist tells you how to develop grit – the willpower and fortitude to keep on going. She argues that this is one of the *only* things needed to succeed in any field or endeavor. She's got all kinds of psychological tricks to teach how to develop this thing called grit, too.

Headstrong: The Bulletproof Plan to Activate Untapped Brain Energy to Work Smarter and Think Faster – in Just Two Weeks by Dave Asprey

We're all aware at this point that our brain offers a plethora of untapped ideas, memories, and motivations, but we don't know how to use them. This Silicon Valley entrepreneur tells you the secrets of using more of your mind's potential. His methods are innovative to say the least. He includes ways to biohack your own brain.

High Performance Habits by Brendan Burchard

The world's highest paid high-performance coach shares his secrets for long-term success after two decades of research in the field. If you think you've peaked or plateaued, this is a must-read book. There are six science-backed habits that will utterly transform your life, according to Burchard.

If You're Not First, You're Last by Grant Cardone

An international sales expert tells you how to make the sale in times of economic contraction, or when your competitors are currently breaking your back. He teaches you how to succeed even when no one else is.

The Like Switch: An Ex-FBI Agent's Guide to Influencing, Attracting, and Winning People Over by Jack Shafer

What if you could easily read people and figure out how to influence them – even compel them to like you? An ex-FBI Special Agent tells you how to do it, like flipping a switch. This applies to strangers, friends, and business colleagues, alike.

Make Your Bed: Little Things that Can Change Your Life by William H. Mcraven

Mcraven gives most of it away in the title. It's the small things we do repeatedly that lead to massive change. This book explores that phenomenon more fully and motivates you to make massive change with tiny actions performed consistently.

Man's Search for Meaning by Viktor E. Frankl

Throughout the 1940s, Frankl was a prisoner in several Nazi concentration camps, including Auschwitz. He offers timeless advice on how to make the most of suffering, instead of trying to avoid it. He argues that our primary purpose in life isn't to experience pleasure, but to find meaning in the experiences we do have.

The Motivation Myth by Jeff Haden

Haden explains away a myth – that the Gods of motivation or some great muse must strike us before we can accomplish anything great. He argues that motivation comes from doing, not from waiting. He tells you how to stay motivated, even when you face a writer's block, a great challenge, or some inconceivable obstacle. Here's a hint: the answer is constantly moving forward.

Own the Day, Own Your Life: Optimized Practices for Waking, Working, Learning, Eating, Training, Playing, Sleeping, and Sex by Aubrey Marcus

The incredibly successful CEO of Onnit, a lifestyle brand, shows you how a single day of positive choice can be the beginning of a revolution in your entire life. Marcus offers strategies for improving the mind, body, and spirit.

Peak: Secrets from the New Science of Expertise by Anders Ericsson

This book explores the science behind peak performance. Ericsson is considered the preeminent teacher in mastering new skills or finding new abilities. It doesn't matter if you want to become a violin virtuoso or the first person to break an earnings cap in your company. Ericsson knows how to help you do it.

Power of Habit by Charles Duhigg and Mike Chamberlain

You can reprogram your brain simply by changing your habits. Habits are formed in very specific, and methodical ways. Tools to change bad habits and replace them with good ones are shared by authors Duhigg and Chamberlain so that you can literally transform your life.

Principles by Ray Dalio

Dalio's moving account of how he manages to stay principled in an unprincipled world, and yet still succeed will move you to tears – and motivate you to do the same.

The Rise of Superman by Steven Kotler

If you want to live like a superhero: Laird Hamilton the big wave rider, Jeremy Jones the big mountain snowboarder, or Danny Way the skateboarding great, you've got to know how to accelerate your performance. Kotler tells you how.

Rising Strong by Brene Brown

A preeminent social scientist shares how you can overcome shame and find your true worth to succeed.

Stealing Fire: How Silicon Valley, the Navy SEALs, and Maverick Scientists Are Revolutionizing the Way We Live and Work by Stephen Kotler and Jamie Wheal

This book is an intriguing read. The cross-germination from unlikely corners (Silicon Valley and the Navy Seals!?) in the field of human potential are astounding. This book ignites your passion for your wildest dreams then makes them seem totally doable with all the advances in science, psychology, and human development.

Unbeatable Mind by Mark Divine

Divine gives some hard-to-find advice about how to sharpen your mental resources to achieve astounding things. He advises that mental clarity can help you to achieve elite level performance, and he proves it with ample case studies and real-life examples.

Unbreakable: A Navy Seal's Way of Life by Thom Shea and Brian Troxell

You think your boardroom troubles are rough, but a soldier that was in combat in Afghanistan for years, shares coping skills with you so that you can lead no matter where you are. Thom Shea's private memoir, meant for his children and wife if he didn't return from a war zone, ended up being an amazing manifesto for living life.

Unfuck Yourself by Gary John Bishop

If you've read Bishop's other titles, like *The Life Changing Magic of Not Giving a Fuck*, or *You Are a Badass*, you know that he isn't one to mince words. It's a refreshing approach to life coaching in a world of PC culture. His books are packed full of great information, despite his sailor's mouth. And really, who among us couldn't use a little unfucking sometimes?

The Way of the Seal by Mark Divine

As an ex-Navy Commander Divine knows his way around high stress and tough situations. He shows you how to train your mind to handle the most challenging parts of your life, and to not only survive, but thrive through it all.

What Doesn't Kill Us: How Freezing Water, Extreme Altitude and Environmental Conditioning Will Renew Our Lost Evolutionary Strength by Scott Carney

People who live through extreme conditions learn some amazing lessons about how to perform in life. Our ancestors did amazing things, that many of us wouldn't imagine tackling today like climbing impassable mountains, or swimming across angry oceans. Take what your great-great grandparents learned and apply it to life *now*. Carney shows you how.

That's the list. We hope you are enriched by every word.

17.0 Addendum I: 128 Studies on Animal Consumption and Disease

As these 128 scientific studies below demonstrate, meat-eaters are more likely to get a variety of diseases, including diabetes, cancer and heart disease. What's more, when they have cancer, they may be more likely to die from it.

Overwhelming scientific evidence also shows that people who eat meat and other animal products are more likely to have high blood pressure and to suffer a heart attack or stroke.

Animal-eaters are also more likely to be overweight or obese, which themselves are risk factors for disease. And in young girls, eating red meat may lead to earlier puberty, which increases their chances of getting breast cancer, cardiovascular disease and becoming obese.

Scientists are looking at a number of reasons why eating animal products might cause diseases. Just a few possible factors include compounds formed when meat is processed, the way our bodies break down animal products during digestion, and the changes that animal products cause in our gut microbiomes.

Check out this list of 128 scientific journal articles (with summaries) that have linked eating animals with disease.

Lung cancer risk and red meat consumption among Iowa women.

Alavanja MC, Field RW, Sinha R, Brus CP, Shavers VL, Fisher EL, Curtain J, Lynch CF
https://www.ncbi.nlm.nih.gov/pubmed/11557111
This case-control study of over 900 people found that consumption of red meat was associated with an increased risk of lung cancer even after controlling for total fat, saturated fat, cholesterol, fruit, yellow-green vegetable consumption and smoking history

Dairy products, calcium, and prostate cancer risk: a systematic review and meta-analysis of cohort studies.

Aune D, Navarro Rosenblatt DA, Chan DS, Vieira AR, Vieira R, Greenwood DC, Vatten LJ, Norat T
https://www.ncbi.nlm.nih.gov/pubmed/25527754
This meta-analysis of 32 studies concluded that high intakes of dairy products, milk, low-fat milk, cheese, and total, dietary, and dairy calcium, but not supplemental or nondairy calcium, may increase total prostate cancer risk.

Meat consumption and the risk of type 2 diabetes: a systematic review and meta-analysis of cohort studies.

Aune D, Ursin G, Veierød MB
https://www.ncbi.nlm.nih.gov/pubmed/19662376/
The results from this meta-analysis of 12 cohort studies suggest that meat consumption increases the risk of type 2 diabetes.

Red Meat and Colorectal Cancer.

Aykan NF
https://www.ncbi.nlm.nih.gov/pubmed/26779313
This review of meta-analyses reported that red and processed meats significantly but moderately increase colorectal cancer risk by 20-30%.

The Strong Heart Study: adding biological plausibility to the red meat-cardiovascular disease association.

Banegas JR, Rodríguez-Artalejo F
http://journals.lww.com/jhypertension/Fulltext/2017/09000/The_Strong_Heart_Study___adding_biological.9.aspx
The authors review evidence of the effects of red and processed meat on subclinical cardiovascular disease (CVD). They conclude that a low red-meat diet prevents preclinical and also symptomatic CVD.

Consumptions of Meat, Dietary Fat, and Fatty-acids and Prevalence of Overweight/Obesity in Children and Adolescents-a Cross-sectional Survey in Chengdu

Bao YX, Duan RN, Yang MZ, Chen YR, Tian G, Luo J, Cheng G
https://www.ncbi.nlm.nih.gov/pubmed/28612567
In this cross-sectional study of 1800 children in Chengdu, China, consumption of red meat was associated with overweight/obesity of girls aged 7-15 years.

Meat consumption as a risk factor for type 2 diabetes.

Barnard N, Levin S, Trapp C
https://www.ncbi.nlm.nih.gov/pmc/articles/PMC3942738/
The authors of this study reviewed evidence regarding eating meat as a risk factor for type 2 diabetes. They stated that meat-eaters had significantly higher risk of developing diabetes, compared with people who avoided meat. The effect of meat on increasing the risk of diabetes appears to be due to its saturated fat and heme iron, among other factors.

Health Risks Associated with Meat Consumption: A Review of Epidemiological Studies.

Battaglia Richi E, Baumer B, Conrad B, Darioli R, Schmid A, Keller U

https://www.ncbi.nlm.nih.gov/pubmed/26780279
This article discusses recent evidence from large prospective US and European cohort studies and from meta-analyses of epidemiological studies indicates that the long-term consumption of increasing amounts of red meat and particularly of processed meat is associated with an increased risk of total mortality, cardiovascular disease, colorectal cancer and type 2 diabetes. The authors conclude that recommendations for the consumption of unprocessed red meat and particularly of processed red meat should be more restrictive than existing recommendations.

Association between dietary meat consumption and incident type 2 diabetes: the EPIC-InterAct study.

Bendinelli B, Palli D, Masala G, Sharp SJ, Schulze MB, Guevara M, van der AD, Sera F, Amiano P, Balkau B, Barricarte A, Boeing H, Crowe FL, Dahm CC, Dalmeijer G, de Lauzon-Guillain B, Egeberg R, Fagherazzi G, Franks PW, Krogh V, Huerta JM, Jakszyn P, Khaw KT, Li K, Mattiello A, Nilsson PM, Overvad K, Ricceri F, Rolandsson O, Sánchez MJ, Slimani N, Sluijs I, Spijkerman AM, Teucher B, Tjonneland A, Tumino R, van den Berg SW, Forouhi NG, Langeberg C, Feskens EJ, Riboli E, Wareham NJ.
https://www.ncbi.nlm.nih.gov/pubmed/22983636
This prospective study in a large cohort of European adults found that those who eat high amounts of meat overall and red meat in particular have a greater risk of type 2 diabetes.

Processed and Unprocessed Red Meat and Risk of Colorectal Cancer: Analysis by Tumor Location and Modification by Time.

Bernstein AM, Song M, Zhang X, Pan A, Wang M, Fuchs CS, Le N, Chan AT, Willett WC, Ogino S, Giovannucci EL, Wu K
https://www.ncbi.nlm.nih.gov/pubmed/26305323
In these two large cohorts of US health professionals, processed meat intake was

positively associated with risk of CRC, particularly distal colon cancer.

Major dietary protein sources and risk of coronary heart disease in women.

Bernstein AM, Sun Q, Hu FB, Stampfer MJ, Manson JE, Willett WC
https://www.ncbi.nlm.nih.gov/pubmed/20713902
The data from this large prospective cohort study suggests that high red meat intake increases risk of coronary heart disease (CHD) and that CHD risk may be reduced importantly by shifting sources of protein in the US diet.

The impact of red and processed meat consumption on cardiovascular disease risk in women.

Bovalino S, Charleson G, Szoeke C
https://www.ncbi.nlm.nih.gov/pubmed/26732834
The results from this analysis of two cohorts support an association between red and processed meat consumption and CVD risk in women and suggest that the association is stronger for processed meat alone.

Consumption of animal products, olive oil and dietary fat and results from the Belgian case-control study on bladder cancer risk.

Brinkman MT, Buntinx F, Kellen E, Van Dongen MC, Dagnelie PC, Muls E, Zeegers MP
https://www.ncbi.nlm.nih.gov/pubmed/20947337
This European case-control study found a 50% increased risk of bladder cancer among those who ate the most cheese.

Health-related behaviors as predictors of mortality and morbidity in Australian Aborigines.

Burke V, Zhao Y, Lee AH, Hunter E, Spargo RM, Gracey M, Smith RM, Beilin LJ, Puddey IB

https://www.ncbi.nlm.nih.gov/pubmed/17069878/
In this cross-sectional study of Western Australian Aborigines, risk of coronary heart disease rose with consumption of processed meats >once/week, and with eggs >twice/week.

Meat subtypes and their association with colorectal cancer: Systematic review and meta-analysis.

Carr PR, Walter V, Brenner H, Hoffmeister M
https://www.ncbi.nlm.nih.gov/pubmed/25583132
This meta-analysis suggests that redmeat subtypes differ in their association with colorectal cancer and its subtypes. Beef and lamb were both associated with higher risk of colorectal cancer. Beef was also associated with higher risk of colon cancer.

A Systematic Review of the Effects of Plant Compared with Animal Protein Sources on Features of Metabolic Syndrome.

Chalvon-Demersay T, Azzout-Marniche D, Arfsten J, Egli L, Gaudichon C, Karagounis LG, Tomé D
https://www.ncbi.nlm.nih.gov/pubmed/28122929
This literature review reported that soy protein consumption (with isoflavones), but not soy protein alone (without isoflavones) or other plant proteins (pea and lupine proteins, wheat gluten), leads to a 3% greater decrease in both total and LDL cholesterol compared with animal-sourced protein ingestion, especially in individuals with high fasting cholesterol concentrations.

Dairy products, calcium, and prostate cancer risk in the Physicians' Health Study.

Chan JM, Stampfer MJ, Ma J, Gann PH, Gaziano JM, Giovannucci EL
https://www.ncbi.nlm.nih.gov/pubmed/11566656
This prospective cohort study concluded that dairy products and calcium are associated with

a greater risk of prostate cancer. Compared with men consuming < or =150 mg Ca/d from dairy products, men consuming >600 mg/d had a 32% higher risk of prostate cancer.

Red and processed meat consumption and risk of stroke: a meta-analysis of prospective cohort studies.

Chen GC, Lv DB, Pang Z, Liu QF
https://www.ncbi.nlm.nih.gov/
pubmed/23169473
Findings from this meta-analysis indicate that consumption of red and/or processed meat increase risk of stroke, in particular, ischemic stroke.

Relationship between dietary factors and the number of altered metabolic syndrome components in Chinese adults: a cross-sectional study using data from the China Health and Nutrition Survey.

Cheng M, Wang H, Wang Z, Du W, Ouyang Y, Zhang B
https://www.ncbi.nlm.nih.gov/
pubmed/28554922
This cross-sectional study of about 6,000 Chinese adults reported that risk factors for altered metabolic syndrome components include higher intake of meat, fish/seafood, and milk/dairy products.

Taiwanese vegetarians and omnivores: dietary composition, prevalence of diabetes and IFG.

Chiu TH, Huang HY, Chiu YF, Pan WH, Kao HY, Chiu JP, Lin MN, Lin CL
https://www.ncbi.nlm.nih.gov/
pubmed/24523914
This Taiwanese study of over 4,300 Buddhist adults reported that women who avoided all meat reduced their risk of diabetes by 70% compared to those who ate meat; men reduced their risk by 45%.

Red Meat Intake and Risk of Breast Cancer Among Premenopausal Women.

Cho E, Chen WY, Hunter DJ, Stampfer MJ, Colditz GA, Hankinson SE, Willett WC
https://www.ncbi.nlm.nih.gov/
pubmed/17101944
The authors of this large prospective cohort study concluded that higher red meat intake may be a risk factor for estrogen and progesterone receptor positive breast cancer among premenopausal women. Those who ate the most red meat had almost twice the risk of those who ate the least red meat.

Egg consumption and coronary artery calcification in asymptomatic men and women.

Choi Y, Chang Y, Lee JE, Chun S, Cho J, Sung E, Suh BS, Rampal S, Zhao D, Zhang Y, Pastor-Barriuso R, Lima JA, Shin H, Ryu S, Guallar E
https://www.ncbi.nlm.nih.gov/
pubmed/26062990
In this study, participants who ate the most eggs, compared with those who ate the least, had 80% higher coronary artery calcium scores, which is a measure of heart disease risk.

Consumption of red and processed meat and esophageal cancer risk: meta-analysis.

Choi Y, Song S, Song Y, Lee JE
https://www.ncbi.nlm.nih.gov/
pubmed/23467465
Findings from this meta-analysis suggested that a higher consumption of red meat was associated with a greater risk of esophageal cancer.

Socioeconomic and demographic drivers of red and processed meat consumption: implications for health and environmental sustainability.

Clonan A, Roberts KE, Holdsworth M
https://www.ncbi.nlm.nih.gov/

pubmed/27021468
This report states that consumption of meat is increasing in lower-income countries across Latin American and East Asia, increasing the risk in those countries for non-communicable diseases such as diabetes, heart disease, and obesity.

A case-control study of galactose consumption and metabolism in relation to ovarian cancer.

Cramer DW, Greenberg ER, Titus-Ernstoff L, Liberman RF, Welch WR, Li E, Ng WG
https://www.ncbi.nlm.nih.gov/pubmed/10667469
This case-control study of the effects of dairy sugar on ovarian cancer risk suggested that certain genetic or biochemical features of dairy sugar metabolism may influence disease risk for particular types of ovarian cancer.

Diet rapidly and reproducibly alters the human gut microbiome.

David LA, Maurice CF, Carmody RN, Gootenberg DB, Button JE, Wolfe BE, Ling AV, Devlin AS, Varma Y, Fischbach MA, Biddinger SB, Dutton RJ, Turnbaugh PJ
https://www.ncbi.nlm.nih.gov/pubmed/24336217
This study demonstrated that eating meats, eggs and cheese even for a short time (5 days) caused measureable changes in the types and varieties of gut microbes. Animal foods increased the numbers of Bilophila organisms which may trigger inflammatory bowel disease.

Red and processed meat intake and cancer risk: Results from the prospective NutriNet-Santé cohort study.

Diallo A, Deschasaux M, Latino-Martel P, Hercberg S, Galan P, Fassier P, Allès B, Guéraud F, Pierre FH, Touvier M
https://www.ncbi.nlm.nih.gov/pubmed/28913916
In this prospective study, red meat intake was associated with significantly increased risk of overall cancers and breast cancer.

Egg consumption and risk of type 2 diabetes: a meta-analysis of prospective studies.

Djoussé L, Khawaja OA, Gaziano JM
https://www.ncbi.nlm.nih.gov/pubmed/26739035
This meta-analysis suggested a modest elevated risk of type 2 diabetes in those who eat more than three eggs per week.

Fatty acid consumption and incident type 2 diabetes: evidence from the E3N cohort study.

Dow C, Mangin M, Balkau B, Affret A, Boutron-Ruault MC, Clavel-Chapelon F, Bonnet F, Fagherazzi G
https://www.ncbi.nlm.nih.gov/pubmed/27842617
In this prospective study of over 71,000 women, those who had the highest level of fat in their diets increased their risk of type 2 diabetes by 26% compared to those who ate the least. Two specific types of fat, which are mostly found in meat, fish, and eggs, almost doubled the risk.

Associations between red meat and risks for colon and rectal cancer depend on the type of red meat consumed.

Egeberg R, Olsen A, Christensen J, Halkjær J, Jakobsen MU, Overvad K, Tjønneland A
https://www.ncbi.nlm.nih.gov/pubmed/23427329
In this Danish cohort study, the risk for colon cancer was significantly elevated in people who ate higher amounts of lamb. Risk for rectal cancer was elevated for those who ate the most pork.

Mortality from different causes associated with meat, heme iron, nitrates, and nitrites in the NIH-AARP Diet and Health Study: population based cohort study.

Etemadi A, Sinha R, Ward MH, Graubard BI, Inoue-Choi M, Dawsey SM, Abnet CC

https://www.ncbi.nlm.nih.gov/pubmed/28487287
This cohort study showed increased risks of death from any cause, as well as increased death due to nine different causes associated with both processed and unprocessed red meat. The authors stated that this risk was accounted for, in part, by heme iron and nitrate/nitrite from processed meat.

Adolescent meat intake and breast cancer risk.

Farvid MS, Cho E, Chen WY, Eliassen AH, Willett WC
https://www.ncbi.nlm.nih.gov/pubmed/25220168
This prospective study of over 44,000 women found that those who consumed the most total red meat during childhood were at 43% increased risk for developing premenopausal breast cancer, compared with women who consumed the least.

Dietary protein sources in early adulthood and breast cancer incidence: prospective cohort study.

Farvid MS, Cho E, Chen WY, Eliassen AH, Willett WC
https://www.ncbi.nlm.nih.gov/pubmed/24916719
This large prospective cohort study concluded that higher red meat intake in early adulthood may be a risk factor for breast cancer.

Meat consumption, diabetes, and its complications.

Feskens EJ, Sluik D, van Woudenbergh GJ
https://www.ncbi.nlm.nih.gov/pubmed/23354681
This review and meta-analysis reports that eating high amounts of processed red meat raised risk of type 2 diabetes by 32%. The authors also review evidence which has found that eating processed meat increases risk of coronary heart disease, and that eating processed and fresh red meat increase risk of stroke.

Associations of processed meat and unprocessed red meat intake with incident diabetes: the Strong Heart Family Study.

Fretts AM, Howard BV, McKnight B, Duncan GE, Beresford SA, Mete M, Eilat-Adar S, Zhang Y, Siscovick DS
https://www.ncbi.nlm.nih.gov/pubmed/22277554
This prospective cohort study of American Indians reported that the consumption of processed meat was associated with higher risk of diabetes.

Dietary patterns, meat intake, and the risk of type 2 diabetes in women.

Fung TT, Schulze M, Manson JE, Willett WC, Hu FB
https://www.ncbi.nlm.nih.gov/pubmed/15534160/
The authors of this study concluded that the Western pattern of eating, especially a diet high in processed meats, may increase risk of type 2 diabetes in women. Higher risk of diabetes was seen for high intakes of red meat, total processed meats, bacon and hot dogs.

Dairy products and ovarian cancer: a pooled analysis of 12 cohort studies.

Genkinger JM, Hunter DJ, Spiegelman D, Anderson KE, Arslan A, Beeson WL, Buring JE, Fraser GE, Freudenheim JL, Goldbohm RA, Hankinson SE, Jacobs DR Jr, Koushik A, Lacey JV Jr, Larsson SC, Leitzmann M, McCullough ML, Miller AB, Rodriguez C, Rohan TE, Schouten LJ, Shore R, Smit E, Wolk A, Zhang SM, Smith-Warner SA.
https://www.ncbi.nlm.nih.gov/pubmed/16492930
This pooled analysis of 12 cohort studies reported a higher risk of ovarian cancer among women with high intakes of lactose, the primary sugar in dairy milk. Those who consumed the

equivalent of 3 or more servings of milk per day increased their risk of ovarian cancer by 19%.

Dairy consumption and 10-y total and cardiovascular mortality: a prospective cohort study in the Netherlands.

Goldbohm RA, Chorus AM, Galindo Garre F, Schouten LJ, van den Brandt PA
https://www.ncbi.nlm.nih.gov/pubmed/21270377/
In this cohort study of older adults in the Netherlands, dairy fat intake was associated with slightly increased all-cause and ischemic heart disease mortality among women.

Relation of time of introduction of cow milk protein to an infant and risk of type 1 diabetes mellitus.

Goldfarb MF
https://www.ncbi.nlm.nih.gov/pubmed/18410136
This paper reviews several studies of infant feeding that show a causal relationship between time of introduction of formula containing cow milk protein and risk of type-1 diabetes.

Using multicountry ecological and observational studies to determine dietary risk factors for Alzheimer's disease.

Grant WB
https://www.ncbi.nlm.nih.gov/pubmed/27454859
This review of evidence concluded that the most important dietary link to Alzheimer's Disease appears to be meat consumption, with eggs and high-fat dairy also contributing.

Trends in diet and Alzheimer's disease during the nutrition transition in Japan and developing countries.

Grant WB
https://www.ncbi.nlm.nih.gov/pubmed/24037034

This study using data from populations in Japan, India, China and Brazil found that as animal fat and calorie consumption increased, so did obesity rates and prevalence of Alzheimer's disease.

Health risk factors associated with meat, fruit and vegetable consumption in cohort studies: A comprehensive meta-analysis.

Grosso G, Micek A, Godos J, Pajak A, Sciacca S, Galvano F, Boffetta P
https://www.ncbi.nlm.nih.gov/pubmed/28850610
This meta-analysis of 20 studies reported that people who eat more red meat are more likely to have high body mass index, and to be overweight or obese than those who eat less red meat.

Dairy products do not lead to alterations in body weight or fat mass in young women in a 1-y intervention.

Gunther CW, Legowski PA, Lyle RM, McCabe GP, Eagan MS, Peacock M, Teegarden D
https://www.ncbi.nlm.nih.gov/pubmed/15817848
Results from this randomized intervention study counter the recent notion that dairy products encourage weight loss. In fact, participants assigned to a high dairy intake group gained more weight over the course of a year than those in the medium dairy or usual diet groups.

Association of dietary protein consumption with incident silent cerebral infarcts and stroke: the ARIC study.

Haring B, Misialek JR, Rebholz CM, Petruski-Ivleva N, Gottesman RF, Mosley TH, Alonso A
https://www.ncbi.nlm.nih.gov/pubmed/26514185
This prospective cohort study reported that consumption of red meat may increase the risk of ischemic stroke. Individuals who ate the most

red meat had a 47% increased risk for ischemic stroke, compared with those who ate the least. Those who ate the most eggs had a 41% increased risk for hemorrhagic stroke, compared with those who ate the least.

Association of meat and dairy consumption with normal weight metabolic obesity in men: the Qazvin Metabolic Diseases Study.

Hashemipour S, Esmailzadehha N, Mohammadzadeh M, Ziaee A
https://www.ncbi.nlm.nih.gov/pubmed/26729428
In this cross-sectional study of Iranian men, higher meat consumption was associated with visceral (around the abdomen) fat accumulation in normal weight individuals. Visceral fat is strongly associated with obesity-related complications like type 2 diabetes and coronary artery disease.

Red and processed meat intake and risk of esophageal adenocarcinoma: a meta-analysis of observational studies.

Huang W, Han Y, Xu J, Zhu W, Li Z
https://www.ncbi.nlm.nih.gov/pubmed/23179661
This meta-analysis indicates that eating red and processed meat may be associated with increased risk of esophageal adenocarcinoma (EAC). Those who ate the most red meat were 31% more likely to get EAC; those who ate the most processed meat were 41% more likely.

Dietary iron intake and body iron stores are associated with risk of coronary heart disease in a meta-analysis of prospective cohort studies.

Hunnicutt J, He K, Xun P
http://jn.nutrition.org/content/early/2014/01/07/jn.113.185124
In this meta-analysis looking at iron and heart disease, diets high in heme iron (found in meat) increased risk of coronary heart disease (CHD)

by 57%. Diets high in non-heme iron (found in plants) did not increase risk of CHD.

Intolerance of cow's milk and chronic constipation in children.

Iacono G, Cavataio F, Montalto G, Florena A, Tumminello M, Soresi M, Notarbartolo A, Carroccio A
https://www.ncbi.nlm.nih.gov/pubmed/9770556
This double-blind cross-over study found that cow's milk can cause constipation in children with milk intolerance.

Dietary Patterns and Type 2 Diabetes: A Systematic Literature Review and Meta-Analysis of Prospective Studies.

Jannasch F, Kröger J, Schulze MB
https://www.ncbi.nlm.nih.gov/pubmed/28424256
This meta-analysis reported that eating patterns characterized by red and processed meat, refined grains, high-fat dairy, eggs, and fried products were positively associated with diabetes.

Higher childhood red meat intake frequency is associated with earlier age at menarche.

Jansen EC, Marín C, Mora-Plazas M, Villamor E
https://www.ncbi.nlm.nih.gov/pubmed/26962195
This study found that red meat intake during childhood leads to earlier onset of puberty in adolescent girls. The researchers emphasized that earlier menarche negatively affects disease risk for breast cancer, obesity, cardiovascular disease, and other chronic conditions later in life.

Cow's milk challenge through human milk evoked immune responses in infants with cow's milk allergy.

Järvinen KM, Mäkinen-Kiljunen S, Suomalainen H
https://www.ncbi.nlm.nih.gov/pubmed/10518086

This study showed that cow's milk can cause an allergic response in breastfed infants whose mothers consume milk.

Meta-analyses of colorectal cancer risk factors.

Johnson CM, Wei C, Ensor JE, Smolenski DJ, Amos CI, Levin B, Berry DA
https://www.ncbi.nlm.nih.gov/pubmed/23563998/
This meta-analysis found a significant positive correlation between colorectal cancer and red meat consumption. Those who ate 5 servings per week had a 13% greater risk of the cancer.

Processed and unprocessed red meat consumption and risk of heart failure: prospective study of men.

Kaluza J, Akesson A, Wolk A
https://www.ncbi.nlm.nih.gov/pubmed/24926039
Findings from this prospective study of men showed that eating low to moderate amounts of processed red meat was associated with an increased risk of heart failure.

Long-term processed and unprocessed red meat consumption and risk of heart failure: A prospective cohort study of women.

Kaluza J, Åkesson A, Wolk A
https://www.ncbi.nlm.nih.gov/pubmed/26005173
This prospective study of more than 44,000 Swedish women found that eating processed red meat was associated with higher risk of heart failure.

Long-chain omega-3 fatty acids, fish intake, and the risk of type 2 diabetes mellitus.

Kaushik M, Mozaffarian D, Spiegelman D, Manson JE, Willett WC, Hu FB
https://www.ncbi.nlm.nih.gov/pubmed/19625683

This prospective cohort study reported that eating high amounts of fish may modestly increase risk of type 2 diabetes.Women who ate fish at least 5 times per week increased their risk of diabetes by 22%, compared to those who ate it less than once per month.

Red meat, poultry, fish intake and breast cancer risk among Hispanic and Non-Hispanic white women: The Breast Cancer Health Disparities Study.

Kim AE, Lundgreen A, Wolff RK, Fejerman L, John EM, Torres-Mejía G, Ingles SA, Boone SD, Connor AE, Hines LM, Baumgartner KB, Giuliano A, Joshi AD, Slattery ML, Stern MC
https://www.ncbi.nlm.nih.gov/pubmed/26898200
This case-control study found that, among Hispanic women, those who ate the highest amounts of red and processed meat increased their risk for breast cancer by 42%, compared with those who ate the least. Non-Hispanic women with the highest intakes of tuna increased their risk of breast cancer by 25%, compared with those who ate the least amount of tuna.

A review of potential metabolic etiologies of the observed association between red meatconsumption and development of type 2 diabetes mellitus.

Kim Y, Keogh J, Clifton P
https://www.ncbi.nlm.nih.gov/pubmed/25838035
This review of the effect of red and processed meat on type 2 diabetes stated saturated fat, high sodium levels, carcinogens, nitrates, heme iron, and other compounds found in red and processed meats may all contribute to decreased insulin sensitivity and other risk factors for type 2 diabetes.

Short-term exclusive breastfeeding predisposes young children with increased genetic risk of type I diabetes to progressive beta-cell autoimmunity.

Kimpimäki T, Erkkola M, Korhonen S, Kupila A, Virtanen SM, Ilonen J, Simell O, Knip M
https://www.ncbi.nlm.nih.gov/pubmed/11206413
This study in Finland of 3,000 infants with genetically increased risk for developing diabetes showed that early introduction of cow's milk increased susceptibility to type 1 diabetes.

Meat, fish, and ovarian cancer risk: Results from 2 Australian case-control studies, a systematic review, and meta-analysis.

Kolahdooz F, van der Pols JC, Bain CJ, Marks GC, Hughes MC, Whiteman DC, Webb PM; Australian Cancer Study (Ovarian Cancer) and the Australian Ovarian Cancer Study Group
https://www.ncbi.nlm.nih.gov/pubmed/20392889
This study reported that in two case-control studies, with a combination of over 4,000 female participants, those who ate the most processed meat were 18% more likely to get ovarian cancer.

Relationship between meat intake and the development of acute coronary syndromes: the CARDIO2000 case-control study.
Kontogianni MD1, Panagiotakos DB, Pitsavos C, Chrysohoou C, Stefanadis C.
https://www.ncbi.nlm.nih.gov/pubmed/17356558/
In this randomized, case-control study, those who ate the highest amounts of red meat were more likely to have cardiac disease. White meat consumption showed less prominent results.

High and low-fat dairy intake, recurrence, and mortality after breast cancer diagnosis.

Kroenke CH, Kwan ML, Sweeney C, Castillo A, Caan BJ
https://www.ncbi.nlm.nih.gov/pubmed/23492346
In this cohort study of about 1800 women, eating high-fat dairy was related to a higher risk of death after breast cancer diagnosis.

Red meat consumption is associated with the risk of type 2 diabetes in men but not in women: a Japan Public Health Center-based Prospective Study.

Kurotani K, Nanri A, Goto A, Mizoue T, Noda M, Oba S, Kato M, Matsushita Y, Inoue M, Tsugane S; Japan Public Health Center-based Prospective Study Group
https://www.ncbi.nlm.nih.gov/pubmed/23651531
This prospective cohort study of over 63,000 Japanese adults found that eating high amounts of red meat is associated with higher risk of type 2 diabetes, as compared to those who ate less red meat.

Prospective study of diet and ovarian cancer.

Kushi LH, Mink PJ, Folsom AR, Anderson KE, Zheng W, Lazovich D, Sellers TA
https://www.ncbi.nlm.nih.gov/pubmed/9883790
In this prospective cohort study of over 29,000 postmenopausal women, lactose (the sugar found in milk) moderately elevated risk of epithelial ovarian cancer. Eating eggs also increased risk of ovarian cancer.

Processed and unprocessed red meat consumption and hypertension in women.

Lajous M, Bijon A, Fagherazzi G, Rossignol E, Boutron-Ruault MC, Clavel-Chapelon F
https://www.ncbi.nlm.nih.gov/pubmed/25080454/
In a cohort of over 44,000 French women, researchers observed that those who ate the most processed red meat were more likely to get hypertension (high blood pressure). Those who ate ≥5 servings of processed red meat per week had a 17% higher rate of hypertension than that of women who consumed less than one serving per week.

Milk and lactose intakes and ovarian cancer risk in the Swedish Mammography Cohort.

Larsson SC, Bergkvist L, Wolk A
https://www.ncbi.nlm.nih.gov/
pubmed/15531686
In this cohort study, women who drank 2 or more glasses of milk per day had twice this risk of serous ovarian cancer as those who drank it seldom or never.

Red meat and processed meat consumption and all-cause mortality: a meta-analysis.

Larsson SC, Orsini N
https://www.ncbi.nlm.nih.gov/
pubmed/24148709
In this meta-analysis, those who ate red meat and processed meat were more likely to die from any cause.

The cooked meat-derived mammary carcinogen 2-amino-1-methyl-6-phenylimidazo[4,5-b]pyridine promotes invasive behaviour of breast cancer cells. Toxicology.

Lauber SN, Gooderham NJ
https://www.ncbi.nlm.nih.gov/
pubmed/20951759
This study concluded that a carcinogen from cooked meat could increase the likelihood that breast cancer cells will become metastatic, worsening existing disease.

Avoiding milk is associated with a reduced risk of insulin resistance and the metabolic syndrome: findings from the British Women's Heart and Health Study.

Lawlor DA, Ebrahim S, Timpson N, Davey Smith G
https://www.ncbi.nlm.nih.gov/
pubmed/15910636
This study of over 4,000 postmenopausal British women reported that those who had never drank milk had lower indicators of insulin resistance, lower body mass index, higher high-density lipoprotein cholesterol, and lower incidence of type 2 diabetes than women who drank milk.

Low protein intake is associated with a major reduction in IGF-1, cancer, and overall mortality in the 65 and younger but not older population.

Levine ME, Suarez JA, Brandhorst S, Balasubramanian P, Cheng CW, Madia F, Fontana L, Mirisola MG, Guevara-Aguirre J, Wan J, Passarino G, Kennedy BK, Wei M, Cohen P, Crimmins EM, Longo VD
https://www.ncbi.nlm.nih.gov/
pubmed/24606898
This study of over 6,300 American adults found that those who eat the most animal protein are more likely to die at a younger age. Those who ate the most animal protein increased their risk of dying from diabetes five-fold.

Red meat intake and risk of ESRD.

Lew QJ, Jafar TH, Koh HW, Jin A, Chow KY, Yuan JM, Koh WP
https://www.ncbi.nlm.nih.gov/
pubmed/27416946
The authors of this prospective cohort study of over 63,000 Chinese adults reported that eating red meat may increase the risk of end-stage renal disease (ESRD) in the general population. In this study, replacing a single serving of red meat with another source of protein, such as soy products or legumes, cut the risk for disease by over 60%.

Associations between red meat intake and biomarkers of inflammation and glucose metabolism in women.

Ley SH, Sun Q, Willett WC, Eliassen AH, Wu K, Pan A, Grodstein F, Hu FB
https://www.ncbi.nlm.nih.gov/pmc/articles/
PMC3893727/
An analysis of the diets and blood of over 3,600 women found that as total red meat consumption increased, biomarkers for disease risk also increased. These included C-reactive protein (a biomarker of infections and diseases including heart disease and cancer), hemoglobin A1c (an indicator of diabetes risk), and stored

iron (a mineral which in excess is associated with heart disease, cancer, and diabetes). Weight also increased with increasing meat consumption.

Egg consumption and risk of cardiovascular diseases and diabetes: A meta-analysis.

Li Y, Zhou C, Zhou X, Li L
https://www.ncbi.nlm.nih.gov/pubmed/23643053
This meta-analysis suggests that people who eat higher amounts of eggs increase their risk of cardiovascular disease and diabetes. People who ate the most eggs had a 19% increased risk of cardiovascular disease (CVD) and 68% increased risk of diabetes, compared with those who ate the fewest eggs. Among people who already had diabetes, those who ate the most eggs had an 83% higher risk of CVD than those who ate the fewest eggs.

Meat consumption, N-acetyl transferase 1 and 2 polymorphism and risk of breast cancer in Danish postmenopausal women.

Lilla C, Verla-Tebit E, Risch A, Jäger B, Hoffmeister M, Brenner H, Chang-Claude J
https://www.ncbi.nlm.nih.gov/pubmed/18090909
This study of over 24,000 Danish women reported that those who ate more meat (red meat, poultry, fish, and processed meat) had a significantly higher risk of breast cancer. Every 25 gram increase in total meat, red meat, and processed meat led to a 9, 15, and 23% increase in risk of breast cancer, respectively.

Cured meat, vegetables, and bean-curd foods in relation to childhood acute leukemia risk: A population based case-control study.

Liu CY, Hsu YH, Wu MT, Pan PC, Ho CK, Su L, Xu X, Li Y, Christiani DC; Kaohsiung Leukemia Research Group.
https://www.ncbi.nlm.nih.gov/pubmed/19144145
In this case-control study in China, eating cured or smoked meat and fish more than once a week was associated with a 74% increased risk of acute leukemia.

Dairy products intake and cancer mortality risk: a meta-analysis of 11 population-based cohort studies.

Lu W, Chen H, Niu Y, Wu H, Xia D, Wu Y
https://www.ncbi.nlm.nih.gov/pmc/articles/PMC5073921/
In this large meta-analysis, whole milk intake in men contributed to significantly elevated risk of death from prostate cancer. The higher the amount of whole milk that men typically drank, the higher their risk of death from prostate cancer.

Dietary protein intake and risk of type 2 diabetes in US men and women.

Malik VS, Li Y, Tobias DK, Pan A, Hu FB
https://www.ncbi.nlm.nih.gov/pubmed/27022032
This prospective cohort study of over 200,000 adults reported that those who consumed the most animal protein increased their risk for type 2 diabetes by 13%, compared with those who consumed the least animal protein.

Association between pre-pregnancy consumption of meat, iron intake, and the risk of gestational diabetes: the SUN project.

Marí-Sanchis A, Díaz-Jurado G, Basterra-Gortari FJ, de la Fuente-Arrillaga C, Martínez-González MA, Bes-Rastrollo M
https://www.ncbi.nlm.nih.gov/pubmed/28285431
This prospective study of over 3,200 Spanish women found that those who ate higher amounts of meat, especially red and processed meat, before pregnancy were significantly more likely to get gestational diabetes during pregnancy.

Low-fat yoghurt intake in pregnancy associated with increased child asthma and allergic rhinitis risk: a prospective cohort study.

Maslova E, Halldorsson TI, Strøm M, Olsen SF
https://www.ncbi.nlm.nih.gov/pmc/articles/PMC3582227/
This prospective cohort study of over 61,000 pregnant mothers and their children reported that mothers who ate yogurt during pregnancy were more likely to have children who later developed asthma and allergic rhinitis.

Usual consumption of specific dairy foods is associated with breast cancer in the Roswell Park Cancer Institute Databank and BioRepository.

McCann SE, Hays J, Baumgart CW, Weiss EH, Yao S, Ambrosone CB
http://cdn.nutrition.org/content/1/3/e000422
This case-control study found that higher intakes of American, cheddar, and cream cheeses were associated with an increased risk of breast cancer. Participants who drank milk were more likely than those who did not to have estrogen receptor-negative breast cancer.

Unprocessed red and processed meats and risk of coronary artery disease and type 2 diabetes—an updated review of the evidence.

Micha R, Michas G, Mozaffarian D
https://www.ncbi.nlm.nih.gov/pubmed/23001745
In this meta-analysis of cohort studies, significantly higher risk of coronary heart disease is seen among people who eat processed meat. Eating both red meat and processed meat were associated with increased risk of type 2 diabetes.

Red and processed meat consumption and risk of incident coronary heart disease, stroke, and diabetes mellitus: a systematic review and meta-analysis.

Micha R, Wallace SK, Mozaffarian D
https://www.ncbi.nlm.nih.gov/pubmed/20479151
This meta-analysis concluded that eating processed meats is associated with higher incidence of coronary heart disease and type 2 diabetes.

Milk intake and risk of mortality and fractures in women and men: cohort studies.

Michaëlsson K, Wolk A, Langenskiöld S, Basu S, Warensjö Lemming E, Melhus H, Byberg L
https://www.ncbi.nlm.nih.gov/pubmed/25352269
This large prospective study in Sweden found that, among people drinking 200 ml of milk per day, there was an increased risk of death from cardiovascular disease.

Associations of red and processed meat with survival among patients with cancers of the upper aerodigestive tract and lung.

Miles FL, Chang SC, Morgenstern H, Tashkin D, Rao JY, Cozen W, Mack T, Lu QY, Zhang ZF
https://www.ncbi.nlm.nih.gov/pubmed/27188908
This analysis of patients with cancers of the upper aerodigestive tract (UADT) found that those who ate the highest amounts of red or processed meats were more likely to die from their cancer. Similarly, among patients with lung cancer, there was also some increased risk of dying from the cancer among those who ate the most processed or red meats.

A prospective study of dietary calcium, dairy products and prostate cancer risk

Mitrou PN, Albanes D, Weinstein SJ, Pietinen P, Taylor PR, Virtamo J, Leitzmann MF
https://www.ncbi.nlm.nih.gov/pubmed/17278090
The results from this large prospective study suggest that intake of calcium or some related component contained in dairy foods is associated with increased risk of prostate cancer.

Adherence to cancer prevention recommendations and antioxidant and inflammatory status in premenopausal women.

Morimoto Y, Beckford F, Cooney RV, Franke AA, Maskarinec G
https://www.ncbi.nlm.nih.gov/pubmed/26051510
This cross-sectional study of 275 women reported that those who avoid red meat are more likely to be at a healthy weight and have lower levels of chronic inflammation and oxidative stress than those who eat red meat.

Meat, fish, and colorectal cancer risk: the European Prospective Investigation into cancer and nutrition.

Norat T, Bingham S, Ferrari P, Slimani N, Jenab M, Mazuir M, Overvad K, Olsen A, Tjønneland A, Clavel F, Boutron-Ruault MC, Kesse E, Boeing H, Bergmann MM, Nieters A, Linseisen J, Trichopoulou A, Trichopoulos D, Tountas Y, Berrino F, Palli D, Panico S, Tumino R, Vineis P, Bueno-de-Mesquita HB, Peeters PH, Engeset D, Lund E, Skeie G, Ardanaz E, González C, Navarro C, Quirós JR, Sanchez MJ, Berglund G, Mattisson I, Hallmans G, Palmqvist R, Day NE, Khaw KT, Key TJ, San Joaquin M, Hémon B, Saracci R, Kaaks R, Riboli E
https://www.ncbi.nlm.nih.gov/pubmed/15956652
This prospective cohort study of over 470,000 European adults found that risk of colorectal cancer is higher among those who eat high amounts of red and processed meat .

Dairy products and breast cancer: the IGF-1, estrogen, and bGH hypothesis.

Outwater JL, Nicholson A, Barnard N
https://www.ncbi.nlm.nih.gov/pubmed/9247884
This article discusses the hormones, growth factors, fat and various chemical contaminants found in dairy products that have been implicated in the proliferation of human breast cancer cells.

Changes in red meat consumption and subsequent risk of type 2 diabetes mellitus: three cohorts of US men and women.

Pan A, Sun Q, Bernstein AM, Manson JE, Willett WC, Hu FB
https://www.ncbi.nlm.nih.gov/pubmed/23779232
By tracking diet and health of participants over 4 years, this large study found that eating more than 1/2 serving of red meat per day was associated with a 48% elevated risk of diabetes. Reducing red meat was associated with a 14% lower risk of diabetes.

Meat consumption and colorectal cancer risk: an evaluation based on a systematic review of epidemiologic evidence among the Japanese population.

Pham NM, Mizoue T, Tanaka K, Tsuji I, Tamakoshi A, Matsuo K, Wakai K, Nagata C, Inoue M, Tsugane S, Sasazuki S; Research Group for the Development and Evaluation of Cancer Prevention Strategies in Japan.
https://www.ncbi.nlm.nih.gov/pubmed/24842864
This systematic review of 19 studies concluded that eating high amounts of red meat and processed meat may increase risk of colorectal cancer or colon cancer among the Japanese population.

Dairy, calcium, vitamin D and ovarian cancer risk in African–American women.

Qin B, Moorman PG, Alberg AJ, Barnholtz-Sloan JS, Bondy M, Cote ML, Funkhouser E, Peters ES, Schwartz AG, Terry P, Schildkraut JM, Bandera EV
https://www.ncbi.nlm.nih.gov/pubmed/27632371
In this case-control study of African-American women, those who drank whole milk were more likely to have ovarian cancer.

Milk consumption is a risk factor for prostate cancer: meta-analysis of case-control studies.

Qin LQ, Xu JY, Wang PY, Kaneko T, Hoshi K, Sato A
https://www.ncbi.nlm.nih.gov/pubmed/15203374
This meta-analysis of 11 case-control studies determined milk consumption was positively associated with prostate cancer.

Milk consumption is a risk factor for prostate cancer in Western countries: evidence from cohortstudies.

Qin LQ, Xu JY, Wang PY, Tong J, Hoshi K
https://www.ncbi.nlm.nih.gov/pubmed/17704029
This meta-analysis suggests that drinking milk and eating dairy products may increase the risk of prostate cancer.

Egg, red meat, poultry intake and risk of lethal prostate cancer in the prostate specific antigen-era: incidence and survival.

Richman EL, Kenfield SA, Stampfer MJ, Giovannucci EL, Chan JM
https://www.ncbi.nlm.nih.gov/pubmed/21930800
In this prospective study of more than 27,000 men, those who ate 2.5 eggs per week, increased their risk for a deadly form of prostate cancer by 81%, compared with men who consumed less than half an egg per week.

Processed Meat and Colorectal Cancer Risk: A Pooled Analysis of Three Italian Case-Control Studies.

Rosato V, Tavani A, Negri E, Serraino D, Montella M, Decarli A, La Vecchia C, Ferraroni M
https://www.ncbi.nlm.nih.gov/pubmed/28426250
This study analyzed the results from three case-control studies of meat consumption and gastric cancer in Southern Europe. Participants who ate the most processed meat were significantly more likely to get colon cancer, and particularly proximal colon cancer.

Is there a relationship between red or processed meat intake and obesity? A systematic review and meta-analysis of observational studies.

Rouhani MH, Salehi-Abargouei A, Surkan PJ, Azadbakht L
https://www.ncbi.nlm.nih.gov/pubmed/24815945
This meta-analysis revealed that red and processed meat intake is directly associated with risk of obesity, and higher body mass index and waist circumference.

Meat, fish, and esophageal cancer risk: a systematic review and dose-response meta-analysis.

Salehi M, Moradi-Lakeh M, Salehi MH, Nojomi M, Kolahdooz F
https://www.ncbi.nlm.nih.gov/pubmed/23590703
This literature review found that people who ate the highest levels of red meat and processed meat had significantly increased risk of esophageal cancers.

Red and processed meat consumption and risk of glioma in adults: A systematic review and meta-analysis of observational studies.

Saneei P, Willett W, Esmaillzadeh A
https://www.ncbi.nlm.nih.gov/pubmed/26600837
In this meta-analysis of 18 observational studies, researchers reported that those who ate higher amounts of unprocessed red meat were somewhat more likely to have gliomas.

Significance of cow's milk protein antibodies as risk factor for childhood IDDM: interaction with dietary cow's milk intake and HLA-DQB1 genotype.

Saukkonen T, Virtanen SM, Karppinen M, Reijonen H, Ilonen J, Räsänen L, Akerblom HK, Savilahti E
https://www.ncbi.nlm.nih.gov/pubmed/9498633
In this case-control study, children with type 1 diabetes (IDDM) have higher levels of cow's milk protein antibodies than their sibling controls, and these high levels of antibodies are independent risk markers for IDDM.

Intake of animal products and stroke mortality in the Hiroshima/Nagasaki Life Span Study.

Sauvaget C, Nagano J, Allen N, Grant EJ, Beral V
https://www.ncbi.nlm.nih.gov/pubmed/12913025/
This study of 40,349 people showed no protection from stroke through the consumption of animal products.

Processed meat intake and incidence of type 2 diabetes in younger and middle-aged women.

Schulze MB, Manson JE, Willett WC, Hu FB
https://www.ncbi.nlm.nih.gov/pubmed/14576980/
In this prospective cohort study of over 91,000 American women, those who ate meat 5 or more times per week were 91% more likely to get type 2 diabetes than those who ate meat less than once per week. Frequent consumption of bacon, hot dogs, and sausage was each associated with an increased risk of diabetes.

Food groups and risk of type 2 diabetes mellitus: a systematic review and meta-analysis of prospective studies.

Schwingshackl L, Hoffmann G, Lampousi AM, Knüppel K, Iqbal K, Schwedhelm C, Bechthold A, Schlesinger S, Boeing H

https://www.ncbi.nlm.nih.gov/pubmed/28397016
This meta-analysis of prospective studies found increased risk of type 2 diabetes with increasing consumption of red meat and processed meat.

Dietary protein from different food sources, incident metabolic syndrome and changes in its components: An 11-year longitudinal study in healthy community-dwelling adults.

Shang X, Scott D, Hodge A, English DR, Giles GG, Ebeling PR, Sanders KM
https://www.ncbi.nlm.nih.gov/pubmed/27746001
In this cohort study of over 5,300 participants who were tracked for over 11 years, those who ate the most chicken and red meat were more likely to get metabolic syndrome.

Meat intake and mortality: a prospective study of over half a million people.

Sinha R, Cross AJ, Graubard BI, Leitzmann MF, Schatzkin A
https://www.ncbi.nlm.nih.gov/pubmed/19307518
This prospective cohort study of over 500,000 people found that eating red and processed meat was associated with modest increases in death from any cause, death from cancer, and death from cardiovascular disease.

Dietary intake of total, animal, and vegetable protein and risk of type 2 diabetes in the European Prospective Investigation into Cancer and Nutrition (EPIC)-NL study.

Sluijs I, Beulens JW, van der A DL, Spijkerman AM, Grobbee DE, van der Schouw YT
https://www.ncbi.nlm.nih.gov/pubmed/19825820
This prospective cohort study of over 38,000 European adults reported a more than two-fold increase in risk of type 2 diabetes for those who ate the most animal protein.The authors

concluded that diets high in animal protein are associated with an increased diabetes risk.

Whole milk intake is associated with prostate cancer-specific mortality among U.S. male physicians.

Song Y, Chavarro JE, Cao Y, Qiu W, Mucci L, Sesso HD, Stampfer MJ, Giovannucci E, Pollak M, Liu S, Ma J
https://www.ncbi.nlm.nih.gov/pubmed/23256145
In this prospective cohort study of over 21,000 men, those who drank whole milk were more likely to get prostate cancer. Among men with prostate cancer already, those who drank whole milk were more likely to die from prostate cancer. Those who drank skim and low-fat milk were more likely to get non-aggressive prostate cancer.

A prospective study of red meat consumption and type 2 diabetes in middle-aged and elderly women: the women's health study.

Song Y, Manson JE, Buring JE, Liu S
https://www.ncbi.nlm.nih.gov/pubmed/15333470/
The data from this prospective cohort study indicates that eating high amounts of red meat, especially processed meats, may increase risk of developing type 2 diabetes in women. Those who ate processed meat at least 5 times per week were almost one and a half times more likely to get diabetes than those who ate processed meat less than once per month.

Fish Intake in Pregnancy and Child Growth: A Pooled Analysis of 15 European and US Birth Cohorts.

Stratakis N, Roumeliotaki T, Oken E, Barros H, Basterrechea M, Charles MA, Eggesbø M, Forastiere F, Gaillard R, Gehring U, Govarts E, Hanke W, Heude B, Iszatt N, Jaddoe VW, Kelleher C, Mommers M, Murcia M, Oliveira A, Pizzi C, Polańska K, Porta D, Richiardi L, Rifas-Shiman S, Schoeters G, Sunyer J, Thijs C, Viljoen K, Vrijheid M, Vrijkotte TG, Wijga AH, Zeegers MP, Kogevinas M, Chatzi L
https://www.ncbi.nlm.nih.gov/pubmed/26882542
In this very large study, mothers who ate a lot of fish during pregnancy were more likely to have children who would later become obese. Those who ate fish more than three times per week had children with higher body mass indexes through early childhood when compared to those who ate less fish per week. Researchers suspect chemical pollutants found in fish may alter fat metabolism and contribute to weight gain.

Red meat intake may increase the risk of colon cancer in Japanese, a population with relatively low red meat consumption.

Takachi R, Tsubono Y, Baba K, Inoue M, Sasazuki S, Iwasaki M, Tsugane S; Japan Public Health Center-Based Prospective Study Group
https://www.ncbi.nlm.nih.gov/pubmed/22094846
In this prospective cohort study, women who ate higher amounts of red meat and men who ate higher amounts of any type of meat were significantly more likely to get colon cancer.

Meat, dietary heme Iron, and risk of type 2 diabetes mellitus: the Singapore Chinese Health Study.

Talaei M, Wang YL, Yuan JM, Pan A, Koh WP
https://www.ncbi.nlm.nih.gov/pubmed/28535164
In this prospective cohort study in China of over 63,000 adults, red meat (pork, beef, lamb), poultry and fish intake were associated with an increased risk of type 2 diabetes. Those who ate the most red meat increased their risk by 23%.

Fish Consumption, Mercury Levels, and Amyotrophic Lateral Sclerosis (ALS)

Tessman R, Uher M
https://www.aan.com/PressRoom/Home/

GetDigitalAsset/12339
This case-control study found that high mercury levels in the body associated with fish and shellfish consumption increased risk for developing Lou Gehrig's disease (amyotrophic lateral sclerosis [ALS]).

Type of Vegetarian Diet, Body Weight, and Prevalence of type 2 diabetes

Tonstad S, Butler T, Yan R, Fraser GE
https://www.ncbi.nlm.nih.gov/pubmed/19351712
This prospective study compared vegans, lacto-ovo-vegetarians, semi-vegetarians, pesco-tarians and non-vegetarians. The more animal products, such as red meat and fish, that were included in the diet, the greater the risk of type 2 diabetes.

American Cancer Society (ACS) Nutrition and Physical Activity Guidelines after colon cancer diagnosis and disease-free (DFS), recurrence-free (RFS), and overall survival (OS) in CALGB 89803 (Alliance).

Van Blarigan E, Fuchs CS, Niedzwiecki D.
http://ascopubs.org/doi/abs/10.1200/JCO.2017.35.15_suppl.10006
Among patients with stage 3 colon cancer, those with a healthy body mass index who exercised and followed a diet high in fruits, vegetables, and whole grains and low in red/processed meats had longer overall survival and disease-free survival rates, compared with patients who did not meet these parameters.

Dietary fat and meat intake in relation to risk of type 2 diabetes in men.

van Dam RM, Willett WC, Rimm EB, Stampfer MJ, Hu FB
https://www.ncbi.nlm.nih.gov/pubmed/11874924/
This prospective cohort study of over 42,000 males found that frequent consumption of processed meat was associated with a higher risk for type 2 diabetes

Prospective Study of Cured Meats Consumption and Risk of Chronic Obstructive Pulmonary Disease in Men.

Varraso R, Jiang R, Barr RG, Willett WC, Camargo CA Jr
https://www.ncbi.nlm.nih.gov/pubmed/17785711
This prospective study of over 42,000 men found that those who ate cured meats daily had more than two and half times the risk of Chronic Obstructive Pulmonary Disease (COPD) compared with those who ate these products rarely or never.

The association of meat intake and the risk of type 2 diabetes may be modified by body weight.

Villegas R, Shu XO, Gao YT, Yang G, Cai H, Li H, Zheng W
https://www.ncbi.nlm.nih.gov/pubmed/17088942/
In this prospective cohort study of Chinese women, processed meat intake was positively associated with the risk of type 2 diabetes.

Maternal Western dietary patterns and the risk of developing a cleft lip with or without a cleft palate.

Vujkovic M, Ocke MC, van der Spek PJ, Yazdanpanah N, Steegers EA, Steegers-Theunissen RP
https://www.ncbi.nlm.nih.gov/pubmed/17666614
In this case-control study of women in the Netherlands, those women with a "Western dietary pattern," (high intakes of organ meat, red meat, processed meat, pizza, legumes, potatoes, French fries, condiments, and mayonnaise, but low intakes of fruits) had an approximately two-fold higher risk of a cleft lip or cleft palate among their offspring.

Meat consumption and colorectal cancer risk in Japan: The Takayama study.

Wada K, Oba S, Tsuji M, Tamura T, Konishi K, Goto Y, Mizuta F, Koda S, Hori A, Tanabashi S, Matsushita S, Tokimitsu N, Nagata C
https://www.ncbi.nlm.nih.gov/pubmed/28256076
This prospective cohort study of over 30,000 adults in Japan found that those who ate the most meat were 36% more likely to get colorectal cancer than those who ate the least meat. Red meat similarly increased risk by 44%. The authors concluded that abstaining from excessive consumption of meat might be protective against developing colorectal cancer.

Red meat intake is positively associated with non-fatal acute myocardial infarction in the Costa Rica Heart Study.

Wang D, Campos H, Baylin A
https://www.ncbi.nlm.nih.gov/pubmed/28875869
This case-control study of over 4,000 people found that the odds of acute MI (heart attack) increased significantly with increasing consumption of red meat and cured meat.

Red and processed meat consumption and mortality: dose-response meta-analysis of prospective cohort studies.
Wang X, Lin X, Ouyang YY, Liu J, Zhao G, Pan A, Hu FB
https://www.ncbi.nlm.nih.gov/pubmed/26143683
This meta-analysis indicated that eating higher amounts of red meat and processed meat is associated with an increased risk of death from any cause, death from cardiovascular disease and death from cancer.

Prognostic value of elevated levels of intestinal microbe-generated metabolite trimethylamine-n-oxide in patients with heart failure: refining the gut hypothesis.

Wilson Tang WH, Wang Z, Fan Y, Levison B, Hazen JE, Donahue LM, Wu Y, Hazen SL
https://www.ncbi.nlm.nih.gov/pmc/articles/PMC4254529/
In a study that tracked 720 patients who had previously been treated for heart failure, those with the highest levels of trimethylamine N-oxide (TMAO) in their blood had a 3.4-fold increase risk of dying, compared with those with the lowest levels. TMAO is produced during digestion of certain foods, including organ meats, red meat, and eggs. Its levels in the blood are also affected by other factors, including gut microbiota.

Potential health hazards of eating red meat.

Wolk A
https://www.ncbi.nlm.nih.gov/pubmed/27597529
This article analyzes six prospective cohort studies. It reports that eating 100 grams of red meat per day increased the risk for stroke and for breast cancer, death from heart disease, colorectal cancer, and advanced prostate cancer.

Dietary Protein Sources and Incidence of Breast Cancer: A Dose-Response Meta-Analysis of Prospective Studies.

Wu J, Zeng R, Huang J, Li X, Zhang J, Ho JC, Zheng Y
https://www.ncbi.nlm.nih.gov/pubmed/27869663
In this meta-analysis, increasing consumption of red meat, fresh red meat and processed meat was associated with increasing risk of breast cancer.

Nutritional factors in relation to endometrial cancer: a report from a population-based case-control study in Shanghai, China.

Xu WH, Dai Q, Xiang YB, Zhao GM, Ruan ZX, Cheng JR, Zheng W, Shu XO

https://www.ncbi.nlm.nih.gov/pubmed/17230528
This case-control study of endometrial cancer found that people who ate the most animal products had nearly four times the risk of cancer, compared with those who ate the least animal products. Cancer risk increased as protein and fat from animal products was increased.

Red Meat Consumption and the Risk of Stroke: A Dose-Response Meta-analysis of Prospective Cohort Studies.

Yang C, Pan L, Sun C, Xi Y, Wang L, Li D
https://www.ncbi.nlm.nih.gov/pubmed/26935118
The findings from this study indicate that high consumption of red meat, especially processed red meat, increases the risk of stroke.

Red and processed meat consumption and gastric cancer risk: a systematic review and meta-analysis.

Zhao Z, Yin Z, Zhao Q
https://www.ncbi.nlm.nih.gov/

pubmed/28430644
This meta-analysis found that those who ate the most red meat were 1.67 times more likely to have gastric cancer than those who ate the least red meat. Those who ate the most processed meat were 1.76 times more likely to have gastric cancer than those who ate the least processed meat.

Meat consumption is associated with esophageal cancer risk in a meat- and cancer-histological-type dependent manner.

Zhu HC, Yang X, Xu LP, Zhao LJ, Tao GZ, Zhang C, Qin Q, Cai J, Ma JX, Mao WD, Zhang XZ, Cheng HY, Sun XC
https://www.ncbi.nlm.nih.gov/pubmed/24395380
This meta-analysis reported that high intake of red meat was associated with an increased risk of esophageal squamous cell carcinoma. High meat intake, especially processed meat, is likely to increase esophageal adenocarcinoma risk.

18.0 Addendum II: Citations and References

1 Andrews, B.R. *Habit*. The American Journal of Psychology. https://books.google.com/books. . .

2 Sklar, Aesal Y. et. Al. *Reading and Doing Arithmetic Nonconsciously*. PNAS. https://www.ncbi.nlm.nih.gov/pmc/articles/PMC3511729/

3 Borreli, Lizette. *The Human Brain: The Subconscious Mind Processes Thoughts to Feel Like Second Nature*. Medical Daily. https://www.medicaldaily.com/pulse/human-brain-your-subconscious-mind-processes-habits-feel-second-nature-343538

4 Prochaska, James and Di Clementa, Carlo. *Transtheoretical Theory: Toward a More Integrative Model of Change*. https://www.researchgate.net/profile/James_Prochaska/publication/232461028_Trans-Theoretical_Therapy_-_Toward_A_More_Integrative_Model_of_Change/links/02e7e52d6d-b5ee1110000000.pdf

5 Scholl, Jesse. *The Stages of Change*. Experience Life. https://experiencelife.com/article/the-stages-of-change/

6 Duhugg, Charles. *How Habits Work*. Charles Duhigg. http://charlesduhigg.com/how-habits-work/

7 Lipton, Bruce. *The Biology of Belief*. https://www.brucelipton.com/books/biology-of-belief

8 The 8 Unusual Habits of Famous and Successful People (Infographic). Entrepreneur. https://www.entrepreneur.com/article/297580

9 *Brain Waves and Meditation*. The Norwegian University of Science and Technology. https://www.sciencedaily.com/releases/2010/03/100319210631.htm

10 *Alpha State of Mind: What it Is, Why You Want it, And How to Get There*. Mind to Succeed. https://www.mindtosucceed.com/alpha-state-of-mind.html

11 *Forget Setting Goals Focus On This Instead*. Entrepreneur. https://www.entrepreneur.com/article/230333

12 *This Day in History*. History. https://www.history.com/this-day-in-history/hillary-and-tenzing-reach-everest-summit

13 Taleb, Nassim. *Fooled by Randomness*. Nassim Nicholas Taleb's Home Page. http://www.fooledbyrandomness.com

14 Weinberger, Matt and Canales, Katie. *The incredible story of Elon Musk, from getting bullied in school to the most interesting man in tech*. Business Insider. http://www.businessinsider.com/the-rise-of-elon-musk-2016-7

15 Slayback, Zacharay. *3 Ways to Develop a Bias for Action*. Praxis. http://discoverpraxis.com/start-now-3-ways-to-develop-a-bias-for-action/

16 Robaton, Anna. *Why So Many American Hate Their Jobs*. CBS News. https://www.cbsnews.com/news/why-so-many-americans-hate-their-jobs/

17 Emily. *Interviews: Prep it Now to Nail It Later, Lesson from Yo Yo Ma*. Refresh Your Step. https://refreshyourstep.com/interviews-prep-it-now-nail-it-later-a-lesson-from-yo-yo-ma/

18 Elkins, Kathleen. *Self-Made Millionaires Agree on How Many Hours You Should Be Working to Succeed*. CNBC. https://www.cnbc.com/2017/06/15/self-made-millionaires-agree-on-how-many-hours-you-should-be-working.html

19 Lang, Susan S. *Mindless Autopilot Drives People to Dramatically Underestimate How Many Daily Food Decisions They Make.* Cornell Chronicle. http://www.news.cornell.edu/stories/2006/12/mindless-autopilot-drives-people-underestimate-food-decisions

20 *Ketchup as a Vegetable.* http://en.wikipedia.org/wiki/Ketchup_as_a_vegetable

21 Kessler, Daniel. *Jamie Oliver Meets Some First Graders Who Don't Know Fruits and Vegetables.* Treehugger. https://www.treehugger.com/corporate-responsibility/jamie-oliver-meets-some-first-graders-who-dont-know-fruits-and-vegetables.html

22 Myles, Ian. A. *Fast food forever: reviewing the impacts of the Western diet on immunity.* Nutritional Journal. https://www.ncbi.nlm.nih.gov/pmc/articles/PMC4074336/

23 Aggawal, Bharat. B. PhD. *Chronic Disease Caused by Chronic Inflammation Require Chronic Treatment" Anti-Inflammatory Role of Spices.* https://www.omicsonline.org/open-access/chronic-diseases-caused-by-chronic-inflammation-require-chronic-treatment-2155-9899.1000238.php?aid=28021

24 Manzel, Amdt. *Role of Western Diet in Auto-Inflammatory Disease.* Current Allergy Asthma Rep. https://www.ncbi.nlm.nih.gov/pmc/articles/PMC4034518/

25 Giugliano, D. et al. *The Effects of Diet on Inflammation.* Pub Med https://www.ncbi.nlm.nih.gov/pubmed/16904534

26 Minniehane, Anne M. *Low-grade inflammation, diet, composition and health.* R J. Nutrition. https://www.ncbi.nlm.nih.gov/pmc/articles/PMC4579563/

27 Welsh A. Jean. *Consumption of added sugars is decreasing in the United States.* The American Journal of Clinical Nutrition. http://ajcn.nutrition.org/content/94/3/726.full

28 Griffin, R. Morgan. *Obesity Epidemic Astronomical.* Web MD. http://www.webmd.com/diet/obesity/features/obesity-epidemic-astronomical#1

29 *Added Sugar is Hiding in 74% of Packaged Foods.* Sugar Science. http://sugarscience.ucsf.edu/hidden-in-plain-sight/#.WwDB7y-OZMdV

30 Danger of Carbohydrates. (n.d.). Retrieved from https://www.diabetes.co.uk/features/danger-of-carbohydrates.html

31 Bruske, Ed. Grist. Scientists say carbs – not fat – are the biggest problem with America's diet. https://grist.org/article/food-2010-12-20-scientists-say-carbs-not-fat-are-the-biggest-problem-with/

32 Pereira, M. A., & Liu, S. (2003). Types of Carbohydrates and Risk of Cardiovascular Disease. *Journal of Women's Health*, 12(2), 115-122. doi:10.1089/154099903321576501

33 The Hidden Dangers Of A Low Carbohydrate Diet. (2017, September 30). Retrieved from https://bengreenfieldfitness.com/article/low-carb-ketogenic-diet-articles/the-hidden-dangers-of-a-low-carbohydrate-diet/

34 Liu, A. G., Ford, N. A., Hu, F. B., Zelman, K. M., Mozaffarian, D., & Kris-Etherton, P. M. (2017). A healthy approach to dietary fats: understanding the science and taking action to reduce consumer confusion. *Nutrition Journal*, 16(1). doi:10.1186/s12937-017-0271-4

35 Holecek, M. (2012). Side Effects of Long-Term Glutamine Supplementation. *Journal of Parenteral and Enteral Nutrition*, 37(5), 607-616. doi:10.1177/0148607112460682

36 Jacobsen, C. (2004). Developing polyunsaturated fatty acids as functional ingredients. *Functional Foods, Cardiovascular Disease and Diabetes*, 307-332. doi:10.1533/9781855739499.3.307

37 Da Boit, M., Hunter, A. M., & Gray, S. R. (2017). Fit with good fat? The role of n-3 polyunsaturated fatty acids on exercise performance. *Metabolism*, 66, 45-54. doi:10.1016/j.metabol.2016.10.007

38 684 Hepatic steatosis and insulin resistance (IR): Does the etiology makes the difference? (2005). *Journal of Hepatology*, 42, 249-250. doi:10.1016/s0168-8278(05)82094-x

39 Kim, Y., Keogh, J., & Clifton, P. (2016). Differential Effects of Red Meat/Refined Grain

Diet and Dairy/Chicken/Nuts/Whole Grain Diet on Glucose, Insulin and Triglyceride in a Randomized Crossover Study. *Nutrients*, *8*(11), 687. doi:10.3390/nu8110687

40 Low Carbohydrate Diet. *The Nutrition Source*. Harvard T.H. Chan. https://www.hsph.harvard.edu/nutritionsource/carbohydrates/low carbohydrate-diets

41 Krebs, N. F., Gao, D., Gralla, J., Collins, J. S., & Johnson, S. L. (2010). Efficacy and Safety of a High Protein, Low Carbohydrate Diet for Weight Loss in Severely Obese Adolescents. *The Journal of Pediatrics*, *157*(2), 252-258. doi:10.1016/j.jpeds.2010.02.010

42 Low Carb Diets and Sleep Quality | SimplyShredded.com. (2010, February 1). Retrieved from http://www.simplyshredded.com/low-carb-diets-and-sleep-quality.html

43 Low carbohydrate diet to achieve weight loss and improve HbA1c in type 2 diabetes and pre-diabetes: experience from one general practice - Unwin - 2014 - Practical Diabetes - Wiley Online Library. (2014). Retrieved from http://onlinelibrary.wiley.com/doi/10.1002/pdi.1835/abstract

44 Eugene J Fine, E. J. (2016). Part 2: Can low carbohydrate ketogenic diets inhibit cancers? doi:10.18258/7344

45 Hu, T., Mills, K. T., Yao, L., Demanelis, K., Eloustaz, M., Yancy, W. S., ... Bazzano, L. A. (2012). Effects of Low-Carbohydrate Diets Versus Low-Fat Diets on Metabolic Risk Factors: A Meta-Analysis of Randomized Controlled Clinical Trials. *American Journal of Epidemiology*, *176*(suppl_7), S44-S54. doi:10.1093/aje/kws264

46 Harvard Health Publishing. (2017, August 7). Halt heart disease with a plant-based, oil-free diet - Harvard Health. Retrieved from https://www.health.harvard.edu/heart-health/halt-heart-disease-with-a-plant-based-oil-free-diet-

47 How Does Your Mouth Affect Your health? (n.d.). Retrieved from https://www.webmd.com/oral-health/plaque-on-teeth#1

48 Roberts, R. O., Roberts, L. A., Geda, Y. E., Cha, R. H., Pankratz, V. S., O'Connor, H. M., ... Petersen, R. C. (2012). Relative Intake of Macronutrients Impacts Risk of Mild Cognitive Impairment or Dementia. *Journal of Alzheimer's Disease*, *32*(2), 329-339. doi:10.3233/jad-2012-120862

49 Longland, T. M., Oikawa, S. Y., Mitchell, C. J., Devries, M. C., & Phillips, S. M. (2016). Higher compared with lower dietary protein during an energy deficit combined with intense exercise promotes greater lean mass gain and fat mass loss: a randomized trial. *The American Journal of Clinical Nutrition*, *103*(3), 738-746. doi:10.3945/ajcn.115.119339

50 Eat Fat, Live Longer? (2017, September 12). Retrieved from https://www.ucdavis.edu/news/eat-fat-live-longer

51 Alexandre, Misoto. *95% of Diets Fail, Except This*. FitWirr. https://www.fitwirr.com/health/tips/why-diets-fail

52 Neuman Fredric, M.D. *Why Diets Fail*. Psychology Today. https://www.psychologytoday.com/blog/fighting-fear/201310/why-diets-fail

53 Bernard J. Luskin, Ed.D., LMFT. *The Habit Replacement Loop*. https://www.psychologytoday.com/us/blog/the-media-psychology-effect/201705/the-habit-replacement-loop.

54 *Sustainable Behavior: Changing the habit by changing the context*. Colorado State University. http://blog.sustainability.colostate.edu/?q=node/59

55 Moghaddam, Elham. *The Effects of Fat and Protein on Glycemic Responses in Nondiabetic Humans Vary with Waist Circumference, Fasting Plasma Insulin, and Dietary Fiber Intake*. http://jn.nutrition.org/content/136/10/2506.full?_ga=2.57361962.1885303565.1505428947-364750831.1505428947

56 Baltazar, Amanda. *Can Vegan or Vegetarian Diets Help Reduce Arthritis Inflammation?* Arthritis Foundation. http://www.arthritis.org/living-with-arthritis/arthritis-diet/anti-inflammatory/vegan-and-vegetarian-diets.php

57 *The Vegetarian Food Pyramid*. Loma Linda University. http://www.vegetariannutrition.org/6icvn/food-pyramid.pdf

58 Prevention Research Centers | Yale University Yale-Griffin Prevention Research Center | PRC. (2015, October 5). Retrieved from https://www.cdc.gov/prc/center-descriptions/yale-university.htm

59 The China Study - T. Colin Campbell Center for Nutrition Studies. (n.d.). Retrieved from https://nutritionstudies.org/the-china-study/

60 Why Processed Foods May Promote Gut Inflammation. (23, May). Retrieved from https://www.livescience.com/54839-food-additives-gut-bacteria.html

61 Diets Avoiding Dry-Cooked Foods Can Protect Against Diabetes, Say Mount Sinai Researchers | Mount Sinai - New York. (2016, August 23). Retrieved from http://www.mountsinai.org/about-us/newsroom/press-releases/diets-avoiding-dry-cooked-foods-can-protect-against-diabetes-say-mount-sinai-researchers

62 What happens to your body when you give up meat. (2017, July 15). Retrieved from http://www.independent.co.uk/life-style/health-and-families/features/how-cutting-meat-out-of-your-diet-changes-your-body-vegetarian-vegan-a6825631.html

63 Annex C: Use of Phosphate Salts and Nitrites in the Preparation of Meat Products - Canadian Food Inspection Agency. (2016, December 22). Retrieved from http://www.inspection.gc.ca/food/meat-and-poultry-products/manual-of-procedures/chapter-4/annex-c/eng/1370525150531/1370525354148

64 Allred, C. D. (2001). Dietary genistin stimulates growth of estrogen-dependent breast cancer tumors similar to that observed with genistein. *Carcinogenesis*, 22(10), 1667-1673. doi:10.1093/carcin/22.10.1667

65 Miraghajani, M. S., Esmaillzadeh, A., Najafabadi, M. M., Mirlohi, M., & Azadbakht, L. (2012). Soy Milk Consumption, Inflammation, Coagulation, and Oxidative Stress Among Type 2 Diabetic Patients With Nephropathy. *Diabetes Care*, 35(10), 1981-1985. doi:10.2337/dc12-0250

66 The Right Start — Tell Clients Breakfast Can Promote Weight Loss and Provide Other Great Benefits. (n.d.). Retrieved from http://www.todaysdietitian.com/newarchives/070113p24.shtml

67 Veggies at Breakfast. (n.d.). Retrieved from http://www.todaysdietitian.com/newarchives/070114p40.shtml

68 10 Low-Glycemic Fruits for Diabetes. (n.d.). Retrieved from http://www.healthline.com/health/diabetes/low-glycemic-fruits-for-diabetes

69 Could grapefruit juice protect against diabetes? (2014, October 9). Retrieved from https://www.nhs.uk/news/diabetes/could-grapefruit-juice-protect-against-diabetes/

70 Incidence of the Paradox. (n.d.). *Cycles and Social Choice*, 24-37. doi:10.1017/9781316848371.003

71 Micronutrients in Cancer Prevention. (2010). *Micronutrients in Health and Disease*, 103-131. doi:10.1201/ebk1439821060-8

72 Digestive Issues. American Nutrition Magazine. http://americannutritionassociation.org/newsletter/digestive-issues

73 AGRAWAL, A., & WHORWELL, P. J. (2007). Review article: abdominal bloating and distension in functional gastrointestinal disorders - epidemiology and exploration of possible mechanisms. *Alimentary Pharmacology & Therapeutics*, 27(1), 2-10. doi:10.1111/j.1365-2036.2007.03549.x

74 Gerritsen, J., Smidt, H., Rijkers, G. T., & De Vos, W. M. (2011). Intestinal microbiota in human health and disease: the impact of probiotics. *Genes & Nutrition*, 6(3), 209-240. doi:10.1007/s12263-011-0229-7

75 Harvard Health Publishing. (2018, February 22). The benefits of probiotics bacteria - Harvard Health. Retrieved from https://www.health.harvard.edu/staying-healthy/the-benefits-of-probiotics

76 Digesting Fat, Optimizing Your Health, and My Daily Supplements - Dr. Mark Hyman. (2017, April 28). Retrieved from http://

drhyman.com/blog/2017/04/28/digesting-fat-optimizing-health-daily-supplements/

77 Probiotics for the prevention antibiotic-associated diarrhea in children | Cochrane. (n.d.). Retrieved from http://www.cochrane.org/CD004827/IBD_probiotics-prevention-antibiotic-associated-diarrhea-children

78 Aslani, A., Ghannadi, A., & Rostami, F. (2016). Design, formulation, and evaluation of ginger medicated chewing gum. *Advanced Biomedical Research*, 5(1), 130. doi:10.4103/2277-9175.187011

79 Hu, M. (2011). Effect of ginger on gastric motility and symptoms of functional dyspepsia. *World Journal of Gastroenterology*, 17(1), 105. doi:10.3748/wjg.v17.i1.105

80 Wu, K., Rayner, C. K., Chuah, S., Changchien, C., Lu, S., Chiu, Y., ... Lee, C. (2008). Effects of ginger on gastric emptying and motility in healthy humans. *European Journal of Gastroenterology & Hepatology*, 20(5), 436-440. doi:10.1097/meg.0b013e3282f4b224

81 Makhdoomi Arzati, M., Mohammadzadeh Honarvar, N., Saedisomeolia, A., Anvari, S., Effatpanah, M., Makhdoomi Arzati, R., ... Djalali, M. (2017). The Effects of Ginger on Fasting Blood Sugar, Hemoglobin A1c, and Lipid Profiles in Patients with Type 2 Diabetes. *International Journal of Endocrinology and Metabolism*, In Press(In Press). doi:10.5812/ijem.57927

82 Hewlings, S., & Kalman, D. (2017). Curcumin: A Review of Its' Effects on Human Health. *Foods*, 6(10), 92. doi:10.3390/foods6100092

83 Secretion of Bile and the Role of Bile Acids In Digestion. (n.d.). Retrieved from http://www.vivo.colostate.edu/hbooks/pathphys/digestion/liver/bile.html

84 Hegde, K., Haniadka, R., Alva, A., Periera-Colaco, M., & Baliga, M. (2013). Turmeric (Curcuma longa L.) the Golden Curry Spice as a Nontoxic Gastroprotective Agent. *Bioactive Food as Dietary Interventions for Liver and Gastrointestinal Disease*, 337-348. doi:10.1016/b978-0-12-397154-8.00040-3

85 Park, W., Amin, A. R., Chen, Z. G., & Shin, D. M. (2013). New Perspectives of Curcumin in Cancer Prevention. *Cancer Prevention Research*, 6(5), 387-400. doi:10.1158/1940-6207.capr-12-0410

86 Shanmugam, M., Rane, G., Kanchi, M., Arfuso, F., Chinnathambi, A., Zayed, M., ... Sethi, G. (2015). The Multifaceted Role of Curcumin in Cancer Prevention and Treatment. *Molecules*, 20(2), 2728-2769. doi:10.3390/molecules20022728

87 Wilken, R., Veena, M. S., Wang, M. B., & Srivatsan, E. S. (2011). Curcumin: A review of anti-cancer properties and therapeutic activity in head and neck squamous cell carcinoma. *Molecular Cancer*, 10(1), 12. doi:10.1186/1476-4598-10-12

88 Soleimani, V., Sahebkar, A., & Hosseinzadeh, H. (2018). Turmeric (Curcuma longa) and its major constituent (curcumin) as nontoxic and safe substances: Review. *Phytotherapy Research*. doi:10.1002/ptr.6054

89 Raggi, P. (2016). Inflammation, depression and atherosclerosis or depression, inflammation and atherosclerosis? *Atherosclerosis*, 251, 542-543. doi:10.1016/j.atherosclerosis.2016.07.902

90 Inflammation and Cancer. (2017). doi:10.3390/books978-3-03842-609-7

91 JCI -Inflammatory links between obesity and metabolic disease. (2011, June 1). Retrieved from https://www.jci.org/articles/view/57132

92 Daily, J. W., Yang, M., & Park, S. (2016). Efficacy of Turmeric Extracts and Curcumin for Alleviating the Symptoms of Joint Arthritis: A Systematic Review and Meta-Analysis of Randomized Clinical Trials. *Journal of Medicinal Food*, 19(8), 717-729. doi:10.1089/jmf.2016.3705

93 Where Do You Get Your Fiber? | NutritionFacts.org. (2015, September 29). Retrieved from https://nutritionfacts.org/2015/09/29/where-do-you-get-your-fiber/

94 Improve Your Gut Health With Fiber. (n.d.). Retrieved from http://www.webmd.com/diet/features/fiber-digestion

95 Fibre. (n.d.). Retrieved from http://www.diabetes.ca/diabetes-and-you/healthy-living-resources/diet-nutrition/fibre

96 Slavin, J. (2013). Fiber and Prebiotics: Mechanisms and Health Benefits. *Nutrients, 5*(4), 1417-1435. doi:10.3390/nu5041417

97 Soluble vs. insoluble fiber: MedlinePlus Medical Encyclopedia. (n.d.). Retrieved from https://medlineplus.gov/ency/article/002136.htm

98 USGS; The Water In You; https://water.usgs.gov/edu/propertyyou.html

99 University of California-Davis; Your Brain on H2O; https://shcs.ucdavis.edu/blog/healthy-habits/your-brain-h2o; Last accessed June 18, 2017

100 Frontiers in Human Neuroscience; Subjective thirst moderates changes in speed of responding associated with water consumption; journal.frontiersin.org/article/10.3389/fnhum.2013.00363/full; July 16, 2013

101 Nutrients; Dehydration Influences Mood and Cognition: A Plausible Hypothesis?; https://www.ncbi.nlm.nih.gov/pmc/articles/PMC3257694/; May 2011

102 USDA; Dehydration Affects Mood; https://www.ars.usda.gov/news-events/news/research-news/2009/dehydration-affects-mood-not-just-motor-skills/; November 23, 2009

103 Benefits Of Drinking Water: H2O Nourishes The Digestive System, Helps With Fluid Balance. (n.d.). Retrieved from http://www.medicaldaily.com/health-benefits-drinking-water-digestive-system-fluid-balance-391799

104 Edelman, D. (2017, April 19). How Water Impacts Blood Sugars. Retrieved from https://www.diabetesdaily.com/blog/2011/02/how-water-impacts-blood-sugars/

105 75% of Americans May Suffer From Chronic Dehydration, According to Doctors. (n.d.). Retrieved from https://www.medicaldaily.com/75-americans-may-suffer-chronic-dehydration-according-doctors-247393

106 Food Ingredients that Cause Inflammation | Slideshows. (n.d.). Retrieved from http://www.arthritis.org/living-with-arthritis/arthritis-diet/foods-to-avoid-limit/food-ingredients-and-inflammation-2.php

107 DiNicolantonio, James J. *Sugar Addiction is It Real? A narrative review* British Journal of Sports Medicine. http://bjsm.bmj.com/content/early/2017/08/23/bjsports-2017-097971

108 Roberto A. Ferdman. (2015). Where people around the world eat the most sugar and fat. Retrieved from https://www.washingtonpost.com/news/wonk/wp/2015/02/05/where-people-around-the-world-eat-the-most-sugar-and-fat/

109 Roberto A. Ferdman. (2015). Where people around the world eat the most sugar and fat. Retrieved from https://www.washingtonpost.com/news/wonk/wp/2015/02/05/where-people-around-the-world-eat-the-most-sugar-and-fat/

110 Ferdman, Roberto A. *Where people around the world eat the most sugar and fat.* Washington Post. https://www.washingtonpost.com/news/wonk/wp/2015/02/05/where-people-around-the-world-eat-the-most-sugar-and-fat/?utm_term=.ef244185915f

111 FastStats. (2017, May 3). Retrieved from https://www.cdc.gov/nchs/fastats/diet.htm

112 Effects of Fat and Protein on Glycemic Responses in Nondiabetic Humans Vary with Waist Circumference, Fasting Plasma Insulin, and Dietary Fiber Intake | The Journal of Nutrition | Oxford Academic. (2006, October 1). Retrieved from http://jn.nutrition.org/content/136/10/2506.full?_ga=2.57361962.1885303565.1505428947-364750831.1505428947

113 increase in dietary protein improves the blood glucose response in persons with type 2 diabetes | The American Journal of Clinical Nutrition | Oxford Academic. (2003, October 1). Retrieved from http://ajcn.nutrition.org/content/78/4/734.full?_ga=2.251847305.1885303565.1505428947-364750831.1505428947

114 Simple Steps to Preventing Diabetes. (2016, July 25). Retrieved from https://www.hsph.harvard.edu/nutritionsource/diabetes-prevention/preventing-diabetes-full-story

115 Begnoche, T. (2018, March 9). List Of High Glycemic Index Fruits And Vegetables. Retrieved from https://www.curejoy.com/content/high-glycemic-index-fruits-and-vegetables/

116 How I Learned to Regulate My Blood Sugar With a Plant-Based Diet - One Green Planet. (2014, October 7). Retrieved from http://www.onegreenplanet.org/natural-health/how-i-learned-to-regulate-my-blood-sugar-with-a-plant-based-diet

117 Swanson, D., Block, R., & Mousa, S. A. (2012). Omega-3 Fatty Acids EPA and DHA: Health Benefits Throughout Life. *Advances in Nutrition*, *3*(1), 1-7. doi:10.3945/an.111.000893

118 Solon-Biet, S., McMahon, A., Ballard, J., Ruohonen, K., Wu, L., Cogger, V., … Simpson, S. (2014). The Ratio of Macronutrients, Not Caloric Intake, Dictates Cardiometabolic Health, Aging, and Longevity in Ad Libitum-Fed Mice. *Cell Metabolism*, *19*(3), 418-430. doi:10.1016/j.cmet.2014.02.009

119 Zinn, C., Wood, M., Williden, M., Chatterton, S., & Maunder, E. (2017). Ketogenic diet benefits body composition and well-being but not performance in a pilot case study of New Zealand endurance athletes. *Journal of the International Society of Sports Nutrition*, *14*(1). doi:10.1186/s12970-017-0180-0

120 Evangeliou, A., Vlachonikolis, I., Mihailidou, H., Spilioti, M., Skarpalezou, A., Makaronas, N., … Smeitink, J. (2003). Application of a Ketogenic Diet in Children With Autistic Behavior: Pilot Study. *Journal of Child Neurology*, *18*(2), 113-118. doi:10.1177/08830738030180020501

121 Wyker, B. A., & Davison, K. K. (2013). Plant-Based Diet Theory of Planned Behavior Measure. *PsycTESTS Dataset*. doi:10.1037/t22871-000

122 Fogelholm, M. (2008). Faculty of 1000 evaluation for The effects of high-intensity intermittent exercise training on fat loss and fasting insulin levels of young women. *F1000 - Post-publication peer review of the biomedical literature*. doi:10.3410/f.1108284.564309

123 Aly, S. M. (2014). Role of Intermittent Fasting on Improving Health and Reducing Diseases. *International Journal of Health Sciences*, *8*(3), v-vi. doi:10.12816/0023985

124 Arnason, T. G., Bowen, M. W., & Mansell, K. D. (2017). Effects of intermittent fasting on health markers in those with type 2 diabetes: A pilot study. *World Journal of Diabetes*, *8*(4), 154. doi:10.4239/wjd.v8.i4.154

125 Byrne, N. M., Sainsbury, A., King, N. A., Hills, A. P., & Wood, R. E. (2017). Intermittent energy restriction improves weight loss efficiency in obese men: the MATADOR study. *International Journal of Obesity*, *42*(2), 129-138. doi:10.1038/ijo.2017.206

126 10 Evidence-Based Health Benefits of Intermittent Fasting. (n.d.). Retrieved from https://www.healthline.com/nutrition/10-health-benefits-of-intermittent-fasting

127 The Benefits Of Intermittent Fasting - Dr Brian Mowll. (2018, April 30). Retrieved from https://drmowll.com/the-benefits-of-intermittent-fasting/

128 Young, Dr. Scott. A Focus on Weight Management. The Permanente Journal. http://kpcmi.org/files/PermJournal_Weight_Mgmt_Supplement.pdf

129 Collier, R. (2013). Intermittent fasting: the science of going without. *Canadian Medical Association Journal*, *185*(9), E363-E364. doi:10.1503/cmaj.109-4451

130 Circadian Rhythms - Fasting 19. (2018, April 25). Retrieved from https://idmprogram.com/circadian-rhythms-fasting-19/

131 Flood, J. E., & Rolls, B. J. (2007). Soup preloads in a variety of forms reduce meal energy intake. *Appetite*, *49*(3), 626-634. doi:10.1016/j.appet.2007.04.002

132 Varady, K. A., Bhutani, S., Klempel, M. C., Kroeger, C. M., Trepanowski, J. F., Haus, J. M., … Calvo, Y. (2013). Alternate day fasting for weight loss in normal weight and overweight subjects: a randomized

controlled trial. *Nutrition Journal, 12*(1). doi:10.1186/1475-2891-12-146

133 Johnson, J. B., Summer, W., Cutler, R. G., Martin, B., Hyun, D., Dixit, V. D., ... Mattson, M. P. (2007). Corrigendum to "Alternate day calorie restriction improves clinical findings and reduces markers of oxidative stress and inflammation in overweight adults with moderate asthma" [Free Radic. Biol. Med. 42 (2007) 665–674]. *Free Radical Biology and Medicine, 43*(9), 1348. doi:10.1016/j.freeradbiomed.2007.06.008

134 Bhutani, S., Klempel, M. C., Kroeger, C. M., Trepanowski, J. F., & Varady, K. A. (2013). Alternate day fasting and endurance exercise combine to reduce body weight and favorably alter plasma lipids in obese humans. *Obesity, 21*(7), 1370-1379. doi:10.1002/oby.20353

135 Hoddy, K. K., Kroeger, C. M., Trepanowski, J. F., Barnosky, A., Bhutani, S., & Varady, K. A. (2014). Meal timing during alternate day fasting: Impact on body weight and cardiovascular disease risk in obese adults. *Obesity*, n/a-n/a. doi:10.1002/oby.20909

136 Longo, V., & Mattson, M. (2014). Fasting: Molecular Mechanisms and Clinical Applications. *Cell Metabolism, 19*(2), 181-192. doi:10.1016/j.cmet.2013.12.008

137 McKiernan, F., Hollis, J. H., McCabe, G. P., & Mattes, R. D. (2009). Thirst-Drinking, Hunger-Eating; Tight Coupling? *Journal of the American Dietetic Association, 109*(3), 486-490. doi:10.1016/j.jada.2008.11.027

138 Martin, C. K., Rosenbaum, D., Han, H., Geiselman, P. J., Wyatt, H. R., Hill, J. O., ... Foster, G. D. (2011). Change in Food Cravings, Food Preferences, and Appetite During a Low-Carbohydrate and Low-Fat Diet. *Obesity, 19*(10), 1963-1970. doi:10.1038/oby.2011.62

139 Hattangadi, V. (2015, February 2). Benefits of drinking water in the morning - Dr. Vidya Hattangadi. Retrieved from http://drvidyahattangadi.com/benefits-of-drinking-water-in-the-morning/

140 Thornton, S. N. (2016). Increased Hydration Can Be Associated with Weight Loss. *Frontiers in Nutrition, 3*. doi:10.3389/fnut.2016.00018

141 Benelam, L.V. Hydration and Health. https://onlinelibrary.wiley.com/doi/abs/10.1111/j.1467-3010.2009.01795.x

142 Herbal Remedies. (n.d.). *SpringerReference*. doi:10.1007/springerreference_188046

143 Jackman, S. R., Witard, O. C., Philp, A., Wallis, G. A., Baar, K., & Tipton, K. D. (2017). Branched-Chain Amino Acid Ingestion Stimulates Muscle Myofibrillar Protein Synthesis following Resistance Exercise in Humans. *Frontiers in Physiology, 8*. doi:10.3389/fphys.2017.00390

144 Yoon, M. (2016). The Emerging Role of Branched-Chain Amino Acids in Insulin Resistance and Metabolism. *Nutrients, 8*(7), 405. doi:10.3390/nu8070405

145 Okimura, Y. (2014). Branched Chain Amino Acids and Muscle Atrophy Protection. *Branched Chain Amino Acids in Clinical Nutrition*, 49-63. doi:10.1007/978-1-4939-1914-7_4

146 Eckel, R. H., Hanson, A. S., Chen, A. Y., Berman, J. N., Yost, T. J., & Brass, E. P. (1992). Dietary substitution of medium-chain triglycerides improves insulin-mediated glucose metabolism in NIDDM subjects. *Diabetes, 41*(5), 641-647. doi:10.2337/diabetes.41.5.641

147 Harvard Health. https://www.health.harvard.edu/blog/nutritional-psychiatry-your-brain-on-food-201511168626

148 T. S. Sathyanarayana Rao, M. R. Asha, B. N. Ramesh, and K. S. Jagannatha Rao. (2008). Retrieved from https://www.ncbi.nlm.nih.gov/pmc/articles/PMC2738337/

149 Shaheen E Lakhan, Karen F Vieira. (2008). Nutritional therapies for mental disorders. Retrieved from https://www.ncbi.nlm.nih.gov/pmc/articles/PMC2248201/

150 Jennifer Remnant, Jean Adams. (2015) The nutritional content and cost of supermarket ready-meals. Cross-sectional analysis, Volume 92, 36-42. Retrieved from https://www.sciencedirect.com/science/article/pii/S0195666315002159

151 Dirt Poor: Have Fruits and Vegetables Become Less Nutritious?. Retrieved from https://www.scientificamerican.com/article/soil-depletion-and-nutrition-loss/

152 Neil Bernard Boyle, Clare Lawton, Louise Dye. (2017). The Effects of Magnesium Supplementation on Subjective Anxiety and Stress—A Systematic Review. Retrieved from https://www.ncbi.nlm.nih.gov/pmc/articles/PMC5452159/

153 What you need to know about magnesium. Retrieved from https://www.dietitians.ca/Your-Health/Nutrition-A-Z/Minerals/Food-Sources-of-Magnesium.aspx

154 Rapid recovery from major depression using magnesium treatment. Retrieved from https://www.ncbi.nlm.nih.gov/pubmed/16542786

155 Emily Deans M.D. (2013). Zinc: an Antidepressant. Retrieved from https://www.psychologytoday.com/blog/evolutionary-psychiatry/201309/zinc-antidepressant

156 Swardfager W, Herrmann N, McIntyre RS, Mazereeuw G, Goldberger K, Cha DS, Schwartz Y, Lanctôt KL. (2013). Potential roles of zinc in the pathophysiology and treatment of major depressive disorder. Retrieved from https://www.ncbi.nlm.nih.gov/pubmed/23567517

157 Robert J. Cousins. (2013). Gastrointestinal Factors Influencing Zinc Absorption and Homeostasis. Retrieved from https://www.ncbi.nlm.nih.gov/pmc/articles/PMC3777256/

158 Jurowski, K., Szewczyk, B., Nowak, G., & Piekoszewski, W. (2014). Biological consequences of zinc deficiency in the pathomechanisms of selected diseases. *JBIC Journal of Biological Inorganic Chemistry*, *19*(7), 1069-1079. doi:10.1007/s00775-014-1139-0

159 Catherine Shaffer, Ph.D. (2018). Vitamin B Function in the Body. Retrieved from https://www.news-medical.net/health/Vitamin-B-Function-in-the-Body.aspx

160 Retrieved from https://www.umm.edu/health/medical/altmed/supplement/vitamin-b6-pyridoxine

161 Retrieved from https://www.umm.edu/health/medical/altmed/supplement/vitamin-b9-folic-acid

162 Retrieved from https://www.umm.edu/health/medical/altmed/supplement/vitamin-b12-cobalamin

163 Scott, K. R., & Barrett, A. M. (2007). Dementia syndromes: evaluation and treatment. *Expert Review of Neurotherapeutics*, *7*(4), 407-422. doi:10.1586/14737175.7.4.407

164 Kamal. (2018). L-Tyrosine. Retrieved from https://examine.com/supplements/l-tyrosine/

165 James Lake, MD. (2017). L-tryptophan and 5-hydroxytryptophan in Mental Health Care. Retrieved from https://www.psychologytoday.com/blog/integrative-mental-health-care/201709/l-tryptophan-and-5-hydroxytryptophan-in-mental-health

166 Peet M, Stokes C. (2005). Omega-3 fatty acids in the treatment of psychiatric disorders. Retrieved from https://www.ncbi.nlm.nih.gov/pubmed/15907142

167 Dr. James L. Wilson's. Sleep Disruptions. Retrieved from http://adrenalfatigue.org/sleep-disruptions/

168 Cherie L. Marvel, PhD, Sergio Paradiso, MD, PhD. (2008). Cognitive and neurological impairment in mood disorders. Retrieved from https://www.ncbi.nlm.nih.gov/pmc/articles/PMC2570029/

169 (2018). Understanding the stress response. Retrieved from https://www.health.harvard.edu/staying-healthy/understanding-the-stress-response

170 April Kahn. (2016). What Causes Irritable Mood?. Retrieved from https://www.healthline.com/symptom/irritable-mood#modal-close

171 Cornish, S., & Mehl-Madrona, L. (2008). The Role of Vitamins and Minerals in Psychiatry. *Integrative Medicine Insights*, *3*, 117863370800300. doi:10.4137/117863370800300003

172 Cavaye, J. (2018, March 1). Why nutritional psychiatry is the future of mental

health treatment. Retrieved from https://theconversation.com/why-nutritional-psychiatry-is-the-future-of-mental-health-treatment-92545

173 Scull, A. (2015, April 16). Mad Science: The Treatment of Mental Illness Fails to Progress [Excerpt]. Retrieved from https://www.scientificamerican.com/article/mad-science-the-treatment-of-mental-illness-fails-to-progress-excerpt/

174 Cavaye, J. (2018, March 1). Why nutritional psychiatry is the future of mental health treatment. Retrieved from https://theconversation.com/why-nutritional-psychiatry-is-the-future-of-mental-health-treatment-92545

175 Anthony L. Komaroff. The gut-brain connection. Retrieved from https://www.health.harvard.edu/diseases-and-conditions/the-gut-brain-connection

176 Fawne Hansen. HPA Axis Dysfunction. Retrieved from https://adrenalfatiguesolution.com/hpa-axis/

177 The Brain and Mental Illness. Retrieved from https://www.webmd.com/mental-health/brain-mental-illness

178 Sonnenburg, Justin. Scientific American Excerpt from the Good Gut https://www.scientificamerican.com/article/gut-feelings-the-second-brain-in-our-gastrointestinal-systems-excerpt/

179 Tim Taylor, . Intestines. Retrieved from http://www.innerbody.com/image/dige08.html

180 Gunnar C. Hansson. (2013). Role of mucus layers in gut infection and inflammation. Retrieved from https://www.ncbi.nlm.nih.gov/pmc/articles/PMC3716454/

181 Retrieved from http://www.gutmicrobiotaforhealth.com/en/about-gut-microbita-info/

182 (2016). Interaction Between the Brain and the Digestive System. Retrieved from https://www.ncbi.nlm.nih.gov/books/NBK279994/

183 Retrieved from http://www.aboutyourgut.com/digestion-system-functions.aspx

184 Petrus R. de Jong, José M. González-Navajas, Nicolaas J. G. Jansen. (2016). The digestive tract as the origin of systemic inflammation. Retrieved from https://ccforum.biomedcentral.com/articles/10.1186/s13054-016-1458-3

185 Monsen ER. Iron nutrition and absorption: dietary factors which impact iron bioavailability.. Retrieved from https://www.ncbi.nlm.nih.gov/pubmed/3290310

186 Katherine R. Groschwitz, BS, Simon P. Hogan, PhD. (2016). Intestinal Barrier Function: Molecular Regulation and Disease Pathogenesis. Retrieved from https://www.ncbi.nlm.nih.gov/pmc/articles/PMC4266989/

187 Stephan C Bischoff, Giovanni Barbara, Wim Buurman, Theo Ockhuizen, Jörg-Dieter Schulzke, Matteo Serino Herbert Tilg, Alastair Watson, Jerry M Wells. (2014). Intestinal permeability – a new target for disease prevention and therapy. Retrieved from https://www.ncbi.nlm.nih.gov/pmc/articles/PMC4253991/

188 Marilia Carabotti, Annunziata Scirocco, Maria Antonietta Maselli, Carola Severi. (2015). The gut-brain axis: interactions between enteric microbiota, central and enteric nervous systems. Retrieved from https://www.ncbi.nlm.nih.gov/pmc/articles/PMC4367209/

189 Zhu, X., Han, Y., Du, J., Liu, R., Jin, K., & Yi, W. (2017). Microbiota-gut-brain axis and the central nervous system. Oncotarget, 8(32). doi:10.18632/oncotarget.17754

190 Geuking MB, Köller Y, Rupp S, McCoy KD. (2014). The interplay between the gut microbiota and the immune system.. Retrieved from https://www.ncbi.nlm.nih.gov/pubmed/24922519

191 Hsin-Jung Wu, Eric Wu. (2012). The role of gut microbiota in immune homeostasis and autoimmunity. Retrieved from https://www.ncbi.nlm.nih.gov/pmc/articles/PMC3337124/

192 (2018). Intestinal gas. Retrieved from https://www.mayoclinic.org/symptoms/intestinal-gas/basics/causes/sym-20050922

193 Maureen Donohue. What Causes Abdominal Bloating?. Retrieved from https://www.

healthline.com/symptom/abdominal-bloating

194 Susan Jara. 7 Stomach Pains and What They Mean. Retrieved from https://www.rd.com/health/conditions/stomach-pain-causes/

195 Amber Angelle. (2017). Irritable Bowel Syndrome: Symptoms, Treatment & Prevention. Retrieved from https://www.livescience.com/34760-irritable-bowel-syndrome-diarrhea-constipation.html

196 Norton J. Greenberger, MD. (2018). Diarrhea in Adults. Retrieved from https://www.merckmanuals.com/home/digestive-disorders/symptoms-of-digestive-disorders/diarrhea-in-adults

197 Norton J. Greenberger, MD. (2018). Constipation in Adults. Retrieved from http://www.merckmanuals.com/home/digestive-disorders/symptoms-of-digestive-disorders/constipation-in-adults

198 Xiqun Zhu, Yong Han, Jing Du, Renzhong Liu, Ketao Jin, Wei Yi. (2017). Microbiota-gut-brain axis and the central nervous system. Retrieved from https://www.ncbi.nlm.nih.gov/pmc/articles/PMC5581153/

199 Jane A.Foster, LindaRinaman, John F.Cryan. (2017). Stress & the gut-brain axis: Regulation by the microbiome. *Neurobiology of Stress*, Volume 7, 124-136. Retrieved from https://www.sciencedirect.com/science/article/pii/S2352289516300509

200 PaulaPerez-Pardo, Tessa Kliest, Hemraj B.Dodiya, Laus M.Broersen, JohanGarssen, Ali Keshavarzian, Aletta D.Kraneveld. (2017). The gut-brain axis in Parkinson's disease: Possibilities for food-based therapies. *European Journal of Pharmacology*, Volume 817, 86-95. Retrieved from https://www.sciencedirect.com/science/article/pii/S0014299917303734

201 Jiang C, Li G, Huang P, Liu Z, Zhao B. (2017). The Gut Microbiota and Alzheimer's Disease.. Retrieved from https://www.ncbi.nlm.nih.gov/pubmed/28372330

202 Helen Tremlett, Emmanuelle Waubant. (2017). The multiple sclerosis microbiome?. Retrieved from https://www.ncbi.nlm.nih.gov/pmc/articles/PMC5326653/

203 Sticherling M. (2016). Psoriasis and autoimmunity.. Retrieved from https://www.ncbi.nlm.nih.gov/pubmed/27639838

204 Rheumatoid arthritis. Retrieved from https://www.mayoclinic.org/diseases-conditions/rheumatoid-arthritis/symptoms-causes/syc-20353648

205 Bavelaar. (2013). "The microbiome-gut?brain?axis in coeliac disease: mechanisms for depression and anxiety co?morbidity. " Retrieved from https://dspace.library.uu.nl/handle/1874/281761

206 Baohong Wang, Mingfei Yao, Longxian Lv, Zongxin Ling, Lanjuan Li. (2017). The Human Microbiota in Health and Disease. *Engineering*, Volume 3, Issue 1, 71-82. Retrieved from https://www.sciencedirect.com/science/article/pii/S2095809917301492

207 Ohland, C. L., & Jobin, C. (2015). Microbial Activities and Intestinal Homeostasis: A Delicate Balance Between Health and Disease. *Cellular and Molecular Gastroenterology and Hepatology*, 1(1), 28-40. doi:10.1016/j.jcmgh.2014.11.004

208 Dr. Karen Scott, Ph.D.. (2017). Prebiotics. Retrieved from https://isappscience.org/prebiotics/

209 Dr. Mary Ellen Sanders, Ph.D.. (2017). Prebiotics. Retrieved from https://isappscience.org/probiotics/

210 Philippe Ducrotté, Prabha Sawant, Venkataraman Jayanthi. (2012). Clinical trial: Lactobacillus plantarum 299v (DSM 9843) improves symptoms of irritable bowel syndrome. Retrieved from https://www.ncbi.nlm.nih.gov/pmc/articles/PMC3419998/

211 C. Ciacci, F. Franceschi, F. Purchiaroni, P. Capone, F. Buccelletti, P. Iacomini, A. Ranaudo, P. Andreozzi, P. Tondi, N. Gentiloni Silveri, A. Gasbarrini, G. Gasbarrini. (2011). Effect of beta-Glucan, Inositol and digestive enzymes in GI symptoms of patients with IBS. Retrieved from http://www.europeanreview.org/article/957

212 RadhaKrishna Rao, Geetha Samak. (2015). Role of Glutamine in Protection of Intestinal

Epithelial Tight Junctions. Retrieved from https://www.ncbi.nlm.nih.gov/pmc/articles/PMC4369670/

213 Murota K, Terao J.. (2003). Antioxidative flavonoid quercetin: implication of its intestinal absorption and metabolism.. Retrieved from https://www.ncbi.nlm.nih.gov/pubmed/12921774

214 Sadiq Yusuf, AbdulkarimAgunu, Mshelia Diana. (2004). The effect of Aloe vera A. Berger (Liliaceae) on gastric acid secretion and acute gastric mucosal injury in rats. *Journal of Ethnopharmacology*, Volume 93, Issue 1, 33-37. Retrieved from https://www.sciencedirect.com/science/article/pii/S0378874104001199

215 Min-Cheol Kang, Seo Young Kima, Yoon Taek Kim, Eun-A. Kim, Seung- Hong Lee, Seok-Chun Ko, W.A.J.P. Wijesinghe, Kalpa W. Samarakoona, Young-Sun Kimb, Jin Hun Cho, Hyeang-Su Jangb, You-Jin Jeona. (2013). In vitro and in vivo antioxidant activities of polysaccharide purified from aloe vera (Aloe barbadensis) gel. *Carbohydrate Polymers*, Volume 99, " 365-371. " Retrieved from https://www.sciencedirect.com/science/article/pii/S0144861713008060

216 Morris T.J., Calcraft B.J., Rhodes J., Hole D., Morton M.S. . (1974). Effect of a Deglycyrrhizinised Liquorice Compound on the Gastric Mucosal Barrier of the Dog. Volume 11, 6-May. Retrieved from https://www.karger.com/Article/Abstract/197603

217 Mark Anthony, Ph.D.. (2012). Is Algae DHA As Healthy as Fish Oil DHA?. Retrieved from https://www.foodprocessing.com/articles/2012/algae-dha-healthy-as-fish-oil/

218 Aiguo Wu Zhe Ying Fernando Gomez-Pinilla. (2004). Dietary Omega-3 Fatty Acids Normalize BDNF Levels, Reduce Oxidative Damage, and Counteract Learning Disability after Traumatic Brain Injury in Rats. Retrieved from http://online.liebertpub.com/doi/abs/10.1089/neu.2004.21.1457

219 Rebecca Wall, R Paul Ross, Gerald F Fitzgerald, Catherine Stanton. (2010). Fatty acids from fish: the anti?inflammatory potential of long?chain omega?3 fatty acids. Retrieved from http://onlinelibrary.wiley.com/doi/10.1111/j.1753-4887.2010.00287.x/full

220 Jessica Porter. (2016). Time to Chew: The Digestive System Starts in Your Mouth. Retrieved from http://nutritionstudies.org/time-chew-digestive-system-starts-mouth/

221 (2010). Stress and the sensitive gut. Retrieved from https://www.health.harvard.edu/newsletter_article/stress-and-the-sensitive-gut

222 Mohd. Razali Salleh. (2008). Life Event, Stress and Illness. Retrieved from https://www.ncbi.nlm.nih.gov/pmc/articles/PMC3341916/

223 Agro Chemicals!. Retrieved from http://www.ecochem.com/t_organic_fert.html

224 Dirt Poor: Have Fruits and Vegetables Become Less Nutritious?. Retrieved from https://www.scientificamerican.com/article/soil-depletion-and-nutrition-loss/

225 Connie M Weaver, Johanna Dwyer, Victor L Fulgoni, III, Janet C King, Gilbert A Leveille, Ruth S MacDonald, Jose Ordovas, David Schnakenberg. (2014). Processed foods: contributions to nutrition. Retrieved from http://ajcn.nutrition.org/content/99/6/1525.full

226 Freezing, Drying, Cooking, and Reheating. Retrieved from http://nutritiondata.self.com/topics/processing

227 (2010). Stress and the sensitive gut. Retrieved from https://www.health.harvard.edu/newsletter_article/stress-and-the-sensitive-gut

228 How Alcohol Affects Nutrition and Endurance. Retrieved from https://wellness.ucsd.edu/studenthealth/resources/health-topics/alcohol-drugs/Pages/alcohol-nutrition-endurance.aspx

229 Nadia Kounang, CNN. (2016). Dangerous chemicals hiding in everyday products. Retrieved from http://edition.cnn.com/2016/07/01/health/everyday-chemicals-we-need-to-reduce-exposure-to/index.html

230 Anemia of Inflammation or Chronic Disease What is anemia of inflammation?. Retrieved

from https://www.niddk.nih.gov/health-in-formation/blood-diseases/anemia-inflammation-chronic-disease

231 (2018). Low Energy Causes May Be Rooted in These 3 Nutritional Deficiencies. Retrieved from https://universityhealthnews.com/daily/energy/3-top-nutritional-deficiencies-as-fatigue-causes/

232 T. S. Sathyanarayana Rao, M. R. Asha, B. N. Ramesh, K. S. Jagannatha Rao. (2008). Understanding nutrition, depression and mental illnesses. Retrieved from https://www.ncbi.nlm.nih.gov/pmc/articles/PMC2738337/

233 Vitamins and Insomnia. Retrieved from https://www.insomnia.net/natural-remedies/vitamins/

234 Melatonin And Sleep. Retrieved from https://sleepfoundation.org/sleep-topics/melatonin-and-sleep

235 Fabrizio Galimberti, MD, PhD, Natasha A. Mesinkovska, MD, PhD. Skin findings associated with nutritional deficiencies. Retrieved from https://www.mdedge.com/ccjm/article/114635/dermatology/skin-findings-associated-nutritional-deficiencies

236 Weisshof R, Chermesh I.. (2015). Micronutrient deficiencies in inflammatory bowel disease.. Retrieved from https://www.ncbi.nlm.nih.gov/pubmed/26418823

237 Gerry K. Schwalfenberg. (2011). The Alkaline Diet: Is There Evidence That an Alkaline pH Diet Benefits Health?. Retrieved from https://www.ncbi.nlm.nih.gov/pmc/articles/PMC3195546/

238 Jean Weininger. Nutritional disease. Retrieved from https://www.britannica.com/science/nutritional-disease

239 Karuna Singh. (2016). Nutrient and Stress Management. Retrieved from https://www.omicsonline.org/open-access/nutrient-and-stress-management-2155-9600-1000528.php?aid=76425

240 McDougall, C. (2013). Plant-Based Diets Are Not Nutritionally Deficient. The Permanente Journal, 93-93. doi:10.7812/tpp/13-111

241 Philippe Rasoanaivo, Colin W Wright, Merlin L Willcox, Ben Gilbert. (2011). Whole plant extracts versus single compounds for the treatment of malaria: synergy and positive interactions. Retrieved from https://www.ncbi.nlm.nih.gov/pmc/articles/PMC3059462/

242 Mary Jane Brown, PhD, RD (UK) . (2016). What is Organic Food, and is it Better Than Non-Organic?. Retrieved from https://www.healthline.com/nutrition/what-is-organic-food#section3

243 Emily Willingham. (2013). Study: Herbal Supplements Full Of Contaminants, Substitutes, And Fillers. Retrieved from https://www.forbes.com/sites/emilywillingham/2013/11/07/study-herbal-supplements-full-of-contaminants-substitutes-and-fillers/#34e83285960f

244 Debra Rose Wilson, PhD, MSN, RN, IBCLC, AHN-BC, CHT. (2017). Should You Remove Carrageenan from Your Diet?. Retrieved from https://www.healthline.com/health/food-nutrition/carrageenan#side-effects

245 Dr. Mercola. (2012). Magnesium Stearate: Does Your Supplement Contain This Potentially Hazardous Ingredient?. Retrieved from https://articles.mercola.com/sites/articles/archive/2012/06/23/whole-food-supplement-dangers.aspx

246 Erika Yigzaw. (2016). 5 Dangerous Ingredients in your Vitamins and Dietary Supplements. Retrieved from http://info.achs.edu/blog/5-dangerous-ingredients-in-your-vitamins-and-dietary-supplements

247 Erika Yigzaw. (2016). 5 Dangerous Ingredients in your Vitamins and Dietary Supplements. Retrieved from http://info.achs.edu/blog/5-dangerous-ingredients-in-your-vitamins-and-dietary-supplements

248 Conlon, M., & Bird, A. (2014). The Impact of Diet and Lifestyle on Gut Microbiota and Human Health. Nutrients, 7(1), 17-44. doi:10.3390/nu7010017

249 NutraChamps Korean Red Panax Ginseng 1000mg - 120 Vegan Capsules Extra Strength Root Extract Powder Supplement w/High Ginsenosides for Energy, Performance & Mental Health Pills for Men & Women. Retrieved from https://www.

amazon.com/gp/product/B01MECVTDY/ref=oh_aui_detailpage_o01_s00?ie=UTF8&psc=1oh_aui_detailpage_o01_s00?ie=UTF8&psc=1

250 Kang, S., & Min, H. (2012). Ginseng, the 'Immunity Boost': The Effects of Panax ginseng on Immune System. *Journal of Ginseng Research, 36*(4), 354-368. doi:10.5142/jgr.2012.36.4.354

251 Viva Naturals Reduced Glutathione Supplement with ALA for Antioxidant Benefits, 500mg, 60 Capsules. Retrieved from https://www.amazon.com/gp/product/B00BW4TG44/ref=oh_aui_detailpage_o03_s01?ie=UTF8&psc=1

252 Wu, G., Fang, Y., Yang, S., Lupton, J. R., & Turner, N. D. (2004). Glutathione Metabolism and Its Implications for Health. *The Journal of Nutrition, 134*(3), 489-492. doi:10.1093/jn/134.3.489

253 What Are Red Blood Cells?. Retrieved from https://www.urmc.rochester.edu/encyclopedia/content.aspx?ContentID=34&ContentTypeID=160

254 CHOLINE BITARTRATE 500 mg | 90 Vegan Capsules | Promotes Healthy Cognitive Function, Mental Focus & Memory | Prenatal Infant Brain Development Supplement | Cardiovascular Health Booster | 100% Non GMO. Retrieved from https://www.amazon.com/gp/product/B01A9WLFZC/ref=oh_aui_detailpage_o03_s02?ie=UTF8&psc=1

255 Parikh, V., & Sarter, M. (2006). Cortical choline transporter function measuredin vivousing choline-sensitive microelectrodes: clearance of endogenous and exogenous choline and effects of removal of cholinergic terminals. *Journal of Neurochemistry, 97*(2), 488-503. doi:10.1111/j.1471-4159.2006.03766.x

256 Does choline have any effect on cholesterol?. Retrieved from http://www.food-info.net/uk/qa/qa-nut1.htm

257 Organic Turmeric Curcumin with Bioperine - 1200mg (120 Capsules) - Extra Strength Pain Relief & Joint Support Supplement - Non-GMO, Made in the USA. Retrieved from https://www.amazon.com/gp/product/B01DVJNK4E/ref=oh_aui_detailpage_o05_s00?ie=UTF8&psc=1

258 Gupta, S. C., Patchva, S., & Aggarwal, B. B. (2012). Therapeutic Roles of Curcumin: Lessons Learned from Clinical Trials. *The AAPS Journal, 15*(1), 195-218. doi:10.1208/s12248-012-9432-8

259 Viva Naturals Organic Maca Root, 500mg, 250 Veggie Capsules, Gelatinized for Enhanced Bioavailability. Retrieved from https://www.amazon.com/gp/product/B0161GAASI/ref=oh_aui_detailpage_o05_s00?ie=UTF8&psc=1

260 Sifuentes-Penagos, G., León-Vásquez, S., & Paucar-Menacho, L. M. (2015). Study of Maca (Lepidium meyenii Walp.), Andean crop with therapeutic properties. *Scientia agropecuaria*, 131-140. doi:10.17268/sci.agropecu.2015.02.06

261 LUNA | #1 Sleep Aid on Amazon | Naturally Sourced Ingredients | 60 Non-Habit Forming Vegan Capsules | Herbal Supplement with Melatonin, Valerian Root, Chamomile, Magnesium | Sleeping Pills for Adults. Retrieved from https://www.amazon.com/gp/product/B00JCO3ALG/ref=oh_aui_detailpage_o07_s00?ie=UTF8&psc=1

262 Luna Melatonin-Free | 60 Capsules | Naturally Sourced Sleep Aid Without Melatonin | Valerian, Chamomile Extract, Lemon Balm, Herbs & More | Gentle Herbal Sleeping Aid Pill | Vegan, Non-GMO Supplement. Retrieved from https://www.amazon.com/gp/product/B074XHY9WG/ref=oh_aui_search_detailpage?ie=UTF8&psc=1

263 GABA. Retrieved from https://examine.com/supplements/gaba/

264 (2018). Theanine. Retrieved from https://examine.com/supplements/theanine/

265 Valerian. Retrieved from http://www.rjwhelan.co.nz/herbs A-Z/valerian.html

266 Retrieved from https://www.amazon.com/gp/product/B00CQ80FRW/ref=oh_aui_detailpage_o09_s00?ie=UTF8&psc=1

267 El-Mostafa K, El Kharrassi Y, Badreddine A, Andreoletti P, Vamecq J, El Kebbaj MS, Latruffe N, Lizard G, Nasser B, Cherkaoui-Malki M. (2014). Nopal cactus (Opuntia

ficus-indica) as a source of bioactive compounds for nutrition, health and disease.. Retrieved from https://www.ncbi.nlm.nih.gov/pubmed/25232708

268 Eduardo Madrigal-Santillán, Fernando García-Melo, José A. Morales-González, Patricia Vázquez-Alvarado, Sergio Muñoz-Juárez, Clara Zuñiga-Pérez, Maria Teresa Sumaya-Martínez, Eduardo Madrigal-Bujaidar, and Alejandra Hernández-Ceruelos. (2013). Antioxidant and Anticlastogenic Capacity of Prickly Pear Juice. Retrieved from https://www.ncbi.nlm.nih.gov/pmc/articles/PMC3820065/

269 El-Mostafa, K., El Kharrassi, Y., Badreddine, A., Andreoletti, P., Vamecq, J., El Kebbaj, M., ... Cherkaoui-Malki, M. (2014). Nopal Cactus (Opuntia ficus-indica) as a Source of Bioactive Compounds for Nutrition, Health and Disease. *Molecules, 19*(9), 14879-14901. doi:10.3390/molecules190914879

270 PrimaForce ZMA Supplement, 180 Capsules – Increases Muscular Strength and Power / Increases Free Testosterone Levels. Retrieved from https://www.amazon.com/gp/product/B00MKSLYW8/ref=oh_aui_detailpage_o07_s00?ie=UTF8&psc=1

271 ZMA. (2007). *Hawley's Condensed Chemical Dictionary*. doi:10.1002/9780470114735.hawley17434

272 Essential Fatty Acids. (n.d.). *SpringerReference*. doi:10.1007/springerreference_32181

273 Your Optimal health. Our Ultimate growth.. Retrieved from https://www.nordicnaturals.com/consumers/

274 Algae Oil Omega-3 DHA+EPA capsules with 450 mg Omega-3. Retrieved from https://www.testa-omega3.com/en_eur/algae-oil

275 Vitamins and Insomnia: Fix Your Sleeplessness with Vitamin Supplements. Retrieved from https://www.insomnia.net/natural-remedies/vitamins/

276 Catherine Jeans. (2017). Soothing menopausal stress with vitamin B. Retrieved from https://www.healthspan.co.uk/advice/soothing-menopausal-stress-with-vitamin-b

277 Morris, M. S. (2012). The Role of B Vitamins in Preventing and Treating Cognitive Impairment and Decline. *Advances in Nutrition, 3*(6), 801-812. doi:10.3945/an.112.002535

278 Garden of Life Vitamin B Complex - Vitamin Code Raw B Vitamin Whole Food Supplement, Vegan, 120 Capsules. Retrieved from https://www.amazon.com/gp/product/B0098U0SQO/ref=oh_aui_detailpage_o01_s00?ie=UTF8&th=1

279 Retrieved from https://www.umm.edu/health/medical/altmed/supplement/vitamin-b6-pyridoxine

280 Bode, A., & Dong, Z. (2011). The Amazing and Mighty Ginger. *Oxidative Stress and Disease*, 131-156. doi:10.1201/b10787-8

281 Matthew J Leach, Saravana Kumar. (2008). The clinical effectiveness of Ginger (Zingiber officinale) in adults with osteoarthritis. Retrieved from http://onlinelibrary.wiley.com/doi/10.1111/j.1744-1609.2008.00106.x/full

282 Raghavendra Haniadka, Antappa Govindaraju Rajeev, Princy L. Palatty, Rajesh Arora, and Manjeshwar S. Baliga. (2012). Zingiber officinale (Ginger) as an Anti-Emetic in Cancer Chemotherapy: A Review. Retrieved from http://online.liebertpub.com/doi/abs/10.1089/acm.2010.0737

283 Borrelli, Francesca PhD; Capasso, Raffaele PharmD; Aviello, Gabriella PharmD; Pittler, Max H. MD, PhD; Izzo, Angelo A. PhD. (2005). Effectiveness and Safety of Ginger in the Treatment of Pregnancy-Induced Nausea and Vomiting. Retrieved from https://journals.lww.com/greenjournal/Abstract/2005/04000/Effectiveness_and_Safety_of_Ginger_in_the.27.aspx

284 MegaFood - MegaFlora Plus, Probiotic Help for Digestion, Intestinal Balance, and Immune Health, 50 Billion CFU, Vegetarian, Gluten-Free, Non-GMO, 60 Capsules. Retrieved from https://www.amazon.com/MegaFood-MegaFlora-Supports-Intestinal-Regularity/dp/B0075A8V0O/ref=sr_1_2_a_it?ie=UTF8&qid=1514082825&sr=8-2&keywords=megafood+probiotic&th=1

285 Mai, V. (2013). Health Benefits Mediated

by Probiotics - How Can we Better Establish Them? *Journal of Probiotics & Health, 01*(03). doi:10.4172/2329-8901.1000e104

286 Ann M O'Hara1, Fergus Shanahan. (2006). The gut flora as a forgotten organ. Retrieved from https://www.ncbi.nlm.nih.gov/pmc/articles/PMC1500832/

287 Garden of Life Organic Chewable Enzyme Supplement - Dr. Formulated Enzymes Organic Digest+, 90 Chewable Tablets. Retrieved from https://www.amazon.com/gp/product/B00Y8MPKVU/ref=oh_aui_search_detailpage?ie=UTF8&psc=1

288 MegaFood - One Daily, Multivitamin Support for Immune and Nervous System Health, Energy Production, and Mood Balance with Folate and B Vitamins, Vegetarian, Gluten-Free, Non-GMO, 180 Tablets (FFP). Retrieved from https://www.amazon.com/MegaFood-Natural-Multivitamin-Support-Well-Being/dp/B00GZ9JTRA/ref=sr_1_3_a_it?ie=UTF8&qid=1514083498&sr=8-3&keywords=megafood+one+daily&th=1

289 Ann M O'Hara1, Fergus Shanahan. (2006). The gut flora as a forgotten organ. Retrieved from https://www.ncbi.nlm.nih.gov/pmc/articles/PMC1500832/

290 Pure Synergy Organic Berry Power (8 oz Powder) 20+ Superfruit Blend for Radiant Health w/Acai, Pomegranate. Retrieved from https://www.amazon.com/gp/product/B00HONEB6A/ref=oh_aui_detailpage_o02_s00?ie=UTF8&psc=1

291 Chambial, S., Dwivedi, S., Shukla, K. K., John, P. J., & Sharma, P. (2013). Vitamin C in Disease Prevention and Cure: An Overview. *Indian Journal of Clinical Biochemistry, 28*(4), 314-328. doi:10.1007/s12291-013-0375-3

292 Toxic Chemicals released by industries - Worldometers. (n.d.). Retrieved from http://www.worldometers.info/view/toxchem/

293 Your detoxification pathway explained. Retrieved from https://artemis.co.nz/your-detox-pathway-explained

294 Toxic Exposure in the Workplace. Retrieved from http://employment.findlaw.com/workplace-safety/toxic-exposure-in-the-workplace.html

295 (2016). Fat Cells and Toxins. Retrieved from https://www.liverdoctor.com/fat-cells-and-toxins/

296 Liver: Anatomy and Functions. Retrieved from https://www.hopkinsmedicine.org/healthlibrary/conditions/liver_biliary_and_pancreatic_disorders/liver_anatomy_and_functions_85,P00676

297 Kidney Detoxification. Retrieved from http://whydetox.net/kidney-detoxification

298 (1993). Cutaneous Toxicity: Toxic Effects On Skin. Retrieved from http://pmep.cce.cornell.edu/profiles/extoxnet/TIB/cutaneous-tox.html

299 Kenichiro Yasutake, Motoyuki Kohjima, Manabu Nakashima, Kazuhiro Kotoh, Makoto Nakamuta, Munechika Enjoji. Nutrition Therapy for Liver Diseases Based on the Status of Nutritional Intake. Retrieved from https://www.hindawi.com/journals/grp/2012/859697/

300 San-Nan Yang, Chong-Chao Hsieh, Hsuan-Fu Kuo, Min-Sheng Lee, Ming-Yii Huang, Chang-Hung Kuo, Chih-Hsing Hung. (2014). The Effects of Environmental Toxins on Allergic Inflammation. Retrieved from https://www.ncbi.nlm.nih.gov/pmc/articles/PMC4214967/

301 Handzel, Z. T. (2000). Effects of Environmental Pollutants on Airways, Allergic Inflammation, and the Immune Response. *Reviews on Environmental Health, 15*(3). doi:10.1515/reveh.2000.15.3.325

302 Dalene Barton-Schuster . (2018). Normal Symptoms of Detox During a Cleanse. Retrieved from http://natural-fertility-info.com/symptoms-of-detox.html

303 Mitch Leslie. (2015). Short-term fasting may improve health. Retrieved from http://www.sciencemag.org/news/2015/06/short-term-fasting-may-improve-health

304 Ana Sandoiu . (2017). Leafy greens may contribute to a healthy heart. Retrieved from https://www.medicalnewstoday.com/articles/319645.php

305 Joe Bowman, Rachel Nall. (2017). The Ben-

efits of Chlorophyll. Retrieved from https://www.healthline.com/health/liquid-chlorophyll-benefits-risks

306 Peer Review #1 of "Chlorophyll enhances oxidative stress tolerance in Caenorhabditis elegans and extends its lifespan (v0.1)". (2016). doi:10.7287/peerj.1879v0.1/reviews/1

307 Retrieved from https://www.nottingham.ac.uk/nmp/sonet/rlos/bioproc/liverphysiology/6.html

308 Portal vein. Retrieved from https://www.britannica.com/science/portal-vein

309 John T Piper, Sharad S Singhal ab, Mohammad S Salameha, Robert T Torman, Yogesh C Awasthi, Sanjay Awasthi. (1998). Mechanisms of anticarcinogenic properties of curcumin: the effect of curcumin on glutathione linked detoxification enzymes in rat liver. *The International Journal of Biochemistry & Cell Biology*, Volume 30, Issue 4, 423-546 . Retrieved from https://www.sciencedirect.com/science/article/pii/S1357272598000156

310 S. Melino, R. Sabelli, M. Paci. (2010). Allyl sulfur compounds and cellular detoxification system: effects and perspectives in cancer therapy. Retrieved from https://link.springer.com/article/10.1007/s00726-010-0522-6

311 D Labadarios, J E Rossouw, J B McConnell, M Davis, R Williams. Vitamin B6 deficiency in chronic liver disease--evidence for increased degradation of pyridoxal-5'-phosphate.. Retrieved from http://gut.bmj.com/content/18/1/23.long

312 Seaman DR. (2016). Toxins, Toxicity, and Endotoxemia: A Historical and Clinical Perspective for Chiropractors.. Retrieved from https://www.ncbi.nlm.nih.gov/pubmed/27920621

313 Jarisch–Herxheimer reaction. (2018, March 9). Retrieved from https://en.wikipedia.org/wiki/Jarisch–Herxheimer_reaction

314 Dr. Mercola. (2013). This Is What Happens to Your Body When You Exercise. Retrieved from https://fitness.mercola.com/sites/fitness/archive/2013/09/20/exercise-health-benefits.aspx

315 Neville Owen,PhD, Phillip B. Sparling,EdD, Geneviève N. Healy,PhD, David W. Dunstan,PhD, Charles E. Matthews,PhD. (2010). Sedentary Behavior: Emerging Evidence for a New Health Risk. Retrieved from https://www.ncbi.nlm.nih.gov/pmc/articles/PMC2996155/

316 National 5 Biology. Retrieved from http://www.bbc.co.uk/bitesize/standard/biology/the_body_in_action/changing_levels_of_performance/revision/4/

317 Homeostasis in humans. Retrieved from http://www.bbc.co.uk/schools/gcsebitesize/science/add_aqa_pre_2011/homeo/homeostasis1.shtml

318 Trefts, E., Williams, A. S., & Wasserman, D. H. (2015). Exercise and the Regulation of Hepatic Metabolism. *Progress in Molecular Biology and Translational Science*, 203-225. doi:10.1016/bs.pmbts.2015.07.010

319 Science Waste disposal. Retrieved from http://www.bbc.co.uk/schools/gcsebitesize/science/triple_ocr_gateway/the_living_body/waste_disposal/revision/2/

320 Robert Ross, PhD; Damon Dagnone, MSc; Peter J.H. Jones, PhD; Heidi Smith, BSc, RD; Anne Paddags, MSc; Robert Hudson, MD, PhD; Ian Janssen, MSc. (2000). Reduction in Obesity and Related Comorbid Conditions after Diet-Induced Weight Loss or Exercise-Induced Weight Loss in Men: A Randomized, Controlled Trial. Retrieved from http://annals.org/aim/article-abstract/713672/reduction-obesity-related-comorbid-conditions-after-diet-induced-weight-loss

321 Ersilia Nigro, Olga Scudiero, Maria Ludovica Monaco, Alessia Palmieri, Gennaro Mazzarella, Ciro Costagliola, Andrea Bianco, Aurora Daniele. (2014). New Insight into Adiponectin Role in Obesity and Obesity-Related Diseases. Retrieved from https://www.ncbi.nlm.nih.gov/pmc/articles/PMC4109424/

322 Young sub Kwon, M.S.; Len Kravitz, Ph.D.. How do muscles grow?. Retrieved from https://www.unm.edu/~lkravitz/Article folder/musclesgrowLK.html

323 Grossman, A. (1984). Endorphins and exercise. *Clinical Cardiology*, 7(5), 255-260. doi:10.1002/clc.4960070502

324 Harber VJ, Sutton JR.. (1984). Endorphins and exercise.. Retrieved from https://www.ncbi.nlm.nih.gov/pubmed/6091217

325 (2018). Exercising to relax. Retrieved from https://www.health.harvard.edu/staying-healthy/exercising-to-relax

326 (2018). Exercising to relax. Retrieved from https://www.health.harvard.edu/staying-healthy/exercising-to-relax clii (2002). Fuel Choice During Exercise Is Determined by Intensity and Duration of Activity. *Biochemistry*, Retrieved from https://www.ncbi.nlm.nih.gov/books/NBK22417/

327 Edward R. Laskowski, M.D.. (2016). Which is better — 30 minutes of aerobic exercise every day or one hour of aerobic exercise three times a week?. Retrieved from https://www.mayoclinic.org/healthy-lifestyle/fitness/expert-answers/aerobic-exercise/faq-20058561

328 Professor David Pyne. (2014). Should you avoid exercise when you've got a cold?. Retrieved from http://www.abc.net.au/health/talkinghealth/factbuster/stories/2014/09/02/4079324.htm

329 Shashi K Agarwal. (2012). Cardiovascular benefits of exercise. Retrieved from https://www.ncbi.nlm.nih.gov/pmc/articles/PMC3396114/

330 Gerald T Mangine, Jay R Hoffman, Adam M Gonzalez, Jeremy R Townsend, Adam J Wells, Adam R Jajtner, Kyle S Beyer, Carleigh H Boone, Amelia A Miramonti, Ran Wang, Michael B LaMonica, David H Fukuda, Nicholas A Ratamess, and Jeffrey R Stout. (2015). The effect of training volume and intensity on improvements in muscular strength and size in resistance-trained men. Retrieved from https://www.ncbi.nlm.nih.gov/pmc/articles/PMC4562558/

331 Versey NG, Halson SL, Dawson BT.. (2013). Water immersion recovery for athletes: effect on exercise performance and practical recommendations.. Retrieved from https://www.ncbi.nlm.nih.gov/pubmed/23743793

332 Joseph C. Maroon, Jeffrey W. Bost and Adara Maroon. (2010). Natural anti-inflammatory agents for pain relief. Retrieved from https://www.ncbi.nlm.nih.gov/pmc/articles/PMC3011108/

333 McConigal, Kelly. The Science of Compassion and The Willpower Instinct http://kellymcgonigal.com

334 Currey, Masson. Daily Rituals: How Artists Work. https://www.amazon.com/Daily-Rituals-How-Artists-Work/dp/0307273601

335 How 8 of the world's most successful people start their morning. (2015, October 9). Retrieved from https://www.independent.co.uk/news/business/news/from-steve-jobs-obama-jeff-bezos-mark-zuckerberg-how-8-of-the-world-s-most-successful-people-start-a6686466.html

336 Understanding the 24 hour Chi Cycle. (2017, August 13). Retrieved from https://upliftconnect.com/24-hour-chi-cycle/

337 Crawford, B. (2011, May 11). How Does Exercise Affect Your Self-Esteem? Retrieved from https://www.livestrong.com/article/438937-how-does-exercise-affect-your-self-esteem/

338 BYU study says exercise may reduce motivation for food. (n.d.). Retrieved from https://news.byu.edu/news/byu-study-says-exercise-may-reduce-motivation-food

339 13 Health Benefits of Coffee, Based on Science. (n.d.). Retrieved from https://www.healthline.com/nutrition/top-13-evidence-based-health-benefits-of-coffee

340 Lisa Berkman. (n.d.). Retrieved from https://www.hsph.harvard.edu/lisa-berkman/

341 Lauren F Friedman, Kevin Loria, Tech Insider. (2016, April 22). 11 scientific reasons you should be spending more time outside. Retrieved from https://www.businessinsider.com/scientific-benefits-of-nature-outdoors-2016-4#11-reduced-risk-of-early-death-11

342 CDC Press Releases. (2016, February 16). Retrieved from https://www.cdc.gov/media/releases/2016/p0215-enough-sleep.html

343 What Happens When You Sleep?. Retrieved from https://sleepfoundation.org/how-sleep-works/what-happens-when-you-sleep

344 What Happens When You Sleep? (n.d.). Retrieved from https://sleepfoundation.org/how-sleep-works/what-happens-when-you-sleep

345 (2016). Why you're stiff in the morning: Your body suppresses inflammation when you sleep at night. Retrieved from https://www.sciencedaily.com/releases/2016/08/160805115204.htm

346 Why you're stiff in the morning: Your body suppresses inflammation when you sleep at night. (2018, May 21). Retrieved from https://www.sciencedaily.com/releases/2016/08/160805115204.htm

347 Sarah DiGiulio. (2017). What Happens in Your Body and Brain While You Sleep. Retrieved from https://www.nbcnews.com/better/health/what-happens-your-body-brain-while-you-sleep-ncna805276

348 Peter Crosta. (2017). Insomnia: Everything you need to know. Retrieved from https://www.medicalnewstoday.com/articles/9155.php

349 Miller, M., & Cappuccio, F. (2010). Sleep, inflammation, and disease. *Sleep, Health and Society*, 239-268. doi:10.1093/acprof:oso/9780199566594.003.0011

350 Hwan Seok Park, Eun Yeon Joo, and Seung Bong Hong. (2009). Sleep onset Insomnia. Retrieved from https://www.e-jsm.org/journal/view.php?number=97

351 Retrieved from http://www.umm.edu/health/medical/altmed/supplement/melatonin

352 (2018). Melatonin. Retrieved from http://www.yourhormones.info/hormones/melatonin/

353 Stephen N. Haynes, Augustus Adams, Michael Franzen. (1982). The effects of presleep stress on sleep-onset insomnia. Retrieved from https://www.researchgate.net/publication/15879430_The_effects_of_presleep_stress_on_sleep-onset_insomnia

354 Vitamins and Insomnia. Retrieved from https://www.insomnia.net/natural-remedies/vitamins/

355 Caffeine and Sleep. Retrieved from https://sleepfoundation.org/sleep-topics/caffeine-and-sleep

356 Randall Lee Oliver, MD, April Taylor, RN, BSN, CDE and Rebecca Oliver. (2017). Chronic Insomnia and Pain. Volume 2, Retrieved from https://www.practicalpainmanagement.com/pain/other/co-morbidities/chronic-insomnia-pain

357 (2018). The Tart Cherry Juice Sleep Solution: Beat Insomnia With This Natural Remedy. Retrieved from https://universityhealthnews.com/daily/sleep/the-tart-cherry-juice-sleep-solution-tart-cherry-juice-benefits-include-beating-insomnia/

358 The Potential of Phytomelatonin as a Nutraceutical. (2018). *Molecules*, *23*(1), 238. doi:10.3390/molecules23010238

359 Ritamarie Loscalzo. The Role of Liver Detoxification in Hormonal Imbalance. Retrieved from http://drritamarie.com/blog/the-role-of-liver-detoxification-in-hormonal-imbalance/

360 Passion Flower and Sleep. Retrieved from https://88herbs.com/passion-flower-sleep/

361 Craig, C., & Sprang, G. (2010). Compassion satisfaction, compassion fatigue, and burnout in a national sample of trauma treatment therapists. *Anxiety, Stress & Coping*, *23*(3), 319-339. doi:10.1080/10615800903085818

362 Sleep Disruptions. Retrieved from http://adrenalfatigue.org/sleep-disruptions/

363 Sanford, L. D., & Tang, X. (2009). Effect of Stress on Sleep and Its Relationship to Post-Traumatic Stress Disorder. *Post-Traumatic Stress Disorder*, 231-253. doi:10.1007/978-1-60327-329-9_11

364 Jurriaan Plesman BA (Psych). (2011). The Biochemistry of Insomnia. Retrieved from http://www.hypoglycemia.asn.au/2011/the-biochemistry-of-insomnia/

365 Scheen, A. J., Byrne, M. M., Plat, L., Lep-

roult, R., & Van Cauter, E. (1996). Relationships between sleep quality and glucose regulation in normal humans. *American Journal of Physiology-Endocrinology and Metabolism, 271*(2), E261-E270. doi:10.1152/ajpendo.1996.271.2.e261

366 Attarian, H. P. (n.d.). Epidemiology of Sleep Disorders in Women. *Current Clinical Neurology*, 9-17. doi:10.1007/978-1-59745-115-4_2

367 Joyce Walsleben, RN, PhD. Menopause and Insomnia. Retrieved from https://sleepfoundation.org/ask-the-expert/menopause-and-insomnia

368 Stein, M. D., & Friedmann, P. D. (2006). Disturbed Sleep and Its Relationship to Alcohol Use. *Substance Abuse, 26*(1), 1-13. doi:10.1300/j465v26n01_01

369 Nadia Rachdaoui and Dipak K. Sarkar. (2013). Effects of Alcohol on the Endocrine System. Retrieved from https://www.ncbi.nlm.nih.gov/pmc/articles/PMC3767933/

370 Monique Hallee, BScHK, ND and Chris Hergesheimer, BA, MA. (2016). An Unexpected Insomnia Treatment. Retrieved from http://ndnr.com/anxietydepressionmental-health/an-unexpected-insomnia-treatment/

371 PrimaForce ZMA Supplement, 180 Capsules – Increases Muscular Strength and Power / Increases Free Testosterone Level. Retrieved from https://www.amazon.com/gp/product/B00MKSLYW8/ref=oh_aui_search_detailpage?ie=UTF8&psc=1

372 Lirong Zhu, MD, PhD and Phyllis C. Zee, MD, PhD. (2013). Circadian Rhythm Sleep Disorders. Retrieved from https://www.ncbi.nlm.nih.gov/pmc/articles/PMC3523094/

373 Wilson, S., & Nutt, D. (2008). Chapter 6 Circadian rhythm sleep disorders. *Sleep Disorders*. doi:10.1093/med/9780199234332.003.0006

374 How much Sleep do we Really Need?. Retrieved from https://sleepfoundation.org/how-sleep-works/how-much-sleep-do-we-really-need

375 Erin Brodwin. (2016). Here's Why You Should Never Eat Right Before Bed. Retrieved from https://www.sciencealert.com/here-s-why-you-should-never-eat-right-before-bed

376 Sleep disturbance. Retrieved from http://www.emfs.info/health/other-health/sleep/

377 Pall, M. L. (2016). Microwave frequency electromagnetic fields (EMFs) produce widespread neuropsychiatric effects including depression. *Journal of Chemical Neuroanatomy, 75*, 43-51. doi:10.1016/j.jchemneu.2015.08.001

378 Joshua J. Gooley, Kyle Chamberlain, Kurt A. Smith, Sat Bir S. Khalsa, Shantha M. W. Rajaratnam, Eliza Van Reen, Jamie M. Zeitzer, Charles A. Czeisler, and Steven W. Lockley. (2010). Exposure to Room Light before Bedtime Suppresses Melatonin Onset and Shortens Melatonin Duration in Humans. Retrieved from https://www.ncbi.nlm.nih.gov/pmc/articles/PMC3047226/

379 Choosing the Right Light Bulbs for Your Home. Retrieved from https://sleep.org/articles/choosing-lightbulbs/

380 Alina Bradford. (2016). How Blue LEDs Affect Sleep. Retrieved from https://www.livescience.com/53874-blue-light-sleep.html

381 Black Out Curtains, Sleep Shade Gives Cancer Protection ...and more!. Retrieved from http://www.sleep-disorders-gone.com/black-out-curtains.html

382 L-Tryptophan for Insomnia. Retrieved from https://www.insomnia.net/natural-remedies/l-tryptophan/

383 Abbasi B, Kimiagar M, Sadeghniiat K, Shirazi MM, Hedayati M, Rashidkhani B.. (2012). The effect of magnesium supplementation on primary insomnia in elderly: A double-blind placebo-controlled clinical trial.. Retrieved from https://www.ncbi.nlm.nih.gov/pubmed/23853635

384 (2009). Insomnia: Studies Suggest Calcium And Magnesium Effective. Retrieved from https://www.medicalnewstoday.com/releases/163169.php

385 The Definitive Guide to Vitamin B Insomnia and Sleep. Retrieved from https://tired-

feelingtired.com/sleep-aid-ingredients/vitamin-b-insomnia-sleep-guide/

386 PrimaForce ZMA Supplement, 180 Capsules – Increases Muscular Strength and Power / Increases Free Testosterone Levels. Retrieved from https://www.amazon.com/gp/product/B00MKSLYW8/ref=oh_aui_search_detailpage?ie=UTF8&psc=1

387 Luna Melatonin-Free | 60 Capsules | Naturally Sourced Sleep Aid Without Melatonin | Valerian, Chamomile Extract, Lemon Balm, Herbs & More | Gentle Herbal Sleeping Aid Pill | Vegan, Non-GMO Supplement. Retrieved from https://www.amazon.com/gp/product/B074XHY9WG/ref=oh_aui_search_detailpage?ie=UTF8&psc=1

388 Stephen Bent, MD, Amy Padula, MS, Dan Moore, PhD, Michael Patterson, MS, and Wolf Mehling, MD. (2015). Valerian for Sleep: A Systematic Review and Meta-Analysis. Retrieved from https://www.ncbi.nlm.nih.gov/pmc/articles/PMC4394901/

389 Janmejai K Srivastava, Eswar Shankar and Sanjay Gupta. (2011). Chamomile: A herbal medicine of the past with bright future. Retrieved from https://www.ncbi.nlm.nih.gov/pmc/articles/PMC2995283/

390 Retrieved from http://www.umm.edu/health/medical/altmed/herb/lemon-balm

391 Ronnie Corelli. (2016). Thoughts Affect Feelings, Feelings Affect Actions, Actions Determine Happiness. Retrieved from https://www.theodysseyonline.com/thoughts-effect-feelings-feelings-effect-actions-actions-determine-happiness

392 Robert C. Jameson. (2014). Be Careful of Your Thoughts: They Control Your Destiny. Retrieved from https://www.huffingtonpost.com/robert-c-jameson/be-careful-of-your-though_b_5214689.html

393 What is NLP?. Retrieved from http://www.nlp.com/what-is-nlp/

394 Getting Started with Mindfulness. Retrieved from https://www.mindful.org/meditation/mindfulness-getting-started/

395 Cognitive Behavioral Therapy. Retrieved from https://www.psychologytoday.com/us/basics/cognitive-behavioral-therapy

396 Stress effects on the body. Retrieved from http://www.apa.org/helpcenter/stress-body.aspx

397 (2018). Understanding the stress response. Retrieved from https://www.health.harvard.edu/staying-healthy/understanding-the-stress-response

398 Agnese Mariotti. (2015). The effects of chronic stress on health: new insights into the molecular mechanisms of brain–body communication. Retrieved from https://www.ncbi.nlm.nih.gov/pmc/articles/PMC5137920/

399 (2007). Stress and Your Gut. Retrieved from https://www.badgut.org/information-centre/a-z-digestive-topics/stress-and-your-gut/

400 Fawne Hansen. (2018). "Fight or Flight" vs. "Rest and Digest". Retrieved from https://adrenalfatiguesolution.com/fight-or-flight-vs-rest-and-digest/

401 Complementary & Alternative Treatments. Retrieved from https://adaa.org/finding-help/treatment/complementary-alternative-treatment

402 Joaquín. (2017). History of Mindfulness: From East to West and From Religion to Science. Retrieved from https://positivepsychologyprogram.com/history-of-mindfulness/

403 What Is Mindfulness?. Retrieved from https://greatergood.berkeley.edu/topic/mindfulness/definition

404 Marlynn Wei M.D., J.D.. (2015). Yoga for Stress Relief. *Toxicology and Applied Pharmacology*, 104-121. Retrieved from https://www.psychologytoday.com/us/blog/urban-survival/201512/yoga-stress-relief

405 Tai chi: A gentle way to fight stress. Retrieved from https://www.mayoclinic.org/healthy-lifestyle/stress-management/in-depth/tai-chi/art-20045184

406 Physical Activity Reduces Stress. Retrieved from https://adaa.org/understanding-anxiety/related-illnesses/other-related-conditions/stress/physical-activity-reduces-st

407 Rachael Rettner. (2015). Want to Live Longer? Optimal Amount of Exercise Revealed. Retrieved from https://www.livescience.com/50386-exercise-recommendations-longevity.html

408 James M. Ferguson, M.D. (2001). SSRI Antidepressant Medications: Adverse Effects and Tolerability. Retrieved from https://www.ncbi.nlm.nih.gov/pmc/articles/PMC181155/

409 (2012). Well-Known Mechanism Underlies Benzodiazepines' Addictive Properties. Retrieved from https://www.drugabuse.gov/news-events/nida-notes/2012/04/well-known-mechanism-underlies-benzodiazepines-addictive-properties

410 Emily Deans M.D.. (2011). Magnesium and the Brain: The Original Chill Pill. Retrieved from https://www.psychologytoday.com/us/blog/evolutionary-psychiatry/201106/magnesium-and-the-brain-the-original-chill-pill

411 Braet K, Cabooter L, Paemeleire K, Leybaert L.. (2004). Calcium signal communication in the central nervous system. Retrieved from https://www.ncbi.nlm.nih.gov/pubmed/15093130

412 Patak P, Willenberg HS, Bornstein SR.. (2004). Vitamin C is an important cofactor for both adrenal cortex and adrenal medulla.. Retrieved from https://www.ncbi.nlm.nih.gov/pubmed/15666839

413 Con Stough, Tamara Simpson, Justine Lomas, Grace McPhee, Clare Billings, Stephen Myers, Chris Oliver, and Luke A Downey. (2014). Reducing occupational stress with a B-vitamin focussed intervention: a randomized clinical trial: study protocol. Retrieved from https://www.ncbi.nlm.nih.gov/pmc/articles/PMC4290459/

414 Nicola Shubrook. The health benefits of spirulina. Retrieved from https://www.bbcgoodfood.com/howto/guide/health-benefits-spirulina

415 Nicola Shubrook. The health benefits of chlorella. Retrieved from https://www.bbcgoodfood.com/howto/guide/health-benefits-chlorella

416 Winston Craig, MPH, PhD, RD.. (2014). Health Benefits of Green Leafy Vegetables. Retrieved from https://vegetarian-nutrition.info/green-leafy-vegetables/

417 Nutrients and Health Benefits. Retrieved from https://www.choosemyplate.gov/fruits-nutrients-health

418 Omega-3s. Retrieved from https://vegan-health.org/omega-3s/

419 Carolyn Gregoire. (2013). Food And Stress: 8 Of The Worst Picks For When You're Feeling Anxious. Retrieved from https://www.huffingtonpost.com/2013/03/07/worst-foods-stress_n_2773760.html

420 Watkins, P. C., Cruz, L., Holben, H., & Kolts, R. L. (2007). Taking Care of Business?: Grateful Processing of Unpleasant Memories. *PsycEXTRA Dataset*. doi:10.1037/e650032007-001

421 Relationships and the Importance of Reciprocity. (2010, July 12). Retrieved from https://www.goodtherapy.org/blog/relationship-reciprocity/

422 Harvard Health Publishing. (2015, May 20). Giving thanks can make you happier - Harvard Health. Retrieved from https://www.health.harvard.edu/healthbeat/giving-thanks-can-make-you-happier

423 Huffman, J. C., Beale, E. E., Celano, C. M., Beach, S. R., Belcher, A. M., Moore, S. V., … Januzzi, J. L. (2015). Effects of Optimism and Gratitude on Physical Activity, Biomarkers, and Readmissions After an Acute Coronary Syndrome. *Circulation: Cardiovascular Quality and Outcomes*, *9*(1), 55-63. doi:10.1161/circoutcomes.115.002184

424 Evernote. (2017, September 24). Does Gratitude Make Us More Productive? ? Taking Note ? Medium. Retrieved from https://medium.com/taking-note/does-gratitude-make-us-more-productive-fb336bee-af78

425 Altruism. Retrieved from https://www.psychologytoday.com/us/basics/altruism

426 Small Acts of Generosity and the Neuroscience of Gratitude. (2015, October 20). Retrieved from https://www.psychologytoday.com/us/blog/the-athletes-way/201510/

small-acts-generosity-and-the-neuroscience-gratitude

427 7 Surprising Health Benefits of Gratitude. (2017, November 20). Retrieved from http://time.com/5026174/health-benefits-of-gratitude/

428 How to Develop a Gratitude Mindset. (2017, October 30). Retrieved from https://chopra.com/articles/how-to-develop-a-gratitude-mindset

429 Esteve, R., López-Martínez, A. E., Peters, M. L., Serrano-Ibáñez, E. R., Ruiz-Párraga, G. T., & Ramírez-Maestre, C. (2018). Optimism, Positive and Negative Affect, and Goal Adjustment Strategies: Their Relationship to Activity Patterns in Patients with Chronic Musculoskeletal Pain. *Pain Research and Management, 2018*, 1-12. doi:10.1155/2018/6291719

430 Boost Your Health With a Dose of Gratitude. (n.d.). Retrieved from https://www.webmd.com/women/features/gratitute-health-boost#1

431 Jahda Swanborough. (2017). The previous industrial revolutions broke the environment. Can the current one fix it?. Retrieved from https://www.weforum.org/agenda/2017/04/fix-the-environment-there-s-an-app-for-that/

432 The previous industrial revolutions broke the environment. Can the current one fix it? (n.d.). Retrieved from https://www.weforum.org/agenda/2017/04/fix-the-environment-there-s-an-app-for-that/

433 (2017). Introduction to the 2015 TRI National Analysis. Retrieved from https://www.epa.gov/sites/production/files/2017-01/documents/tri_na_2015_complete_english.pdf

434 Michael A. Schmidt. (2002). Tired Or Toxic? Chronic Fatigue Syndrome And Environmental Toxicity. Retrieved from https://www.prohealth.com/library/tired-or-toxic-chronic-fatigue-syndrome-and-environmental-toxicity-20067

435 Introduction to the 2015 TRI National Analysis. Updated January 2017. https://www.epa.gov/sites/production/files/2017-01/documents/tri_na_2015_complete_english.pdf

436 Tired or Toxic? Chronic Fatigue Syndrome and Environmental Toxicity - Prohealth. (2018, March 21). Retrieved from https://www.prohealth.com/library/tired-or-toxic-chronic-fatigue-syndrome-and-environmental-toxicity-20067

437 Interactions in Chemical Mixtures: Additive, Synergistic & Antagonistic. Retrieved from https://study.com/academy/lesson/interactions-in-chemical-mixtures-additive-synergistic-antagonistic.html

438 Interactions in Chemical Mixtures: Additive, Synergistic & Antagonistic - Video & Lesson Transcript | Study.com. (n.d.). Retrieved from https://study.com/academy/lesson/interactions-in-chemical-mixtures-additive-synergistic-antagonistic.html

439 Monitoring Human Tissues for Toxic Substances. (1991). doi:10.17226/1787

440 Monitoring Human Tissues for Toxic Substances. Retrieved from https://www.ncbi.nlm.nih.gov/books/NBK234173/

441 John W. Ludlow, Alexander Kinev, Michael VanKanegan, Ben Buehrer, Nick Trotta and Joydeep Basu. Toxicological Risk Assessment – Proposed Assay Platform Using Stem and Progenitor Cell Differentiation in Response to Environmental Toxicants. *Human Stem Cell Toxicology*, 94 - 123. Retrieved from http://pubs.rsc.org/en/content/chapter/bk9781782624219-00094/978-1-78262-421-9

442 Ludlow, J. W., Kinev, A., VanKanegan, M., Ben Buehrer, B. B., Trotta, N., & Basu, J. (n.d.). Chapter 5. Toxicological Risk Assessment – Proposed Assay Platform Using Stem and Progenitor Cell Differentiation in Response to Environmental Toxicants. *Issues in Toxicology*, 94-123. doi:10.1039/9781782626787-00094

443 Dr. Joseph Mercola. (2017). Roundup And Glyphosate Toxicity Grossly Underestimated. Retrieved from https://www.honeycolony.com/article/roundup-and-glyphosate-toxicity/

444 Roundup And Glyphosate Toxicity Grossly Underestimated | HoneyColony. (2017, March 3). Retrieved from https://www.honeycolony.com/article/roundup-and-glyphosate-toxicity/

445 Dr. Joseph Mercola. (2017). Roundup And Glyphosate Toxicity Grossly Underestimated. Retrieved from https://www.honeycolony.com/article/roundup-and-glyphosate-toxicity/

446 Ruiz, R. (2012, July 11). Industrial Chemicals Lurking In Your Bloodstream. Retrieved from https://www.forbes.com/2010/01/21/toxic-chemicals-bpa-lifestyle-health-endocrine-disruptors.html#790c6974bb91

447 Bethany Winans, Michael C. Humble, and B. Paige Lawrence. (2010). Environmental toxicants and the developing immune system: a missing link in the global battle against infectious disease?. Retrieved from https://www.ncbi.nlm.nih.gov/pmc/articles/PMC3033466/

448 Aristo Vojdani, K. Michael Pollard, and Andrew W. Campbell. (2014). Environmental Triggers and Autoimmunity. Retrieved from https://www.ncbi.nlm.nih.gov/pmc/articles/PMC4290643/

449 Winans, B., Humble, M. C., & Lawrence, B. P. (2011). Environmental toxicants and the developing immune system: A missing link in the global battle against infectious disease? *Reproductive Toxicology*, *31*(3), 327-336. doi:10.1016/j.reprotox.2010.09.004

450 Molina, V., & Shoenfeld, Y. (2005). Infection, vaccines and other environmental triggers of autoimmunity. *Autoimmunity*, *38*(3), 235-245. doi:10.1080/08916930500050277

451 (2015). Cancer-Causing Substances in the Environment. Retrieved from https://www.cancer.gov/about-cancer/causes-prevention/risk/substances

452 Hilary Brueck. (2018). From birth to old age, here's what Americans are most likely to die from at every age. Retrieved from https://www.businessinsider.com/how-youre-most-likely-to-die-at-every-age-2018-6#the-biggest-risk-to-newborns-nascent-lives-from-birth-to-their-first-birthday-is-birth-defects-2

453 Bob Weinhold, MA. (2009). Environmental Factors in Birth Defects: What We Need to Know. Retrieved from https://www.ncbi.nlm.nih.gov/pmc/articles/PMC2897222/

454 Cancer-Causing Substances. (n.d.). Retrieved from https://www.cancer.gov/about-cancer/causes-prevention/risk/substances

455 Brueck, H. (2018, June 17). From birth to old age, here's what Americans are most likely to die from at every age. Retrieved from https://www.businessinsider.com/how-youre-most-likely-to-die-at-every-age-2018-6#the-biggest-risk-to-newborns-nascent-lives-from-birth-to-their-first-birthday-is-birth-defects-2

456 Weinhold, B. (2009). Environmental Factors in Birth Defects: What We Need to Know. *Environmental Health Perspectives*, *117*(10), A440-A447. doi:10.1289/ehp.117-a440

457 Lori A.Dostal, Robert E.Chapin, Steven A.Stefanski, Martha W. Harris and Bernard A. Schwetz. (2005). Testicular toxicity and reduced sertoli cell numbers in neonatal rats by di(2-ethylhexyl) phthalate and the recovery of fertility as adults. Toxicology and Applied Pharmacology, Volume 95, 104-121. Retrieved from https://www.sciencedirect.com/science/article/pii/S0041008X88800127

458 Nicolas Olea and Mariana F Fernandez. (2007). Chemicals in the environment and human male fertility. Retrieved from https://www.ncbi.nlm.nih.gov/pmc/articles/PMC2078473/

459 Hsiao-Ling Lei, Hsiao-Jui Wei, Hsin-Yi Ho, Kai-Wei Liao, and Ling-Chu Chien. (2015). Relationship between risk factors for infertility in women and lead, cadmium, and arsenic blood levels: a cross-sectional study from Taiwan. Retrieved from https://www.ncbi.nlm.nih.gov/pmc/articles/PMC4673771/

460 Rob Stein. (2017). Sperm Counts Plummet In Western Men, Study Finds.

Retrieved from https://www.npr.org/2017/07/31/539517210/sperm-counts-plummet-in-western-men-study-finds

461 (2009). Conditions that affect fertility. Retrieved from https://www.health.harvard.edu/newsletter_article/Conditions-That-Affect-Fertility

462 Testicular toxicity and reduced sertoli cell numbers in neonatal rats by di(2-ethylhexyl) phthalate and the recovery of fertility as adults. (n.d.). Retrieved from https://www.sciencedirect.com/science/article/pii/S0041008X88800127

463 Olea, N., & Fernandez, M. F. (2007). Chemicals in the environment and human male fertility. *Occupational and Environmental Medicine, 64*(7), 430-431. doi:10.1136/oem.2007.033621

464 Sperm Counts Plummet In Western Men, Study Finds. (2017, July 31). Retrieved from https://www.npr.org/2017/07/31/539517210/sperm-counts-plummet-in-western-men-study-finds

465 Harvard Health Publishing. (2015, May 20). Conditions that affect fertility - Harvard Health. Retrieved from https://www.health.harvard.edu/newsletter_article/Conditions-That-Affect-Fertility

466 (2003). Cancer and the Environment. Retrieved from https://www.niehs.nih.gov/health/materials/cancer_and_the_environment_508.pdf

467 Cancer and the Environment. U.S. Department of Health and Human Services. https://www.niehs.nih.gov/health/materials/cancer_and_the_environment_508.pdf

468 James Hamblin. (2014). The Toxins That Threaten Our Brains. Retrieved from https://www.theatlantic.com/health/archive/2014/03/the-toxins-that-threaten-our-brains/284466/

469 (2017). 3 Toxic Chemicals Tied to Depression: Symptoms You Need to Recognize (Part 2 of 3). Retrieved from https://universityhealthnews.com/daily/depression/3-toxic-chemicals-tied-to-depression-symptoms-you-need-to-recognize-part-2-of-3/

470 Hamblin, J. (2014, March 18). The Toxins That Threaten Our Brains. Retrieved from https://www.theatlantic.com/health/archive/2014/03/the-toxins-that-threaten-our-brains/284466/

471 3 Toxic Chemicals Tied to Depression: Symptoms You Need to Recognize (Part 2 of 3). (2017, December 28). Retrieved from https://universityhealthnews.com/daily/depression/3-toxic-chemicals-tied-to-depression-symptoms-you-need-to-recognize-part-2-of-3/

472 Veronica Porterfield. (2017). The Signs of Toxins in Your Body. Retrieved from https://www.livestrong.com/article/67812-signs-toxins-body/

473 Porterfield, V. (2009, December 28). The Signs of Toxins in Your Body. Retrieved from https://www.livestrong.com/article/67812-signs-toxins-body/

474 Cleansing the Body of Candida's Dangerous Toxins. Retrieved from https://bodyecology.com/articles/cleansing-the-body-of-candida's-dangerous-toxins

475 Cleansing the Body of Candida's Dangerous Toxins. (2017, September 13). Retrieved from https://bodyecology.com/articles/cleansing-the-body-of-candida's-dangerous-toxins

476 Patricia B. Hoyer; Jodi A. Flaws. Toxic Responses of the Endocrine System. Retrieved from https://accesspharmacy.mhmedical.com/Content.aspx?bookId=1540&sectionId=92527599

477 Toxic Responses of the Endocrine System | Casarett & Doull's Essentials of Toxicology, 3e | AccessPharmacy | McGraw-Hill Medical. (n.d.). Retrieved from https://accesspharmacy.mhmedical.com/Content.aspx?bookId=1540§ionId=92527599

478 How to Filter Fluoride. Retrieved from https://purewaterfreedom.com/filter-fluoride

479 Developmental Fluoride Neurotoxicity: A Systemic Review and meta-Analysis. Harvard Health. https://dash.harvard.edu/bitstream/handle/1/10579664/3491930.pdf

480 Robert Ferris. (2016). Indoor air can be deadlier than outdoor air, research shows. Retrieved from https://www.cnbc.com/2016/04/22/indoor-air-can-be-deadlier-than-outdoor-air-research-shows.html

481 (2015). 7 Common Indoor Air Pollutants and How To Remove Them. Retrieved from https://www.greenbuildermedia.com/iaq/7-common-air-pollutants-and-how-to-remove-them

482 Choi, Anna L., Guifan Sun, Ying Zhang, and Philippe Grandjean. (2012). Developmental Fluoride Neurotoxicity: A Systematic Review and Meta-Analysis. Retrieved from https://dash.harvard.edu/bitstream/handle/1/10579664/3491930.pdf

483 (2018). The Complete List – 15 Harmful Shampoo Ingredients to Avoid. Retrieved from https://www.nutrafol.com/blog/15-shampoo-ingredients-to-avoid/

484 Cosmetics. Retrieved from https://www.ewg.org/key-issues/consumer-products/cosmetics#.W191UCOZO8U

485 Annalisa Palmer. (2013). Top 10 Dangerous Toxins in Cosmetics. Retrieved from https://www.onegreenplanet.org/lifestyle/top-10-dangerous-toxins-in-cosmetics/

486 MEGAN REDSHAW. (2017). Johnson & Johnson's Baby Bedtime Bath: Is it REALLY Safe?. Retrieved from https://www.livingwhole.org/johnson-johnsons-baby-bedtime-bath-is-it-really-safe/

487 EWG's 2018 Holiday Box: Clean Eating on the Go. Retrieved from https://www.ewg.org/

488 Katherine Baird. (2016). Breast Cancer Awareness Month: For Safe, Nontoxic Personal Care Products, Look Beyond the Pink Ribbon. Retrieved from https://www.ewg.org/cancer/2016/10/safe-nontoxic-personal-care-products-look-beyond-pink-ribbon#.W191PiOZO8U

489 GLOBAL ORGANIC TEXTILE STANDARD. (2018). Retrieved from https://www.global-standard.org/certification.html

490 Certification - Global Standard gGmbH. (2018, June 11). Retrieved from https://www.global-standard.org/certification.html

491 The Shocking Truth About Children's Plastic Toys. Read This Before You Buy Another Toy!. Retrieved from https://safbaby.com/the-shocking-truth-about-childrens-plastic-toys-read-this-before-you-buy-another-toy/

492 (2017). The Ultimate Guide to the Best Non-Toxic Toys. Retrieved from https://www.mommytomax.com/ultimate-guide-best-non-toxic-toys/

493 Katie Wells. (2018). How to Store Food Without Plastic. Retrieved from https://wellnessmama.com/25667/store-food-without-plastic/

494 (2016). Perfluorinated Chemicals (PFCs). Retrieved from https://www.niehs.nih.gov/health/materials/perflourinated_chemicals_508.pdf

495 Maria Janowiak. 9 Air-Cleaning Houseplants That Are Almost Impossible to Kill. Retrieved from https://greatist.com/connect/houseplants-that-clean-air

496 Natural Lawn Care Techniques. Retrieved from https://www.triplepundit.com/podium/toxic-garage-frequent-think/

497 Natural Lawn Care Techniques. Retrieved from https://www.gardeners.com/how-to/natural-lawn-care-techniques/5065.html

Made in the USA
Las Vegas, NV
01 August 2021